Drug
Treatment of
Hyperlipidemia

Fundamental and Clinical Cardiology

Series Editor

Samuel Z. Goldhaber, M.D.

Cardiovascular Division
Department of Medicine
Harvard Medical School
Brigham and Women's Hospital
Boston, Massachusetts

Volume 1 Drug Treatment of Hyperlipidemia
edited by Basil M. Rifkind

Volume 2 Cardiotonic Drugs: A Clinical Review, Second Edition,
Revised and Expanded
edited by Carl V. Leier

Additional Volumes in Preparation

Complications of Coronary Angioplasty
*edited by Alexander J. R. Black, H. Vernon Anderson,
and Stephen G. Ellis*

Drug Treatment of Hyperlipidemia

edited by

Basil M. Rifkind

National Heart, Lung and Blood Institute
National Institutes of Health
Bethesda, Maryland

Marcel Dekker, Inc.   New York • Basel • Hong Kong

This book was edited by Basil M. Rifkind in his private capacity. No official support or endorsement by the National Heart, Lung, and Blood Institute is intended or should be inferred.

Library of Congress Cataloging--in--Publication Data

Drug treatment of hyperlipidemia/edited by Basil M. Rifkind.
     p.   cm.
   Includes bibliographical references and index.
   ISBN 0-8247-8512-6 (alk. paper)
   1. Hyperlipoproteinemia--Chemotherapy. 2. Hyperlipidemia--Chemotherapy. 3. Antilipemic agents. I. Rifkind, Basil M.
   [DNLM: 1. Hyperlipidemia--drug therapy. WD 200.5H8 D794]
RC632.H88D78 1991
616.3'997-- --dc20
DNLM/DLC
for Library of Congress   91-13150
                                        CIP

This book is printed on acid-free paper

MARCEL DEKKER, INC.
270 Madison Avenue, New York, New York 10016

Current printing (last digit):
10 9 8 7 6 5 4 3 2

PRINTED IN THE UNITED STATES OF AMERICA

Series Introduction

Marcel Dekker, Inc., has focused on the development of various series of beautifully produced books in different branches of medicine. These series have facilitated the integration of rapidly advancing information for both the clinical specialist and the researcher.

In this new series, Fundamental and Clinical Cardiology, my goal as Series Editor is to assemble the talents of world-renowned authorities to discuss virtually every area of cardiovascular medicine. In the current monograph, Dr. Rifkind has edited an exceptional collection of chapters written by experts pioneering new efforts in treating hyperlipidemia. Future contributions to this series will include books on molecular biology, interventional cardiology, and clinical management of problems such as coronary artery disease and ventricular arrhythmias.

Samuel Z. Goldhaber

Introduction

Atherosclerosis is not a new condition: we know from the observations of Marc Armand Ruffer that the royal mummies found in Tut-ankh-Amen's tomb exhibited some atherosclerotic lesions. Not until the nineteenth century, however, were atheromas associated with cholesterol or other lipidic substances. In 1847, Julius Vogel described what he saw during an autopsy as follows:

> An old man, aged eighty-four years,—exhibited a deposition—in the arch of the aorta,—of a yellowish-white greasy mass, (atheroma). This soft mass was found to consist of the following elements, when examined under the microscope: of the many tubular colorless crystals of cholesterin, of the ordinary characteristic form—.

It is interesting that it took nearly one hundred years more to establish clearly that the "white greasy mass(es)" found in arteries are nearly always the concomitants or consequences of an elevation of lipids in the plasma. At that time, it was also recognized that blood lipid levels are dependent on the dietary ingestion of fats. Many more years passed before it was demonstrated that lowering blood cholesterol leads to a reduction in the incidence of arterial disease, especially coronary heart disease. Today, we also know that a decrease in blood cholesterol in an individual with atherosclerotic lesions will result in a slowing of the progression of the lesions, if not a significant regression.

Thus, the issue appears simple: keep your blood cholesterol low, or, if it is high, bring it down! In practice, however, lowering blood cholesterol is a complex undertaking that must be carefully planned and executed. Patients differ, and their responses to blood cholesterol-lowering approaches may also vary. Fortunately, physicians have a variety of choices to best meet the needs of their patients.

This volume describes these choices. The first chapters provide the scientific foundation and the rationale for the different options. Then, additional chapters describe the various drug treatments that are available. Despite the volume's title, *Drug Treatment of Hyperlipidemia,* a final chapter on "Dietary Management" is also included.

Dr. Basil Rifkind, the editor of the monograph, brings decades of expertise in the investigation of hyperlipidemia. The authors he has assembled offer a dimension and an experience that only leaders possess. There is no doubt that their viewpoints and explanations will be of great help to practicing physicians addressing the most important public health problem in the United States—the prevention and treatment of atherosclerosis and coronary heart disease.

Claude Lenfant, M.D.
Director
National Heart, Lung, and Blood Institute
National Institutes of Health
Bethesda, Maryland

Preface

Reducing elevated cholesterol and/or triglyceride levels is not an end in itself. Rather it is directed toward preventing or at least delaying the onset of the clinical consequences of such elevations. Most of the clinical burden takes the form of coronary heart disease in its various clinical manifestations and is a consequence of advanced atherosclerosis of the coronary arteries. Other ischemic vascular manifestations include peripheral artery disease and stroke. Occasionally reduction of lipids has the aim of preventing pancreatitis or shrinking xanthomas. The evidence that lowering cholesterol helps to reduce the incidence of coronary heart disease is compelling; corresponding benefits for triglyceride lowering are less well established.

Cholesterol-lowering drugs are being increasingly prescribed. A dramatic fivefold increase in prescriptions dispensed by retail pharmacies occurred between 1983 and 1988. The growing awareness of the importance of reducing elevated cholesterol levels resulting from the activities of the National Cholesterol Education Program and of many other groups, and the introduction of two new drugs, lovastatin and gemfibrozil, account for most of the increase. Further rapid growth can be expected especially as a result of the impact of the Report of the Expert Panel on Detection, Diagnosis and Treatment of High Blood Cholesterol Levels.

Concerns have been expressed that physicians may overprescribe such agents while failing to use adequately the primary approach to cholesterol lowering, namely reduction of dietary saturated fat and cholesterol and, where necessary, excess weight. This volume is designed to assist the physician in the appropriate use of lipid-lowering drugs by providing a comprehensive review of lipid metabolism, of the hyperlipidemias and their management, of the Guidelines of the Expert Panel, and of each of the major classes of lipid-altering agents.

Basil M. Rifkind

Contents

Contributors

H. Bryan Brewer, Jr., M.D. Molecular Disease Branch, National Heart, Lung, and Blood Institute, National Institutes of Health, Bethesda, Maryland

W. Virgil Brown, M.D. Medlantic Research Foundation, Washington, D.C.

Laraine Field Medlantic Research Foundation, Washington, D.C.

Henry N. Ginsberg, M.D. Irving Center for Clinical Research and Department of Medicine, Columbia University College of Physicians and Surgeons, New York, New York

Scott M. Grundy, M.D. Center for Human Nutrition and Departments of Internal Medicine and Biochemistry and Clinical Nutrition, University of Texas Southwestern Medical Center, Dallas, Texas

Jeffrey M. Hoeg, M.D. Molecular Disease Branch, National Heart, Lung, and Blood Institute, National Institutes of Health, Bethesda, Maryland

William James Howard, M.D. Medlantic Research Foundation, Washington, D.C.

Donald B. Hunninghake, M.D. Heart Disease Prevention Clinic, University of Minnesota, Minneapolis, Minnesota

D. Roger Illingworth, M.D. Division of Endocrinology, Metabolism, and Clinical Nutrition, Department of Medicine, Oregon Health Sciences University, Portland, Oregon

Wahida Karmally, M.S., R.D.   Irving Center for Clinical Research and Department of Medicine, Columbia University College of Physicians and Surgeons, New York, New York

John C. LaRosa, M.D.   Lipid Research Clinic, George Washington University Medical Center, Washington, D.C.

Jacques E. Rossouw, M.D.   Lipid Metabolism-Atherogenesis Branch, National Heart, Lung, and Blood Institute, National Institutes of Health, Bethesda, Maryland

Ernst J. Schaefer, M.D.   Department of Medicine, Tufts University School of Medicine; Lipid Clinic, New England Medical Center; Lipid Metabolism Laboratory, USDA Human Nutrition Research Center on Aging at Tufts University, Boston, Massachusetts

Daniel Steinberg, M.D.   Division of Endocrinology and Metabolism, Department of Medicine, University of California, San Diego, La Jolla, California

Joseph L. Witztum, M.D.   Division of Endocrinology and Metabolism, Department of Medicine, University of California, San Diego, La Jolla, California

Drug Treatment of Hyperlipidemia

1

Lipid and Lipoprotein Metabolism

H. Bryan Brewer, Jr.
National Heart, Lung, and Blood Institute
National Institutes of Health
Bethesda, Maryland

I. INTRODUCTION

Plasma lipids in the extracellular fluids are transported by lipoproteins composed of several classes of lipids (including cholesterol, triglycerides, and phospholipids) and proteins designated apolipoproteins. Our understanding of the role of lipoproteins and apolipoproteins in lipid transport has dramatically increased over the last 15 years. The roles of lipoprotein receptors, enzymes, and apolipoproteins in lipoprotein metabolism have been determined, and this new information provides a conceptual framework for understanding lipid transport in normal individuals and subjects with dyslipoproteinemias.

II. CLASSIFICATION OF PLASMA LIPOPROTEINS

In clinical practice, plasma lipoproteins are typically classified on the basis of their electrophoretic mobility and hydrated density (Gofman et al., 1954; Lee and Hatch, 1963). Lipoproteins are separated by electrophoresis into those that remain at the origin, or migrate into the β (β lipoproteins), α_2 (pre-β lipoproteins), or α_1 (α lipoproteins) globulin zones. Five major classes of plasma lipoproteins are separated by hydrated density including chylomicrons, very low density lipoproteins (VLDL), intermediate density lipoproteins (IDL), low density lipoproteins (LDL), and high density lipoproteins (HDL). HDL are further separated into HDL_2 and HDL_3 (Gofman et al., 1954). The lipoproteins which remain at the origin in electrophoresis are equivalent to chylomicrons, the pre-β lipoproteins to VLDL, the β lipoproteins to LDL, and the α lipoproteins to HDL. Triglycerides are transported primarily by chylomicrons and VLDL. Plasma LDL and HDL transport approximately 70 and 20% of plasma cholesterol, respectively. Clinically the concentrations of lipoproteins are most frequently assessed by quantifying the cholesterol moiety of the lipoprotein particle. Apolipoproteins may also be utilized to quantitate lipoproteins and apo B as well as apo A-I have been used to determine LDL and HDL levels, respectively. Thus, either the cholesterol or apolipoprotein component of the lipoprotein particle may be used in the determination of the concentration of plasma lipoproteins.

III. PLASMA APOLIPOPROTEINS

A. Characterization

Ten major human plasma apolipoproteins have been identified and their protein as well as gene structures determined (Table 1) (Osborne and Brewer, 1977; Scanu and Landsberger, 1980; Mahley et al., 1984; Brewer et al., 1988; Breslow, 1989). The six most clinically relevant apolipoproteins are

Table 1 Major Human Plasma Apolipoproteins

Apolipoprotein	Approx. MW (kD)	Major site of synthesis	Major density class
Apo A-I	28	Liver, intestine	HDL
Apo A-II	18	Liver	HDL
Apo A-IV	45	Intestine	Chylomicrons
Apo B-48	250	Intestine	Chylomicrons-VLDL-IDL
Apo B-100	500	Liver	Chylomicrons-VLDL-IDL-LDL
Apo C-I	7	Liver	Chylomicrons-VLDL-IDL
Apo C-II	10	Liver	Chylomicrons-VLDL-IDL
Apo C-III	10	Liver	Chylomicrons-VLDL-IDL
Apo E	34	Liver	VLDL-IDL-LDL
Apo (a)	500	Liver	LDL-HDL

A-I, B-100, B-48, C-II, E, and apo(a). In human plasma, apo B exists as two isoproteins, designated apo B-48 and apo B-100, with apparent molecular weights of 250 and 512 kD, respectively (Kane et al., 1980; Kane, 1983). A novel mechanism for the biosynthesis of apo B-48 and apo B-100 from a single apo B gene has been identified (Law et al., 1985; Blackhart et al., 1986; Powell et al., 1987; Hospattankar et al., 1987; Chen et al., 1987; Higuchi et al., 1988). A single nuclear RNA is transcribed from the single 40 kb gene for apo B on chromosome 2. Apo B-100 contains 4536 amino acids and is translated from the full-length processed 14.1 kb apo B mRNA. Apo B-48 has 2152 amino acids and is synthesized from an apo B mRNA containing a premature in-frame translational stop codon. The premature stop codon is introduced in the RNA by an RNA-editing mechanism by a single base change of a C to U at nucleotide 6666. This C to U base substitution converts the codon CAA, coding for glutamine (amino acid 2153) in apo B-100, to UAA, an in-frame premature stop codon. Translation of the edited mRNA results in the 2152 residue apo B-48 isoprotein. Human liver and intestine contain both the CAA and UAA mRNAs, and apo B-100 and apo B-48 are synthesized by the liver and intestine. However, the major apo B isoproteins synthesized by the human intestine and liver are apo B-48 and apo B-100, respectively. This RNA-editing mechanism represents a unique mechanism for the biosynthesis of two isoproteins from a single gene and a new control mechanism for eukaryotic gene expression.

Apo A-I and apo A-II are the two major apolipoproteins in HDL, and apo A-I has been used in place of cholesterol for HDL quantitation (Osborne and Brewer, 1977; Scanu and Landsberger, 1980). Apo(a) is the unique apolipoprotein of the Lp(a) particle, and elevated levels of Lp(a) are a risk factor for the development of premature cardiovascular disease (Berg et al., 1974; Kostner et al., 1981; Armstrong et al., 1986).

Apo E, a 299 residue apolipoprotein, is primarily associated with HDL and VLDL (for review see Mahley et al., 1984; Davignon et al., 1988; Gregg and Brewer, 1988). Apo E is a genetically determined polymorphic apolipoprotein with three common co-dominantly inherited alleles designated ϵ-2, ϵ-3, and ϵ-4, with relative frequencies of 0.073, 0.783, and 0.143, respectively. The E apolipoproteins coded for these alleles are designated apo E-2, apo E-3, and apo E-4. The structural difference between the common E-2, E-3, and E-4 isoproteins resides in substitution of amino acids at residues 112 and 158. At these two locations apo E-2 contains two cysteines, apo E-3 contains a cysteine and arginine, and apo E-4 two arginines. The charge differences in the apo E isoproteins permits the separation of the common apo E phenotypes by isoelectrofocusing gel electrophoresis. There are three homozygous and

three heterozygous phenotypes resulting in a total of six major plasma phenotypes (Mahley et al., 1984; Davignon et al., 1988; Gregg and Brewer,
1988).

B. Functions of the Plasma Apolipoproteins

Three major physiological functions have been identified for the plasma
apolipoproteins (Table 2).

1. Apolipoproteins function as cofactors or activators of enzymes involved
    in lipid-lipoprotein metabolism. Of particular importance is apo C-II, the
    activator of lipoprotein lipase, which is responsible for the perivascular
    hydrolysis of lipoprotein triglycerides to monoglycerides and free fatty
    acids (LaRosa et al., 1970; Havel et al., 1970). Lipoprotein lipase is
    attached to the capillary endothelium by a heparin-like proteoglycan,
    which permits the direct interaction of the lipoprotein lipase enzyme with
    the circulating triglyceride-rich lipoproteins.
        Apo A-I modulates the enzymic activity of lecithin-cholesterol acyl-
    transferase (LCAT), which catalyzes the esterification of lipoprotein
    cholesterol to cholesteryl esters (Fielding et al., 1972).
2. Apolipoproteins function as structural proteins for the biosynthesis and
    secretion of plasma lipoproteins. Apo A-I has been proposed to be a
    critical structural protein for the ultimate biosynthesis and remodeling of
    HDL (Obsorne and Brewer, 1977; Scanu and Landsberger, 1980). In-

Table 2 Physiological Functions of the Human Plasma Apolipoproteins

Function	Apolipoproteins
I. Structural protein on the lipoprotein particle	
Intestinal chylomicrons	Apo B-48, Apo B-100
Hepatogenous VLDL	Apo B-100
HDL	Apo A-I
II. Ligand on lipoprotein particle for interaction with cellular receptor sites	
Remnant receptor	Apo E
LDL receptor	Apo B-100, Apo E
HDL receptor	Apo A-I, apo A-II
III. Cofactor for enzyme	
Lipoprotein lipase	Apo C-II
Lecithin-cholesterol acyltransferase	Apo A-1

dividuals with a structural defect in the apo A-I gene are unable to synthesize and secrete apo A-I and have a virtual absence of plasma HDL and premature heart disease (Norum et al., 1982; Schaefer et al., 1985). Apo B-100 and apo B-48 are required for the secretion of triglyceride-rich lipoproteins from the liver and intestine. Defects in the biosynthesis or secretion of apo B results in abetalipoproteinemia and homozygous hypobetalipoproteinemia, diseases characterized by the absence of plasma chylomicrons, VLDL, IDL, and LDL, as well as malabsorption, and neurological defects (Herbert et al., 1983).

3. Apolipoproteins function as ligands on lipoprotein particles for interaction with cellular receptors for specific lipoprotein particles. Apo A-I has been proposed as the major apolipoprotein on HDL for interaction with the putative 110 kD HDL receptor. Apo A-I and HDL have been proposed to facilitate the removal of cholesterol from peripheral cells and transport to the liver, where cholesterol is excreted from the body (Oram et al., 1983; Schmitz et al., 1985; Fidge et al., 1989). Apo B-100 interacts with the LDL receptor to initiate absorptive endocytosis and cellular catabolism of LDL (Brown and Goldstein, 1986). Apo E has been proposed to interact with both the LDL receptor and the putative hepatic remnant receptor. Recently a 600 kDa receptor has been cloned and proposed as a potential remnant receptor which facilitates the hepatic removal of lipoprotein remnants secreted by the intestine and liver (Herz et al., 1988).

IV.   LIPOPROTEIN METABOLISM

A.   Apolipoprotein B Cascades

A conceptual overview of the pathway for lipoprotein metabolism of the apo B–containing lipoproteins, including chylomicrons, VLDL, IDL, and LDL, is shown schematically in Figure 1. The metabolism of the major classes of lipoproteins containing apo B-48 and apo B-100 may be considered to consist of two major "apo B metabolic cascades" (for review see Brewer et al., 1988, 1989). The first apo B casade involves the stepwise delipidation of triglyceride rich chylomicrons secreted by the intestine. The primary function of the chylomicron particles is to transport dietary cholesterol and triglycerides from the intestine to peripheral tissues and the liver. Shortly after secretion, chylomicrons acquire apo E and apo C-II, primarily from HDL. As discussed previously, apo C-II activates lipoprotein lipase, which results in triglyceride hydrolysis and remodeling of the triglyceride-rich lipoprotein particles. With triglyceride hydrolysis and remodeling of the lipoprotein

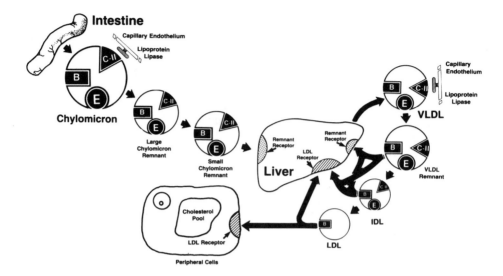

Figure 1   Schematic overview of the metabolism of apo B-containing lipoproteins. Chylomicrons containing apo B are secreted by the intestine and undergo lipolysis by lipoprotein lipase. With triglyceride hydrolysis chylomicron remnant particles are formed with an initial hydrated density of VLDL and finally IDL. The small chylomicron remnants are taken up primarily by the putative remnant receptor. Triglyceride-rich VLDL containing apoB are secreted by the liver, and undergo lipolysis as outlined above for the particles secreted by the intestine. VLDL are initially converted to VLDL remnants, then IDL, and finally to LDL. Some VLDL and IDL particles are removed by the liver via the LDL and putative remnant receptors. LDL particles interact with the LDL receptors on the liver and peripheral cells resulting in LDL endocytosis and catabolism (see text for additional details).

particle, both apolipoproteins as well as lipid constituents are transfered to HDL. With remodeling of the chylomicron particle, the hydrated density of the chylomicron increases and chylomicron remnants are generated with a hydrated density of VLDL and then IDL. Chylomicron remnants have been proposed to be removed primarily by a putative hepatic remnant receptor (Davignon et al., 1988; Herz et al., 1988). A recently cloned 600 kDa lipoprotein receptor, the LDL receptor related protein (LRP), has been proposed as a potential candidate for the remnant receptor (Herz et al., 1988). Further studies will be required to establish the role of the LRP receptor in lipoprotein metabolism.

The second apo B cascade involves triglyceride-rich VLDL containing apo B-100 secreted by the liver. Apo C-II and apo E dissociate from HDL and reassociate with the hepatogeneous triglyceride-rich VLDL following secretion from the liver. Apo C-II activates LDL as outlined above and the VLDL are serially converted to VLDL remnants, IDL, and finally LDL. During the metabolic conversion of VLDL to LDL, approximately 50% of VLDL remnants and IDL are removed from the plasma through interaction of apolipoproteins E and B with the remnant and LDL receptors.

Hepatic lipase, a second lipolytic enzyme, and apo E have been proposed to be necessary for the conversion of IDL to LDL. Hepatic lipase has been proposed to function in lipoprotein particle metabolism as both a phospholipase and triglyceryl hydrolase (Eisenberg, 1984). LDL, the final product of the VLDL cascade, contains virtually only apo B-100 which interacts with the LDL receptor on the plasma membranes of liver, adrenal, and peripheral cells including fibroblasts and smooth muscle cells (Brown and Goldstein, 1986). The interaction of LDL with the LDL receptor initiates receptor-mediated endocytosis and transport of LDL to liposomes where the protein moiety is degraded and cholesteryl esters are hydrolyzed to free cholesterol, which is transferred to the intracellular cholesterol pool. Approximately 50% of plasma LDL is catabolized by the liver and peripheral cells, respectively.

B. HDL Metabolism

HDL are synthesized by four major pathways (Fig. 2) (for reviews see Eisenberg, 1984; Brewer et al., 1988; Brewer et al., 1989). Nascent HDL are synthesized by the liver and intestine primarily in the form of apo A-I phospholipid discs. Nascent HDL acquire cholesterol from tissues via the putative HDL receptor. The free cholesterol present in lipoprotein particles is esterified to cholesteryl esters by the LCAT enzyme. With the increase in lipid content the disc-shaped nascent HDL are converted to spherical lipoproteins with a hydrated density of HDL_3 (d 1.125–1.2 g/ml). HDL_3 lipoproteins are converted to the more buoyant HDL_2 lipoproteins (d 1.063–1.125 g/ml) by the further acquisition of lipid and apolipoproteins released during the stepwise delipidation and remodeling of the triglyceride-rich chylomicrons and VLDL as well as the uptake of cholesterol from peripheral tissues. The free cholesterol is esterified by LCAT, and the cholesteryl esters are transferred to the hydrophilic-lipid core of the HDL particle converting HDL_3 to the larger HDL_2 particles.

HDL_2 particles are converted back to HDL_3 by the removal of cholesteryl esters by the liver and other tissues, and the transfer of HDL cholesteryl esters to VLDL and LDL by the cholesteryl ester transfer protein. In addition, the

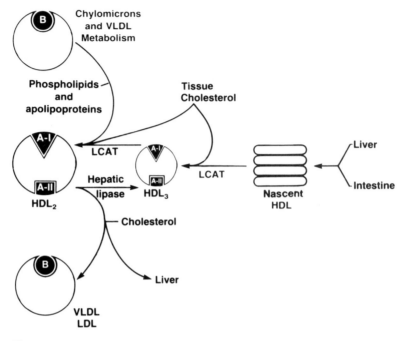

Figure 2 Schematic overview of the synthesis of HDL. Disc-shaped nascent HDL are synthesized by the intestine and liver. Nascent HDL are excellent receptors for cholesterol, and are converted to spherical HDL₃ particles by the esterification of cholesterol to cholesteryl esters as well as the transfer of lipid and apolipoprotein constituents from the delipidation and remodeling of triglyceride-rich chylomicrons and VLDL. HDL₃ are converted to HDL₂ by the further addition of tissue cholesterol and the remodeling of chylomicrons and VLDL.

HDL₂ is converted back to HDL₃ by transfer of cholesterol esters to BLDL and LDL as well as to the liver. The conversion of HDL₂ to HDL is facilitated by the action of hepatic lipase which functions both as a phospholipase and triglyceride hydrolyase. (See text for further details.)

hydrolysis of phospholipids and triglycerides by hepatic lipase is also important in the conversion of HDL₂ to HDL₃.

The overall process of HDL transfer of cholesterol from peripheral cells to the liver has been termed "reverse cholesterol transport" (for reviews see Brewer et al., 1979; Eisenberg, 1984). This still hypothetical process is summarized schematically in Figure 3. VLDL synthesized by the liver is ultimately converted to LDL, the major cholesterol transport lipoprotein. LDL binds to the LDL receptor in the liver and peripheral cells where it

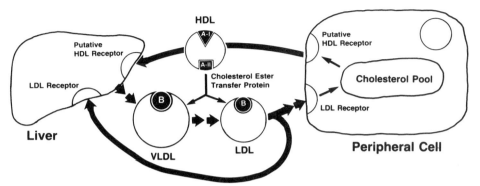

Figure 3 Schematic model of reverse cholesterol transport. VLDL secreted by the liver are ultimately converted to LDL which interact with LDL receptors on the liver and peripheral cells and undergo endocytosis with transport of cholesterol to the intracellular pool. HDL has been proposed to facilitates the removal of excess cholesterol from the peripheral cell by interaction with the putative HDL receptor. Cholesterol within HDL is either transferred to VLDL or LDL by the cholesterol ester exchange protein or transported back to the liver where it interacts with the putative hepatic HDL receptor and is transferred to the cholesterol pool within the hepatocyte. (See text for additional details.)

supplies cholesterol to the intracellular cholesterol pool. Excess cholesterol is removed from the peripheral cells by HDL, presumably by the HDL receptor, which facilitates the transfer of intracellular cholesterol to HDL. HDL transports this cholesterol in plasma and transfers it to VLDL and LDL via the cholesterol transfer protein or delivers the cholesterol to the liver via the putative HDL receptor for removal from the body by direct secretion into the bile or following conversion to bile acids. Cholesteryl esters, therefore, may be transported back to the liver directly by HDL or after exchange to VLDL or LDL. In addition, a variable fraction of tissue cholesterol has been proposed to be transported back to the liver by HDL containing apo E, which may interact with hepatic LDL and remnant receptors (for review see Eisenberg, 1984).

V. ROLE OF LIPOPROTEINS IN ATHEROSCLEROSIS

Decreased plasma levels of HDL (Gordon et al., 1977; Castelli et al., 1977; Miller et al., 1977; Naito, 1980; Yaari et al., 1981) and increased levels of LDL (Gordon et al., 1977; Castelli et al., 1977), β-VLDL (Mahley, 1979; Brewer et al., 1983), and Lp(a) (Berg et al., 1974; Kostner et al., 1981;

Armstrong et al., 1986) have been associated with the development of premature heart disease. The development of the early atherosclerotic lesion is characterized by the formation of foam cells from macrophages and smooth muscle cells (Garrity, 1981a,b; Steinberg, 1983). Blood-derived monocyte-macrophages have been proposed to move into and out of the vessel wall. Smooth muscle cells migrate into the media and both smooth muscle cells and macrophages take up cholesterol-rich lipoproteins by specific cellular receptors and are converted to foam cells. Increased plasma levels of atherogenic lipoproteins have been proposed to result in an increased diffusion of lipoproteins into the media of the vessel wall, which are ultimately taken up by smooth muscle cells and macrophages to form foam cells.

Recent studies have provided new insights into the cellular uptake of LDL. Native LDL is not readily taken up by macrophages in vitro and incubation of LDL with macrophages does not result in the formation of foam cells (Haberland and Fogelman, 1987; Steinberg, 1987). Of particular interest are studies that established that oxidative modification of LDL in vitro markedly enhances the LDL uptake by the scavenger receptor on macrophages with foam cell formation (Steinberg, 1987). Oxidative modification of LDL was observed following in vitro incubation with macrophages, smooth muscle cells, and endothelial cells (Haberland and Fogelman, 1987; Steinberg, 1987) or following modification with malondealdehyde (Fogelman et al., 1980). Malondealdehyde is a metabolic product in the biosynthesis of prostaglandins and is also formed during lipid peroxidation. Based on these interesting observations, it has been proposed that oxidative modification of LDL occurs in vivo and is a prerequisite for the macrophage uptake of LDL and foam cell formation.

β-VLDL remnant lipoproteins are cholesterol-enriched abnormal lipoprotein remnant particles present in patients with dysbetalipoproteinemia (type III hyperlipoproteinemia) and animals fed high fat and cholesterol diets (Brewer et al., 1983; Mahley, 1979). β-VLDL remnant lipoproteins have been proposed to be taken up by macrophages either utilizing a specific macrophage β-VLDL receptor (Van Lenten et al., 1983; Baker et al., 1984) or the LDL receptor (Koo et al., 1988).

Elevated levels of Lp(a) have been reported to be an important independent risk factor for the development of premature cardiovascular disease (Berg et al., 1974; Kostner et al., 1981; Armstrong et al., 1986). Lp(a) is a cholesterol-rich lipoprotein similar to LDL in lipid composition and has a hydrated density (d 1.05–1.1 g/ml) between LDL and HDL. The protein moiety of Lp(a) consists of apo B-100 and a unique 4529 amino acid apolipoprotein, apo(a), linked together by a single disulfide bridge (Taton et al., 1987; McLean et al., 1987). Lp(a) levels in plasma range from <1 to >100 mg/dl

(Utermann, 1987). Lp(a) levels of >30 mg/dl are associated with a twofold increase in the relative risk of coronary artery disease. Elevated levels of both Lp(a) and LDL increase the relative risk of vascular disease approximately fivefold (Armstrong et al., 1986). Patients with the genetic dyslipoproteinemia familial hypercholesterolemia have an approximately threefold increase in Lp(a) levels when compared to normal controls.

As reviewed above, HDL has been proposed to play a major role in decreasing foam cell formation and the development of the atherosclerotic lesion by facilitating the removal of excess cellular cholesterol and the transport of this cholesterol to the liver for removal from the body. In this still hypothetical process, designated reverse cholesterol transport, it is proposed that the efficiency of the HDL transport pathway is directly proportional to the levels of plasma and pericellular HDL. If plasma levels of HDL are low, the removal of cellular cholesterol is inadequate and foam cell formation and atherosclerosis may progress (see Fig. 3).

Plasma levels of triglyceride-rich lipoproteins are not usually considered to be associated with an increased risk of premature heart disease. This concept is based primarily on multivariate statistical analysis of epidemiological studies in which no "independent risk" has been associated with hypertriglyceridemia (Wilhelman et al., 1973; Heyden et al., 1980; Hulley et al., 1980). One note of caution, however, the physician must be careful not to disregard the potential atherogenic risk of triglyceride-rich lipoproteins in patients with established coronary artery disease or in kindreds with a strong family history of premature cardiovascular disease.

The phenomenal growth in our knowledge of lipid transport and plasma lipoprotein metabolism has now provided a unique opportunity to define specific defects in apolipoproteins, lipoprotein receptors, and enzymes in patients with dyslipoproteinemias. This new information will provide the opportunity to identify individuals at risk for the development of early heart disease and to initiate therapy prior to the development of the clinical expression of the disease.

REFERENCES

Armstrong, V. W., Cremer, P., Eberle, E., Manke, A., Schulze, F., Wieland, H., Kreuzer, H., and Seidel, D. (1986). The association between serum Lp(a) concentrations and angiographically assessed coronary atherosclerosis. Dependence on serum LDL levels. *Atherosclerosis* **63**:249–257.

Baker, D. P., VanLenten, B. J., Fogelman, A. M., Edwards, P. A., Kean, C., and Berliner, J. A. (1984). LDL scavenger, and β-VLDL receptors on aortic endothelial cells. *Arteriosclerosis* **4**:248–255.

Berg, K., Dahlen, G., and Frick, M. H. (1974). Lp(a) lipoprotein and pre-β-lipoprotein in patients with coronary heart disease. *Clin. Genet.* **6**:230–235.

Blackhart, B. D., Ludwig, E. M., Pierolli, V. R., Caiati, L., Onasch, M. A., Wallis, S. C., Powell, L., Pease, R., Knott, T. J., Chu, M. L., Mahley, R. W., Scott, J., McCarthy, B. J., and Levy-Wilson, B. (1986). Structure of the human apolipoprotein B gene. *J. Biol. Chem.* **261**:15364–15367.

Breslow, J. L. (1989). Genetic basis of lipoprotein disorders. *J. Clin. Invest.* **84**:373–380.

Brewer, H. B., Jr., Schaefer, E. J., Osborne, J. C., and Zech, L. A. (1979). High density lipoproteins: An overview. Report of the High-Density Lipoprotein Methodology Workshop. Edited by K. Lippel. U.S. Department of Health, Education and Welfare. NIH Publication No. 79-1661, pp. 29–42.

Brewer, H. B., Jr., Zech, L. A., Gregg, R. E., Schwartz, D., and Schaefer, E. J. (1983). Type III hyperlipoproteinemia: Diagnosis, molecular defects, pathology, and treatment. *Ann. Int. Med.* **98**:623–640.

Brewer, H. B., Jr., Gregg, R. E., Hoeg, J. M., and Fojo, S. S. (1988). Apolipoproteins and lipoproteins in human plasma: An overview. *Clin. Chem.* **33**: B4–B8.

Brewer, H. B., Jr. Gregg, R. E., and Hoeg, J. M. (1989). *Apolipoproteins, Lipoproteins, and Atherosclerosis. Heart Disease Update.* Edited by E. Braunwald. W. B. Saunders Co., pp. 121–136.

Castelli, W. P., Doyle, J. T., Gordon, T., Hames, C. G., Hjortland, M. C., Hully, S. B., Kagan, A., and Zukel, W. J. (1977). HDL cholesterol and other lipids in coronary heart disease. The Cooperative Lipoprotein Phenotyping Study. *Circulation* **55**:767–767.

Chen, S. H., Habib, G., Yang, C.-Y., Gu, Z.-W., Lee, B. R., Weng, S.-A., Silberman, S. R., Cai, S. -J., Deslypere, J. P., Rosseneu, M., Gotto, A. M., Li, W. H., and Chan, L. (1987). Apolipoprotein B-48 is the product of a messenger RNA with an organ-specific in-frame stop codon. *Science* **238**:363–366.

Davignon, J., Gregg, R. E., and Sing, C. F. (1988). Apolipoprotein E polymorphism and atherosclerosis (review). *Arteriosclerosis* **8**:1–21.

Eaton, D. L., Fless, G. M., Kohr, W. J., McLean, J. W., Xu, Q.-T., Miller, C. G., Lawn, R. M., and Scanu, A. M. (1987). Partial amino acid sequence of apolipoprotein(a) shows it is homologous to plasminogen. *Proc. Natl. Acad. Sci. USA* **84**:3224–3228.

Eisenberg, S. (1984). High-density lipoprotein metabolism. *J. Lipid Res.* **25**:1017–1058.

Fidge, N. H., Tozuka, M., Ehnholm, C., and Morrison, J. (1989). Studies on the structure and function of cellular HDL binding proteins. *High Density Lipoproteins and Atherosclerosis II.* Edited by N. E. Miller. New York, Excerpta Medica, pp. 219–224.

Fielding, C. J., Shore, V. G., and Fielding, P. E. (1972). A protein cofactor of lecithin:cholesterol acyltransferase. *Biochem. Biophys. Res. Commun.* **46**:1493–1498.

Fogelman, A. M., Shechter, I., Seager, J., Hokom, M., Child, J. S., and Edwards, P. A. (1980). Malondealdehyde alterations of low-density lipoprotein leads to cholesteryl ester accumulation in human monocyte-macrophages. *Proc. Natl. Acad. Sci. USA* **77**:2214–2218.

Gerrity, R. G. (1981a). The role of the monocyte in atherogenesis. I. Transition of blood-borne monocytes into foam cells in fatty lesions. *Am. J. Pathol.* **103**:181–190.

Gerrity, R. G. The role of the monocyte in atherogenesis. II. Migration of foam cells from atherosclerotic lesions. *Am. J. Pathol.* **103**:191–200.

Gofman, J. W., Glazier, F., Tamplin, A., Strisower, B., Delalla, O. (1954). Lipoproteins, coronary artery disease, and atherosclerosis (review). *Physiol. Rev.* **34**:589–607.

Gordon, T., Castelli, W. P., Hjortland, M. C., Kannel, W. B., and Dawber, T. R. (1977). High-density lipoprotein as a protective factor against coronary heart disease: Framingham study. *Am. J. Med.* **62**:707–714.

Gregg, R. E., and Brewer, H. B., Jr. (1988). The role of apolipoprotein E and lipoprotein receptors in modulating the in vivo metabolism of apolipoprotein B-containing lipoproteins in humans. *Clin. Chem.* **33**:B28–B32.

Haberland, M. E., and Fogelman, A. M. (1987). The role of altered lipoproteins in the pathogenesis of atherosclerosis. *Am. Heart J.* **113**:573–577.

Havel, R. J., Shore, V. G., Shore, B., and Bier, D. M. (1970). Role of specific glycopeptides of human serum lipoproteins in the activation of lipoprotein lipase. *Circ. Res.* **27**:595–600.

Herbert, P. N., Assmann, G., Gotto, A. M., Jr., and Fredrickson, D. S. (1983). Familial lipoprotein deficiency: Abetalipoproteinemia, hypobetalipoproteinemia and Tangier disease. In *The Metabolic Basis of Inherited Disease.* Edited by J. B. Stanbury, J. B. Wyngaarden, D. S. Fredrickson, J. L. Goldstein, and M. S. Brown. New York, McGraw-Hill Inc., pp. 605–660.

Herz, J., Hamamn, U., Rogne, S., Myklebost, D., Gausepohl, G., and Stanley, K. K. (1988). Surface location and high affinity for calcium of a 500 kDa liver membrane protein closely related to the LDL receptor suggest a physiological role as lipoprotein receptor. *EMBO J* **7**:4119–4127.

Heyden, S., Heiss, G., Bartel, A., and Hames, C. G. (1980). Fasting triglycerides as predictors of total and CHD mortality in Evans County, Georgia. *J. Chron. Dis.* **33**:275–282.

Higuchi, K., Hospattankar, A. V., Law, S. W., Meglin, N., Cortright, J., and Brewer, H. B., Jr. (1988). Human apolipoprotein B (apoB) mRNA: Identification of two distinct apo B mRNAs, an mRNA with the apo B-100 sequence and an apo B mRNA containing a premature in-frame translational stop codon, in both liver and intestine. *Proc. Natl. Acad. Sci. USA* **85**:1772–1776.

Hiramatsu, K., Rosen, H., Heinecke, J. W., Wolfbauer, G., and Chait, A. (1987). Superoxide initiates oxication of low density lipoproteins by human monocytes. *Arteriosclerosis* **7**:55–60,

Hospattankar, A. V., Higuchi, K., Law, S. W., Meglin, N., and Brewer, H. B., Jr.

(1987). Identification of a novel in-frame translational stop codon in human intestine apo B mRNA. *Biochem. Biophys. Res. Commun.* **148:**279–285.

Hulley, S. B., Rosenman, R. H., Bawol, R. D., and Brand, R. J. (1980). Epidemiology as a guide to clinical decisions: The association between triglyceride and coronary heart disease. *N. Engl. J. Med.* **302:**1383–1389.

Kane, J. P., Hardman, D. A., and Paulus, H. E. (1983). Heterogeneity of apolipoprotein B: Isolation of a new species from human chylomicrons. *Proc. Natl. Acad. Sci. USA* **77:**2465–2469.

Kane, J. P. (1983). Apolipoprotein B: Structural and metabolic heterogeneity. *Ann. Rev. Physicol.* **45:**637–650.

Koo, C., Wernette-Hammonal, M. E., Garcia, Z., Malloy, M. J., Uamy, R., East, C., Bilheimer, D. W., Mahley, R. W., and Innerarity, T. L. (1988). Uptake of cholesterol-rich remnant lipoproteins by human monocyte-derived macrophages is mediated by low-density lipoprotein receptors. *J. Clin. Invest.* **87:**1332–1339.

Kostner, G. M., Avogaro, P., Zazzolato, G., Marth, E., Bittolo-Bon, G., and Quinci, G. B. (1981). Lipoprotein Lp(a) and the risk for myocardial infarction. *Artherosclerosis* **38:**51–61.

LaRosa, J. C., Levy, R. I., Herbert, P., Lux, S. E., and Fredrickson, D. S. (1970). A specific apoprotein activator for lipoprotein lipase. *Biochem. Biophys. Res. Commun.* **41:**57–62.

Law, S. W., Lackner, K. J., Hospattankar, A. V., Anchors, J. M. Sakaguchi, A. Y., Naylor, S. L., and Brewer, H. B., Jr. (1985). Human apolipoprotein B-100: Cloning, analysis of liver mRNA, and assignment of the gene to chromosome 2. *Proc. Natl. Acad. Sci. USA* **82:**8340–8344.

Lee, R. S., and Hatch, F. T. (1963). Sharper separation of lipoprotein species by paper electrophoresis in albumin containing buffer. *J. Lab. Clin. Med.* **61:**518–528.

Mahley, R. W. (1979). Dietary fat, cholesterol, and accelerated atherosclerosis. In *Atherosclerosis Reviews.* Edited by R. Paoletti, and A. M. Gotto, Jr. New York, Raven Press, pp. 1–34.

Mahley, R. W., Innerarity, T. L., Rall, S. C., Jr., and Weisgraber, K. H. (1984). Plasma lipoproteins: Apolipoprotein structure and function. *J. Lipid Res.* **25:**1277–1294.

McLean, J. W., Tomlinson, J. E., Keeany, W.-J., Eaton, D. L., Chen, E. Y., Fless, G. M., Scanu, A. M., and Lawn, R. M. (1987). cDNA sequence of human apolipoprotein(a) is homologous to plasminogen. *Nature* **330:**132–137.

Miller, N. E., Forde, O. H., Thelle, D. S., and Mjos, O. D. (1977). The Tromso heart study. High-density lipoprotein and coronary heart disease: a prospective case-control study. *Lancet* **1:**965–968.

Naito, H. K. (1980). HDL cholesterol concentration and severity of coronary atherosclerosis determined by cine-angiography. *Biochim. Biophys. Acta* **620:**101–105.

Norum, R. A., Lakier, J. B., Goldstein, S., Angel, A., Goldberg, R. B., Block, W. D., Noffze, D. K. Dolphin, P. J., Edelglass, J., Bogorad, D. D., and Alaupovic,

P. (1982). Familial deficiency of apolipoproteins A-I and C-III and precocious coronary-artery disease. *N. Engl. J. Med.* **306:**1513–1519.

Oram, J. F., Brinton, E., and Bierman, E. L. (1983). Regulation of high density lipoprotein receptor activity in cultured human skin fibroblasts and human arterial smooth muscle cells. *J. Clin. Invest.* **72:**1611–1622.

Osborne, J. C., Jr. and Brewer, H. B., Jr. (1977). The plasma lipoproteins. *Adv. Protein Chem.* **31:**253–337.

Powell, L. W., Wallis, S. C., Pease, R. J., Edwards, Y. H., Knott, T. J., and Scott, J. (1987). A novel form of tissue-specific RNA processing produces apolipoprotein-B48 in intestine. *Cell* **50:**831–840.

Scanu, A. M., and Landsberger, F. R. (Eds.) (1980). Lipoprotein structure. *Am. N.Y. Acad. Sci.* **348:**1–436.

Schaefer, E. J., Ordovas, J. M., Law, S. W., Ghiselli, G., Kashyap, M. L., Srivastava, L. S., Heaton, W. H., Albers, J. J., Connor, W. E., Lindgren, F. T., Lemeshev, Y., Segrest, J. P., and Brewer, H. B., Jr. (1985). Familial apolipoprotein A-I and C-III deficiency, variant II. *J. Lipid Res.* **26:**1089–1101.

Schmitz, G., Robenek, H., Lohmann, U., and Assmann, G. (1985). Interaction of high density lipoproteins with cholesteryl ester-laden macrophages: Biochemical and morphological characterization of cell surface binding, endocytosis, and resecretion of high density lipoproteins by macrophages. *EMBO J.* **4:**613–622.

Steinberg, D. (1983). Lipoproteins and atherosclerosis: a look back and a look ahead. *Arteriosclerosis* **3:**283–301.

Steinberg, D. (1987). Lipoproteins and atherosclerosis. Some unanswered questions. *Am. Heart J.* **113:**626–632.

Utermann, G., Menzel, H. J., Kraft, H. G., Duba, H. C., Kemmler, H. G., and Seitz, C. (1987). Lp(a) glycoprotein phenotypes. Inheritance and relation of Lp(a)-lipoprotein concentrations in plasma, *J. Clin. Invest.* **80:**458–465.

Van Lenten, B. J., Fogelman, A. M., Hokom, M. M., Benson, L., Haberland, M. E., and Edwards, P. A. (1983). Regulation of the uptake and degradation of β-VLDL in human monocyte-macrophages. *J. Biol. Chem.* **258:**5151–5157.

Wilhelmsen, L., Wedel, H., and Tibblin, G. 91973). Multivariate analysis of risk factors for coronary heart disease. *Circulation* **48:**950–958.

Yaari, S., Goldbourt, U., Even-Zohar, S., and Neufeld, H. N. (1981). Association of serum high-density lipoprotein and total cholesterol with total, cardiovascular, and cancer mortality in a 7-year prospective study of 10,000 men. *Lancet* **1:**1011–1014.

2

Diagnosis and Management of Lipoprotein Disorders

Ernst J. Schaefer
Tufts University School of Medicine
New England Medical Center
USDA Human Nutrition Research Center on Aging at Tufts University
Boston, Massachusetts

The purpose of this chapter is to provide an overview of the diagnosis and management of lipoprotein disorders. Previous chapters have dealt with lipoprotein metabolism, and subsequent chapters will deal with the dietary management of lipid disorders as well as individual medications used for the treatment of lipoprotein disorders. The current guidelines for the diagnosis and treatment of hypercholesterolemia are also reviewed in a subsequent chapter under the National Cholesterol Education Program guidelines.

I. EVALUATION OF THE PATIENT

An initial approach to the evaluation of patients for the detection of lipoprotein disorders is to measure a plasma or serum cholesterol, triglyceride, and high density lipoprotein (HDL) cholesterol value after an overnight 12–14-hour fast. Plasma values are approximately 3% lower than corresponding serum values. It is important for the physician to ensure that the blood samples are placed on ice or refrigerated expeditiously because at room temperature cholesterol can exchange between particles. In addition the laboratory that carries out these measurements should have coefficients of variation of less than 3% and an accuracy of within 3% of target values based on reference material that can be traced to standards from the Centers for Disease Control Lipid Standardization Program (U.S. Dept. Health and Human Services, 1990). If the fasting triglyceride is below 400 mg/dl, then LDL cholesterol can be calculated by subtracting HDL cholesterol and triglyceride/5 from total cholesterol (Friedewald et al., 1972; McNamara et al., 1990). If the triglyceride value is over 400 mg/dl, then a measurement of lipoproteins following ultracentrifugation is essential for an accurate assessment of LDL cholesterol values (McNamara and Schaefer, 1987; McNamara et al., 1990). More specialized assays of specific protein or lipid constituents within lipoprotein particles or protein isoforms or the activity of various enzymes (apolipoproteins A-I, B, C-II, and E, E isoforms, lipoprotein (a), cholestanol, betasitosterol, lipoprotein lipase, hepatic lipase, or lecithin: cholesterol acyltransferase) will be subsequently discussed and are indicated in special cases. In patients with premature coronary heart disease (CHD), plasma lipoprotein (a) and apo B should also be measured. In patients with severe hypertriglyceridemia presenting in early life in the absence of obesity, apo C-II and lipoprotein lipase should be measured. In patients with marked deficiency of VLDL and LDL, apo B levels and apo B molecular weight should be determined. In patients with marked HDL deficiency (HDL cholesterol < 10 mg/dl), apo A-I levels should be measured. In patients with xanthomas in the presence of normal lipoproteins, plasma cholestanol and betasitosterol should be quantified.

Lipoprotein disorders can be divided into the following categories:

1. Elevated LDL cholesterol only (above the 90th percentile)
2. Elevated LDL cholesterol and triglyceride values (both values above the 90th percentile)
3. Elevated apo B levels (above the 90th percentile, usually ≥ 130 mg/dl)
4. Elevated triglyceride values (above the 90th percentile)
5. Severe hypertriglyceridemia (>1000 mg/dl)
6. Lipoprotein (a) excess (above the 90th percentile, usually ≥ 40 mg/dl)
7. Isolated HDL deficiency (below the 10th percentile)
8. Deficiencies of apolipoprotein B–containing lipoproteins (total cholesterol and LDL cholesterol below the 10th percentile)
9. Xanthomas with normal lipoprotein values

The rationale for screening patients for lipoprotein abnormalities and apolipoprotein abnormalities derives from the fact that elevated plasma LDL cholesterol, lipoprotein (a), apolipoprotein (apo) B, cholestanol, and betasitosterol levels and decreased HDL cholesterol values have been associated with permature CHD, while triglyceride levels above 1000 mg/dl in the fasting state have been shown to be associated with recurrent pancreatitis (Castelli et al., 1977; Miller et al., 1977; Kannel et al., 1979; Sniderman et al., 1982; Schaefer and Levy, 1985; Dahlen et al., 1986; Kannel et al., 1986). In addition, patients with severe deficiencies of VLDL and LDL may develop spinocerebellar ataxia and retinitis pigmentosa (Schaefer and Levy, 1985; Brunzell, 1989; Kane and Havel, 1989). Therefore, screening for lipoprotein and apolipoprotein abnormalities is different than screening just to detect hypercholesterolemia associated with elevated LDL cholesterol values. The current guidelines of the National Cholesterol Education Program were designed to detect individuals with elevated LDL cholesterol values and therefore can initially use nonfasting cholesterol as a screening tool (Expert Panel, 1988). In contrast, in screening patients for lipoprotein abnormalities, initially a fasting cholesterol, triglyceride, and HDL cholesterol value is essential. Other assays are only required in specialized cases.

The current National Cholesterol Education Program (NCEP) guidelines were designed to decrease risk of coronary heart disease in our population by lowering elevated and moderately elevated LDL cholesterol values above the approximate 75th percentile in the normal population (Expert Panel, 1988). However, for a precise diagnosis of lipoprotein abnormalities, one must use age- and gender-specific norms. Such norms, based on the Lipid Research Clinic's population, are provided in Table 1. The major reasons to use such norms are the significant age-related increases in plasma cholesterol, plasma triglyceride, very low density lipoprotein (VLDL), and low density lipoprotein cholesterol levels. In addition, there is a significant gender difference with regard to HDL cholesterol after the age of puberty, which persists throughout the rest of life. Therefore, while approximate cutpoints such as a total cholesterol of $\geq$ 240 mg/dl and an LDL cholesterol $\geq$ 160 mg/dl as well as an HDL cholesterol < 35 mg/dl are all cutpoints associated with increased heart disease risk (Expert Panel, 1988), age- and gender-specific percentile values are more accurate for clearly defining an abnormality, specifically values that are above the 90th or below the 10th percentile of normal (Dept. of Health and Human Services, 1980).

Before considering primary familial lipoprotein disorders, it is important to rule out secondary causes of lipid disturbances in patients. Common secondary causes of lipoprotein abnormalities are shown in Table 2. These can generally be ruled out by a careful history, especially with regard to diet and medication use, as well as an assessment of thyroid function, liver function, renal function, and glucose values. A complete diet history is best carried out

Table 1 Normal Plasma Lipid and Lipoprotein-Cholesterol Concentrations[a]

Age (Yr)	Plasma Cholesterol (mg/dl)			Plasma Triglyceride (mg/dl)			VLDL Cholesterol (mg/dl)			LDL Cholesterol (mg/dl)			HDL Cholesterol (mg/dl)		
	10[b]	50[b]	90[b]	10[b]	50[b]	90[b]	10[b]	50[b]	90[b]	10[b]	50[b]	90[b]	10[b]	50[b]	90[b]
Males															
0–4	125	151	186	33	51	84	—	—	—	—	—	—	—	—	—
5–9	130	159	191	33	51	85	2	7	15	69	90	117	42	54	70
10–14	127	155	190	37	59	102	2	9	18	72	94	122	40	55	71
15–19	120	146	183	43	69	120	3	12	23	68	93	123	34	46	59
20–24	130	165	204	50	86	165	5	12	24	73	101	138	32	45	57
25–29	143	178	227	54	95	199	6	15	31	75	116	157	32	44	58
30–34	148	190	239	58	104	213	8	18	36	88	124	166	32	45	59
35–39	157	197	249	62	113	251	7	19	46	92	131	176	31	43	58
40–44	163	203	250	64	122	248	8	21	43	98	135	173	31	43	60
45–49	169	210	258	68	124	253	8	20	40	106	141	186	33	45	60
50–54	169	210	261	68	124	250	10	23	49	102	143	185	31	44	58
55–59	167	212	262	67	119	235	6	19	39	103	145	191	31	46	64
60–64	171	210	259	68	119	235	4	16	35	106	143	188	34	49	69
65–69	170	210	258	64	112	208	3	16	40	104	146	199	33	49	74
>70	162	205	252	67	111	212	3	15	31	100	142	182	33	48	70

Females															
0–4	120	156	189	38	59	96	—	—	—	—	—	—	—	—	—
5–9	134	163	195	36	55	90	1	9	19	73	98	125	38	52	67
10–14	131	158	190	44	70	114	3	10	20	73	94	126	40	52	64
15–19	126	154	190	44	66	107	4	11	20	67	93	127	38	51	68
20–24	130	160	203	41	64	112	3	10	22	62	98	136	37	50	68
25–29	136	168	209	42	65	116	4	11	22	73	103	141	40	55	73
30–34	139	172	213	44	69	123	2	9	20	76	108	142	40	55	71
35–39	147	182	225	46	73	137	3	13	26	81	116	161	38	52	74
40–44	154	191	235	51	82	155	5	12	26	89	120	164	39	55	78
45–49	161	199	247	53	87	171	4	14	32	90	127	173	39	56	78
50–54	172	215	268	59	97	186	4	14	32	102	141	192	40	59	77
55–59	183	228	282	63	106	204	4	18	40	103	148	204	39	58	82
60–64	186	228	280	64	105	202	3	13	30	105	151	201	43	60	85
65–69	183	229	280	66	112	204	3	15	36	104	156	208	38	60	79
>70	180	226	278	69	111	204	0	13	34	107	146	189	37	60	82

aData are from Lipid Research Clinics population studies in the United States and Canada for white males and females (nonusers of sex hormones). All subjects were tested in the fasting state. Values in the lowest 5th percentile and highest 95th percentile for all age and sex groups (milligrams per deciliter) are: cholesterol, 112 to 303; triglyceride, 29 to 303; VLDL cholesterol, 0 to 62; LDL cholesterol, 60 to 234; and HDL cholesterol, 27 to 91. To convert cholesterol and triglyceride values to millimoles per liter, multiply by 0.02586 and 0.01129, respectively. Dashes indicate that no data are available because there were fewer than 100 subjects in a cell.

bPercentile.

Table 2 Secondary Causes of Lipoprotein Abnormalities

Increased LDL Cholesterol	Increased Triglycerides	Decreased HDL
Hypothyroidism	Obesity	Hypertriglyceridemia
Diabetes mellitus	Diabetes mellitus	Obesity
Nephrotic syndrome	Lack of exercise	Diabetes mellitus
Obstructive liver disease	Alcohol intake	Cigarette smoking
Progestins	Renal insufficiency	Lack of exercise
Anabolic steroids	Estrogens	Beta blockers
	Beta blockers	Progestins
		Anabolic steroids

by a trained dietitian so that estimated dietary intake of calories, saturated fat, and cholesterol can be calculated. In addition the physician should carefully question the patient with regard to medication use, as well as personal and family history of coronary disease, stroke, peripheral vascular disease, and pancreatitis. The age of onset of such disorders should also be ascertained. Information about cigarette smoking, diabetes, and history of hypertension should be obtained. In addition, physical examination is important in evaluating patients with lipid disorders. An accurate assessment of height and weight is important to assess whether obesity is present. The presence of xanthelasmas, tendinous xanthomas, tuberous xanthomas, or eruptive xanthomas may provide important clues as to which type of lipoprotein disorder is present (see Table 3). Whether carotid and femoral bruits are present should be ascertained. All pulses should be checked. A careful eye examination is important to rule out arcus senilis, lipemia retinalis, and corneal opacification. Examination of the heart and abdomen are important to detect murmurs, hepatosplenomegaly, or tenderness over the pancreas. Finally, in high risk individuals it is not unreasonable to carry out an exercise test to determine if cardiac ischemia is present.

II. LIPOPROTEIN DISORDERS

A. Elevated LDL

Familial lipoprotein disorders associated with premature coronary heart disease are shown in Table 4, including those associated with elevated LDL cholesterol values. Elevated LDL cholesterol levels may be due to a diet high in saturated fat and cholesterol or to any of the secondary causes listed in

Table 3 Association of Xanthomas with Familial Lipoprotein Disorders

Xanthelasma	Tendinous xanthomas	Eruptive xanthomas	Tuberous xanthomas	Tuboeruptive xanthomas
Familial hyper-cholesterole-mia	Familial hyper-cholesterole-mia	Familial hyper-triglyceride-mia	Familial dysbe-talipoprotei-nemia	Familial dysbe-talipoprotei-nemia
Familial dysbe-talipoprotei-nemia	Familial dysbe-talipoprotei-nemia	Familial lipo-protein lipase deficiency	Familial hyper-cholesterole-mia	Familial hyper-triglyceride-mia
Phytosterolemia	Phytosterolemia	Familial apo C-II deficiency	Cerebrotendi-nous xantho-matosis	
Cerebrotendi-nous xantho-matosis	Cerebrotendi-nous xantho-matosis			

Table 2. However, values above the 90th percentile (see Table 1) in the absence of secondary causes (see Table 2) in patients that have been placed on an NCEP Step 2 diet (< 7% of calories as saturated fat, < 200 mg of dietary cholesterol per day) are generally associated with a familial lipoprotein disorder. Therefore in such cases it is worthwhile to screen family members to detect additional affected subjects. When family studies are carried out, in some cases no clear genetic pattern is detected, and such cases have been designated as sporadic or polygenic hypercholesterolemia. In other cases, kindreds either have familial combined hyperlipidemia or familial hyper-cholesterolemia.

Familial Combined Hyperlipidemia

Patients with familial combined hyperlipidemia (FCH) may have elevations of plasma LDL cholesterol or triglycerides or both (Goldstein et al., 1973; Hazzard et al., 1973). In order for a kindred to be designated as FCH, at least two family members must be affected, and both elevated LDL cholesterol (> 90th percentile) and elevated triglyceride levels (> 90th percentile) must be documented, although both abnormalities do not need to be present in the same individual (Hazzard et al., 1973). Affected individuals also frequently have decreased HDL cholesterol levels and generally do not have xanthomas (Genest et al., 1989). They are at increased risk for developing premature CHD (Goldstein et al., 1973; Hazzard et al., 1973; Genest et al., 1989) Approximately 10–15% of patients with CHD prior to age 60 years have this

Table 4 Genetic Lipoprotein Disorders Associated with Premature Coronary Heart Disease

Disorder	Estimated frequency in premature CHD	Biochemical abnormality[a]	Metabolic abnormality	Molecular defect
Familial Lp(a) excess	15%	Elevated Lp(a)>40 mg/dl	Unknown	Decreased apo(a) molecular weight, decreased number of kringle 4 repeats, precise defect(s) not known
Familial dyslipidemia	15%	Elevated triglyceride Decreased HDL cholesterol	Increased liver triglyceride synthesis, enhanced HDL apoA-I catabolism	Unknown
Familial combined hyperlipidemia	15%	Elevated triglyceride Increased LDL, often decreased HDL cholesterol	Increased apoB-100 production	Unknown
Hyperapobetalipoproteinemia	5%	Elevated apoB only, apoB > 130 mg/dl	Increased apoB-100 production	Unknown
Familial hypoalphalipoproteinemia	4%	Decreased HDL	Decreased HDL apoA-I synthesis	Unknown
Familial hypercholesterolemia*	3%	Elevated LDL	Delayed LDL apoB fractional catabolism	Mutations within LDL receptor gene or within apoB gene
Familial dysbetalipoproteinemia	0.5%	Elevated VLDL—VLDL cholesterol: triglyceride ratio > 0.3	Delayed VLDL and chylomicron remnant catabolism	ApoE mutations

[a]Defined as above the 90th percentile or below the 10th percentile of normal.

disorder (see Table 3) (Goldstein et al., 1973; Hazzard et al., 1973; Brunzell et al., 1976; Genest et al., 1989). It has been reported that patients with FCH have overproduction of apo B-100 and triglyceride by the liver (Janus et al., 1980; Chait et al., 1980, 1981; Kissebah et al., 1981; Beil et al., 1982; Kesaniemi and Grundy, 1983; Brunzell et al., 1983). The precise defect at the molecular level is not known. Some patients with familial combined hyperlipidemia may also have delayed triglyceride catabolism secondary to heterozygous familial lipoprotein lipase deficiency (Barbirak and Brunzell, 1989).

Patients with FCH are often overweight, hypertensive, diabetic, and frequently have elevated uric acid levels. Treatment consists of an exercise program, avoidance of beta blockers, calorie restriction if the patient is over-weight, and a diet consistent with NCEP Step 2 guidelines (< 7% of calories as saturated fat, < 200 mg/day of dietary cholesterol). Optimal control of diabetes if present with diet and medication should be carried out prior to consideration of cholesterol-lowering drug therapy. In addition, patients on beta blockers for hypertension control should be switched to calcium channel blockers or angiotensin-converting enzyme inhibitors if possible, since beta adrenergic blocking agents have been reported to raise triglyceride levels and decrease HDL cholesterol levels (Fager et al., 1983).

The medication of choice in these patients is niacin if they are not diabetic. If they are diabetic or unable to tolerate niacin, then either gemfibrozil or lovastatin can be used. The goal of therapy in these patients is to lower LDL cholesterol below 130 mg/dl and triglycerides below 200 mg/dl. In patients who do not achieve the LDL cholesterol goal with one agent, combinations can be used such as niacin and an anion exchange resin, gemfibrozil and resin, or lovastatin and resin. In patients with CHD attempts should be made to lower LDL cholesterol to less than 100 mg/dl.

Familial Hypercholesterolemia

Patients with heterozygous familial hypercholesterolemia (FH) often have isolated striking elevations of LDL cholesterol (usually > 250 mg/dl). Triglyceride levels are usually normal, but may be slightly elevated, while HDL cholesterol levels are usually normal. Clinically these patients often have arcus senilis and tendinous xanthomas (see Fig. 1). The diagnosis of this condition can be made based on the finding of marked LDL cholesterol elevation and the presence of tendinous xanthomas in the patient or in another affected kindred member. One of the first signs of tendon xanthomas is thickening of the Achilles tendons, while in the hands an early sign is unevenness or beading of the tendinous surface. Arthritis and tendinitis can occur in the area of xanthomas. These patients are at increased risk of

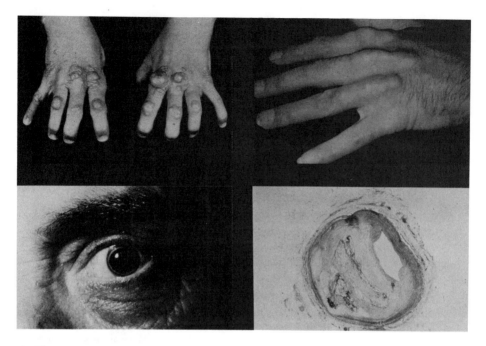

Figure 1 Upper left: tuberous xanthomas in a patient with homozygous familial hypercholesterolemia;
Upper right: tendinous xanthomas in a patient with heterozygous familial hypercholesterolemia;
Lower left: arcus senilis in a patient with heterozygous familial hypercholesterolemia;
Lower right: severe coronary artery atherosclerosis in the left main coronary artery of a patient with heterozygous familial hypercholesterolemia who died suddenly at age 50 years.

developing premature CHD, with the average onset age of disease being 45 years in males and 55 years in females (Stone et al., 1974). These patients may also have a higher prevalence of calcific aortic stenosis even in the presence of a tricuspid aortic value.

Patients with homozygous FH often have LDL cholesterol values > 500 mg/dl and frequently have decreased HDL cholesterol values. In addition to having tendinous xanthomas, these patients often develop tuberous xanthomas over the elbows, hands, and knees (see Fig. 1) (Sprecher et al., 1984). Homozygotes often develop CHD prior to age 20, with males developing disease earlier than females. In addition to atherosclerosis, these patients often develop aortic stenosis secondary to cholesterol deposition within and adjacent to the valve leaflets (Sprecher et al., 1984).

The defect in these patients has been shown to be due to a variety of mutations within the LDL receptor gene on chromosome 19, resulting in lack of expression of receptors or defective receptors (Goldstein and Brown, 1989). Occasional patients may have a defect within apo B-100 resulting in defective binding of LDL to the LDL receptor (Vega and Grundy, 1986; Innerarity et al., 1987). These defects result in a marked decrease in the fractional catabolic rate of LDL and result in increased plasma LDL levels. The overall estimated frequency of this class of mutations in the general population is 1:500 for the heterozygous state, but significantly higher or lower frequencies may be observed in various populations due to genetic variation. In patients with premature CHD the frequency is 1–3% (Goldstein et al., 1973; Genest et al., 1989). Homozygotes may be homozygous for the same defect or may be compound heterozygotes (Goldstein and Brown, 1989). Currently there are no reliable assays for LDL receptor activity that can be performed in a routine clinical chemistry laboratory. Therefore the diagnosis rests on the finding of an elevated LDL cholesterol, (usually > 250 mg/dl) and tendinous xanthomas.

Treatment of heterozygotes consists of a diet consistent with NCEP Step 2 guidelines as well as, in most cases, combined drug therapy. Dietary treatment alone usually results in only small reductions in LDL cholesterol levels in these patients. The initial agent of choice is an anion exchange resin (either cholestyramine or colestipol). In FH heterozygotes who are prepubertal, resins are the only agents that should be used. After the age of puberty the use of most lipid-lowering agents are justified in FH heterozygotes. Resins alone occasionally may be sufficient to lower LDL cholesterol values to less than 160 mg/dl, but usually combination therapy is required (Hashim and VanItallic, 1965; Levy et al., 1973; Shepherd et al., 1980). In patients with established CHD, efforts should be made to lower LDL cholesterol to less than 130 mg/dl, and optimally less than 100 mg/dl. The most effective combination in heterozygotes is an anion exchange resin and lovastatin (Mabuchi et al., 1983; Illingworth, 1984). In patients who cannot tolerate resins, lovastatin alone should be used. The combination of resins and niacin is also extremely effective but is difficult for many patients to tolerate (Kane et al., 1981). Niacin and lovastatin can be used in combination, but the incidence of significant liver enzyme elevation is over 10%. Probucol can be added as a third-line drug in FH heterozygotes and appears to be effective in inducing regression of tendinous xanthomas. Homozygotes generally require plasmaphoresis every 1–2 weeks for effective therapy (Thompson et al., 1985).

B. Elevated Apolipoprotein B

Hyperapobetalipoproteinemia

Familial hyperapobetalipoproteinemia may be a variant of familial combined hyperlipidemia. These patients have plasma apo B values above the 90th percentile of normal (approximately 130 mg/dl) with normal LDL cholesterol values (Sniderman et al., 1982, 1985; Teng et al., 1983). Diagnosis requires the use of a standardized immunoassay for plasma apo B (Ordovas et al., 1987). Their triglyceride values are normal, but they have been reported to have elevated postprandial triglyceride levels as compared to normal subjects (Genest et al., 1986). The etiology of this disorder appears to be due to enhanced production of apo B-100, similar to familial combined hyperlipidemia. These patients generally do not have xanthomas, and the precise molecular defect has not been described.

This disorder is present in approximately 5% of patients with premature CHD (Genest et al., 1989). Treatment of affected individuals involves a diet consistent with NCEP Step 2 guidelines, calorie restriction if the patient is overweight, avoidance of beta blockers if possible, and a regular program of exercise. In patients with established CHD, the use of niacin or lovastatin should be considered to optimize the lipid profile (i.e., LDL cholesterol < 100 mg/dl). More information with regard to effects of diet and drug therapy in these patients is required.

C. Combined Elevations of LDL Cholesterol and Triglyceride

Patients with combined elevations of plasma cholesterol and triglyceride usually have increases in both VLDL and LDL cholesterol levels and are members of familial combined hyperlipidemia kindreds (see previous description). Rarely patients will present with combined cholesterol and triglyceride elevations due to increases in VLDL and intermediate density lipoproteins particles. These patients have dysbetalipoproteinemia.

Familial Dysbetalipoproteinemia

The diagnosis of this disorder requires analysis of plasma lipoproteins following ultracentrifugation. In addition to having markedly elevated plasma cholesterol and triglyceride levels, they have a VLDL cholesterol : triglyceride ratio > 0.3 (normal 0.2) based on quantification of VLDL cholesterol levels following ultracentrifugation (Fredrickson et al., 1967; Hazzard et al., 1975; Morganroth et al., 1975). They also have VLDL that migrates in the beta region instead of the prebeta position on lipoprotein electrophoresis (Frederickson et al., 1967; Hazzard et al., 1975); Morganroth et al., 1975). The diagnosis is confirmed by the finding of the homozygous apo E2/2 phenotype or rarely apo E deficiency on isoelectric focusing of VLDL protein (Utermann et al., 1977; Zannis and Breslow, 1981). These patients may develop tuberous or tubo-eruptive xanthomas (Fig. 2) and are at increased risk for premature CHD and peripheral vascular disease. The defect is due to mutations within the apo E gene resulting in defective apo E or, rarely, absence of the protein (Ghiselli et al., 1981; Weisgraber et al., 1981; Rall et al., 1983; Schaefer et al., 1986; Cladaras et al., 1987). Apo E is necessary for normal receptor-mediated uptake of chylomicron and VLDL remnants (Rall et al., 1983; Schaefer, et al., 1986). These patients have delayed catabolism of these lipoproteins and are also often obese, diabetic, hypertensive, and hyperuricemic.

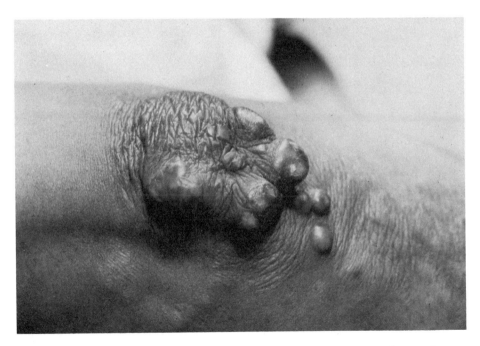

Figure 2 Tuberous xanthomas on the elbow of a patient with dysbetalipoproteine-mia due to familial apolipoprotein E deficiency.

Treatment consists of an NCEP Step 2 diet, caloric restriction if indicated, cessation of beta blockers if possible, and a regular program of exercise. Niacin, gemfibrozil, and lovastatin will lower lipids in these patients, with niacin being the most effective in terms of reducing levels of both cholesterol and triglyceride (Schaefer, 1983). The goal of therapy in such patients is to lower the total cholesterol to less than 240 mg/dl, optimally to less than 200 mg/dl.

D. Elevated Triglycerides

Familial Hypertriglyceridemia and Dyslipidemia

Familial hypertriglyceridemia is a common genetic disorder associated with elevated triglyceride levels (Goldstein et al., 1973). Familial dyslipidemia is a variant of familial hypertriglyceridemia in which affected family members have elevated triglyceride levels or decreased HDL cholesterol levels or both (Genest et al., 1989). Both abnormalities must be present in kindreds in order for a kindred to warrant the latter designation, but affected individuals may have only one abnormality. Other lipoprotein values are normal, and these patients generally do not have xanthelasmas or xanthomas. Patients with these disorders are frequently overweight, with male pattern (truncal) obesity, diabetic with elevated insulin levels, and hypertensive, and often have elevated uric acid levels. Kinetic studies indicate that such patients have increased hepatic triglyceride production, with normal apo B production (Brunzell et al., 1976, 1983; Janus et al., 1980; Chait et al., 1980, 1981; Kissebah et al., 1981; Beil et al., 1982; Kesaniemi and Grundy, 1983). Patients with hypertriglyceridemia have decreased HDL levels associated with enhanced fractional catabolism of apo A-I, the major protein of HDL (Schaefer and Ordovas, 1986).

Familial dyslipidemia is present in approximately 15% of patients with premature CHD, and the precise molecular defect is unknown (Genest et al., 1989). The expression of this disorder is undoubtedly governed by a variety of genetic and environmental factors. Treatment of affected individuals involves a diet consistent with NCEP Step 2 guidelines, calorie restriction if the patient is overweight, avoidance of beta blockers if possible, and a regular program of exercise. In patients with established CHD the use of gemfibrozil, niacin, or lovastatin should be considered to optimize the lipid profile (i.e., LDL cholesterol < 100 mg/dl, triglyceride < 200 mg/dl, and HDL cholesterol > 40 mg/dl). More information about dietary and drug therapy in these patients is needed.

E. Severe Hypertriglyceridemia

Adult Onset Severe Hypertriglyceridemia

Severe hypertriglyceridemia (triglyceride values > 1000 mg/dl) in the fasting state when present is usually observed in middle-aged or elderly individuals who are obese and have glucose intolerance and hyperuricemia. These subjects generally have HDL deficiency and may develop lipemia retinalis and erputive xanthomas (Fig. 3). They are at increased risk for developing pancreatitis due to triglyceride deposition in the pancreas and may have paresthesias and emotional lability (Fredrickson et al., 1967; Greenberg et al., 1977). These patients often have delayed chylomicron and VLDL clearance and excess VLDL apo B production (Sigurdsson et al., 1970). Treatment consists of a calorie-restricted NCEP Step 2 diet. In patients with diabetes mellitus, it is crucial to control the blood glucose as well as possible. Medications that are effective in lowering the triglycerides to less than 500 mg/dl in these patients to reduce their risk of pancreatitis include gemfibrozil

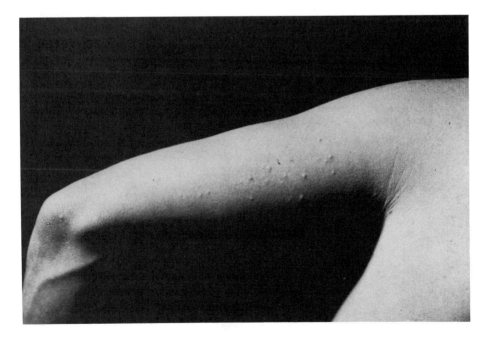

Figure 3 Eruptive xanthomas on the upper arm of a patient with severe hypertriglyceridemia due to familial lipoprotein lipase deficiency.

and/or fish oil capsules (6–10 capsules/day), or the combination (Saku et al., 1985). In nondiabetic patients, niacin can be used.

Juvenile Onset Severe Hypertriglyceridemia

Patients who present with severe hypertriglyceridemia in childhood or early adulthood and who are not obese or diabetic often have a deficiency of the enzyme lipoprotein lipase or its activator protein (apo C-II) resulting in markedly impaired removal of triglyceride (Fredrickson et al., 1967; Krauss et al., 1974; Breckenridge et al., 1978). Therefore, they have a defect in chylomicron and VLDL catabolism. These patients are at increased risk of recurrent pancreatitis and eruptive xanthoma formation, and it is important to restrict their dietary fat to less than 20% of calories. Niacin and/or gemfibrozil are generally ineffective in these patients; however, fish oil capsules may be helpful in certain patients to keep their triglyceride levels below 1000 mg/dl and minimize their risk of pancreatitis.

F. Familial Lp(a) Excess

Lipoprotein (a) is a lipoprotein particle similar to LDL except that it has one molecule of apo(a) attached to it (Berg, 1963; Berg et al., 1979; Fless et al., 1984). Elevated Lp(a) is a highly heritable trait (Berg et al., 1979). A value over the 90th percentile of normal is considered elevated (above 40 mg/dl using assays which assess the level of the entire particle). Elevated levels of Lp(a) are associated with premature CHD (Dahlen et al., 1986). Approximately 15% of patients with premature CHD have familial Lp(a) excess (Genest et al., 1989). These patients do not have xanthomas. Lp(a) appears to promote atherosclerosis and atherothrombosis by two different mechanisms: 1) deposition in the arterial wall and 2) inhibition of fibrinolysis (Dahlen et al., 1986; Hajjar et al., 1989; Loscalzo et al., 1990).

Assays for the measurement of Lp(a) are commercially available. Different isoproteins of apo(a) exist which vary in their molecular weight (Utermann et al., 1987). Decreased apo(a) molecular weight is associated with increased Lp(a) levels. Apo(a) has been shown to contain multiple repeats of a protein domain highly homologous to the kringle 4 domain of plasminogen, and one repeat of a protein domain highly homologous to the kringle 5 domain of plasminogen (McLean et al., 1987). Variability in apo(a) molecular weight appears to be related to a decreased number of kringle 4 repeats (Gavish et al., 1989). Elevated levels of Lp(a) are also observed in patients with heterozygous familial hypercholesterolemia (Seed et al., 1990). Diets and medications (resins, HMG CoA reductase inhibitors) that lower LDL levels have no effect on Lp(a) but niacin administration has been reported to decrease Lp(a) levels (Gurakar et al., 1985) No guidelines for the treatment of Lp(a) excess have been formulated, but treatment with niacin in such patients may be warranted if they have established CHD.

G.   Hypoalphalipoproteinemia

Familial Hypoalphalipoproteinemia

Familial hypoalphalipoproteinemia is characterized by HDL cholesteral levels below the 10th percentile of normal in affected family members, and are usually about 50% of normal. An autosomal dominant mode of inheritance has been reported (Vergani and Bettale, 1981; Third et al., 1984). Other lipoprotein values are within normal limits in these patients, and their triglyceride levels are not elevated. These patients do not have xanthelasmas or xanthomas and generally have normal body weight. No clear association with obesity, hypertension, or glucose intolerance has been reported. Kinetic studies indicate that some of these patients have a decreased HDL apo A-I production rate (Le and Ginzberg, 1988). This disorder is present in approximately 4% of patients with premature coronary heart disease, and the precise molecular defect is not known (Genest et al., 1989). Treatment of affected individuals involves a diet consistent with NCEP Step 2 guidelines, calorie restriction if the patient is overweight, avoidance of beta blockers if possible, and a regular program of exercise. In patients with established CHD, the use of gemfibrozil, niacin, or lovastatin should be considered to optimize their lipid profile (i.e., lower LDL cholesterol to below 100 mg/dl, and raise HDL cholesterol levels to over 40 mg/dl if possible). Generally it is not possible to achieve this latter goal. Additional studies on the effects of these agents in such patients are required.

Severe HDL Deficiency

These rare disorders are characterized by HDL cholesterol levels below 10 mg/dl in the absence of liver disease or severe hypertriglyceridemia, and some, but not all, have been associated with premature CHD.

Apolipoprotein A-I Deficiency States

   Apolipoprotein A-I/C-III/A-IV deficiency: The proband in this kindred from northern Alabama died of severe diffuse coronary atherosclerosis at age 45 years. She had marked HDL deficiency, decreased triglyceride levels, and normal LDL cholesterol values (Schaefer et al., 1982, 1985). She had mild corneal opacification, but no planar xanthomas. She also had evidence of fat malabsorption (vitamin E, K, and essential fatty acid deficiency). Plasma apo A-I and apo C-III were undetectable (Schaefer et al., 1985). Heterozygotes had levels of HDL cholesterol, apo A-I, apo C-III, and apo A-IV that were 50% of normal (Ordovas et al., 1989). The defect has been shown to be due to deletion of the entire apo A-I/C-III/A-IV gene complex (Ordovas et al., 1989). Treatment should consist of optimization of other risk factors including LDL cholesterol levels.

Apolipoprotein A-I and C-III deficiency: A kindred has been reported in which two sisters presented in their late twenties with CHD, planar xanthomas, mild corneal opacification, with marked HDL deficiency, normal LDL cholesterol values, and decreased triglycerides. No evidence of fat malabsorption was noted (Norum et al., 1982, 1986). Plasma apo A-I and apo C-III were not detectable in these homozygotes, and the defect was shown to be due to a DNA rearrangement affecting the adjacent apoA-I and apo C-III genes (Karathanasis and Haddad, 1987). Heterozygotes in this kindred from Detroit had HDL cholesterol, apo A-I, and apo C-III values that were approximately 50% of normal. Treatment is to optimize other CHD risk factors.

Apolipoprotein A-I deficiency: A kindred of Turkish origin has been reported in which the homozygous proband was a child with marked HDL deficiency, planar xanthomas, and undetectable plasma apo A-I (Schmitz and Lackner, 1989). The defect has been shown to be due to a point mutation, resulting in lack of apo A-I gene expression. No evidence of fat malabsorption was noted. Treatment is to optimize other CHD risk factors.

Apolipoprotein A-I variants: Studies examining apo A-I isoforms by isoelectric focusing have led to the discovery of 18 different mutations within the apo A-I sequence. The mutations are at residues 3 (Pro, 2 mutations), 4 (Pro), 89 (Asp), 103 (Asp), 107 (Lys, 2 mutations), 136 (Glu), 139 (Glu), 143 (Pro), 147 (Glu), 158 (Ala), 165 (Pro), 169 (Glu), 173 (Arg), 177 (Arg), 198 (Glu), and 213 (Asp) within the 243 residue apo A-I sequence (Assmann et al., 1989). All subjects detected have been heterozygotes. The residue 173 mutation (Arg-Cys) is known as apo A-I Milano and is associated with mild hypertriglyceridemia and markedly decreased HDL cholesterol levels and no evidence of premature CHD (Weisgraber et al., 1980). Most other variants were found in Germany. The residue 165 mutation (Pro-Arg) has also been associated with decreased HDL cholesterol and apo A-I levels, as has the 143 mutation (Pro-Arg) (Assman et al., 1989). This latter mutation results in decreased ability of apo A-I to activate the enzyme lecithin:cholesterol acyltransferase (Utermann et al., 1984). Other mutations have not been associated with decreased HDL cholesterol, but the mutations at residue 3 (Pro-His or Pro-Arg) result in an increased pro apo A-I:apo A-I ratio in plasma, suggesting reduced conversion of proapo A-I to mature apo A-I in these subjects (Assmann et al., 1989). The incidence of apo A-I variants is rare at 1:1000 in normals as well as in myocardial infarction survivors (Assmann et al., 1989).

Tangier disease: This disease was named after the Chesapeake Bay island home of the original kindred. Homozygotes with this disorder have marked HDL deficiency, mild hypertriglyceridemia, and decreased LDL cholesterol values (Fredrickson et al., 1961; Schaefer et al., 1980). Apo A-I levels are 1% of normal, while apo C-III and apo A-IV values are within normal limits. These patients have lipid-laden macrophages resulting in enlarged orange tonsils, hepatosplenomegaly, and lymphadenopathy (Schaefer et al., 1980). The defect is not known. These patients have hypercatabolism of HDL constituents, but the primary structure of both apo A-I and apo A-II are normal (Schaefer et al., 1978, 1981). Tangier patients appear to have altered processing of HDL by macrophages (Schmitz et al., 1985). Heterozygotes have HDL cholesterol and apo A-I values that are 50% of normal (Schaefer et al., 1980). Homozygotes may develop premature CHD and peripheral neuropathy (Schaefer et al., 1980). Treatment consists of optimization of CHD risk factors.

*Lecithin:Cholesterol Acyltransferase (LCAT) **Deficiency* 17*Familial LCAT deficiency:*   This disorder is due to deficiency of the enzyme LCAT, which is responsible for cholesterol esterification in plasma. Patients with LCAT deficiency have a very high proportion of plasma cholesterol in the unesterified form, marked HDL cholesterol deficiency, hypertriglyceridemia, and increased amounts of free cholesterol-rich VLDL and LDL. They develop marked corneal opacification, anemia, proteinuria, renal insufficiency, and atherosclerosis. Treatment consists of dietary saturated fat and cholesterol restriction and renal dialysis and transplantation if necessary (Norum et al., 1989).

Fish eye disease: This disorder has been associated with mild hypertriglyceridemia and significant HDL deficiency. Patients with fish eye disease develop striking corneal opacification, but have not been reported to have premature CHD. These patients have a deficiency of alpha-LCAT, which differs from beta-LCAT in that it acts only on HDL, whereas beta-LCAT acts on VLDL and LDL. This disorder appears to be a milder variant of LCAT deficiency (Norum et al., 1989).

H. Deficiencies of VLDL and LDL

Abetalipoproteinemia

These patients often present in childhood with diarrhea, fat malabsorption, and failure to gain weight normally. Intestinal biopsy reveals lipid-laden epithelial cells. Untreated, these patients develop spino-cerebellar ataxia and retinitis pigmentosa in their teens and twenties. On laboratory analysis they have plasma cholesterol values of approximately 40 mg/dl, triglyceride levels of 20 mg/dl, and HDL cholesterol of approximately 40 mg/dl (Bassen and Kornzweig, 1950; Gotto et al., 1971). Diagnosis is confirmed by undetectable plasma apo B, and the defect is due to an inability to secrete apo B-containing lipoproteins (chylomicrons, VLDL, and LDL) (Gotto et al., 1971). Intestinal apo B mRNA levels are increased (Lackner et al.). They also have acanthocytosis and deficiencies of fat soluble vitamins and essential fatty acids (Gotto et al., 1971). Supplementation with vitamin A and E is recommended (Muller et al., 1977, 1983; Hegele and Angel, 1985; Kayden and Traber, 1986). Vitamin E replacement appears to prevent the onset of neuropathy (Muller et al., 1977, 1983; Hegele and Angel, 1985). Obligate heterozygotes (parents) have normal lipoproteins. Restriction of dietary fat may be necessary to minimize diarrhea. It is not yet known whether these patients should be supplemented with the essential fatty acids linoleic acid and alpha linolenic acid.

Hypobetalipoproteinemia

The clinical and laboratory picture is the same in these patients as in abetalipoproteinemia (Levy et al., 1970; Cottrill et al., 1974; Berger et al., 1983; Ross et al., 1988). However, obligate heterozygotes in these kindreds have LDL cholesterol and apo B values that are 50% of normal. Treatment is the same as in abetalipoproteinemia and is only indicated in homozygotes. The defect is due to an inability to synthesize normal amounts of apo B protein, and intestinal apo B mRNA levels are decreased (Ross et al., 1988).

Other Forms of Hypobetalipoproteinemia

Normotriglyceridemic Abetalipoproteinemia Cases have been reported in which subjects have normal chylomicron formation, but lack plasma apo B-100 and LDL in plasma. One patient had serum cholesterol levels of 25 mg/dl and triglycerides that increased from 30 mg/dl to 250 mg/dl with fat-feeding. She had mental retardation and marked vitamin E deficiency, as well as ataxia, which improved with vitamin E supplementation. These patients have apo B-48 present in their plasma and have been classified as normotriglyceridemic abetalipoproteinemia (Malloy et al., 1981).

Hypobetalipoproteinemia with Abnormal ApoB Molecular Weight Another variant of these disorders is associated with abnormal apo B molecular weight. These subjects have marked deficiencies of VLDL and LDL and very low plasma apo B levels. The apo B is of abnormal molecular weight as assessed by polyacrylamide gels (Steinberg et al., 1979; Young et al., 1987a, b, 1988; Collins et al., 1988). This disorder has been called hypobetalipoproteinemia with truncated apo B. Cholesterol levels are generally approximately 40 mg/dl, but triglyceride levels can be as high as 100 mg/dl.

Chylomicron Retention Disease Another group of patients with fat malabsorption, diarrhea, and deficiency of fat-soluble vitamins, as well as lipid-laden intestine epithelial cells, has been described. LDL cholesterol and apo B levels are about 50% of normal, and after fat-feeding no significant increase in triglyceride levels are noted (Anderson et al., 1961; Levy et al., 1987). The defect is due to an inability to secrete apo B-48–containing lipoprotein. Only apo B-100 is present in plasma; no apo B-48 is noted. Treatment is similar to abetalipoproteinemia. This disorder has been designated as chylomicron retention disease, or Anderson's disease, and the defect appears to be due to an inability to secrete apo B-48–containing lipoproteins from the intestine (Levy et al., 1987).

I. Xanthomas with Normal Lipoprotein Levels

Cerebrotendinous Xanthomatosis

Cerebrotendinous xanthomatosis (CTX) is a rare familial sterol storage disorder with accumulations of cholestanol and cholesterol in most tissues, in particular in xanthomas and brain. Clinically this disorder is characterized by dementia, spinocerebellar ataxia, tuberous and tendinous xanthomas, early atherosclerosis, and cataracts. The defect in CTX is due to a lack of the hepatic mitochondrial 26-hydroxylase enzyme involved in the normal biosynthesis in bile lipids and bile acids. Patients with CTX have normal plasma lipoprotein levels, except for reduced plasma HDL cholesterol. The diagnosis should be suspected in a patient with tendinous xanthomas in the presence of a normal cholesterol and can be established by documentation of elevated plasma cholestanol levels by gas chromatography. If the diagnosis is established reasonably early, treatment with chenodeoxycholate at a dose of 250 mg three times daily reduces cholestanol levels to normal, and apparently halts the progression of the disease (Bjorkem and Skrede, 1989).

Phytosterolemia

Phytosterolemia is a rare inherited sterol storage disorder characterized by tendinous and tuberous xanthomas and by a strong predisposition to premature coronary athersclerosis (Bjorkem and Skrede, 1989). Increased amounts of phytosterols such as sitosterol and campesterol are found in plasma as well as in various tissues. Increased serum cholesterol and cholestanol levels have also been found in some patients. The basic biochemical defect has not been elucidated. These patients abosrb plant sterols from the intestine in contrast to normal subjects. Phytosterolemia should be suspected in patients who develop xanthomas in early childhood despite normal or only moderately elevated serum cholesterol levels. The diagnosis can easily be established by analysis of plasma sterols. Treatment consists of a diet containing the lowest possible amount of plant sterols with elimination of all sources of vegetable fats as well as all plant foods with a high fat content. Such a diet should not contain vegetable oil, shortening, or margarine, nor should it contain nuts, seeds, chocolate, olives, or avocados. Cholestyramine should be used in addition to diets since this causes a significant reduction in serum phytosterols, cholesterol, and cholestanol. Such treatment presumably will reduce the risk of subsequent atherosclerosis in these patients (Bjorkem and Skrede, 1989).

III. DIET THERAPY

The cornerstone of the treatment of hyperlipidemic states is diet therapy (Expert Panel, 1988). The use of meats rich in saturated fat (beef, lamb, pork) should be restricted, as should whole milk, butter, ice cream, egg yolks, and all food prepared in butter, animal fat, cream, or other sauces rich in saturated fat. The use of oils rich in saturated fat such as coconut oil, palm oil, and palm kernel oil should also be restricted. Instead, it is recommended that poultry (white meat) without skin, fish, skimmed milk, nonfat or low-fat yogurt, and/or low fat cheeses be eaten. The use of fruits and vegatables is encouraged. Oils that can be used are unsaturated vegetable oils such as canola, soybean, olive, or corn oil. Excellent patient dietary phamphlets are available from the American Heart Association as well as the National Cholesterol Education Program on the Step 1 and 2 diets. Patients unable to get an adequate response with diet after being given pamphlets and being counseled by the physician and office nurse can be referred to a registered dietitian for instruction on the Step 2 diet. In most cases, diet therapy should be tried for at least 6 months prior to initiating drug therapy. Diet treatment is more extensively discussed in Chapter 11.

IV. DRUG THERAPY

An overview of available lipid-lowering drugs is provided in Table 5. Lipid-lowering medications can be divided into two general classes: 1) drugs effective in lowering LDL cholesterol (greater than 15% reduction) and 2) drugs effective in lowering triglyceride levels (greater than 25% reduction). There are currently three classes of agents that meet the LDL lowering criteria: 1) anion exchange resins (cholestyramine and colestipol), 2) niacin, and 3) HMG CoA reductase inhibitors (lovastatin and pravastatin). Of these agents, patient acceptance and compliance with the resins and niacin is often poor, while with HMG CoA reductase inhibitors it is generally excellent. At the present time, however, CHD risk reduction and long-term safety has not been documented with these latter agents. Therefore resins and/or niacin remain the drugs of choice for LDL lowering, especially in young patients free of CHD. There are currently two agents that lower triglyceride levels by more than 25%: niacin and gemfibrozil. These agents generally lower LDL levels and raise HDL levels. Both niacin and gemfibrozil have been shown to lower CHD risk prospectively.

For patients with increased LDL cholesterol only, the drugs of choice are cholestyramine or colestipol (resins) (Hashim and VanItallic, 1965; Levy et al., 1973). If patients cannot tolerate resins even at low doses, then niacin should be used. The combination of resins and niacin is also very effective (Kane et al., 1981). For patients who cannot tolerate these agents, lovastatin or pravastatin should be utilized. The combination of a reductase inhibitor and resin is also very effective (Mabuchi et al., 1983; Illingworth, 1984). It should be noted that in postmenopausal women who have had a hysterectomy, estrogen replacement is quite effective in lowering LDL cholesterol and raising HDL cholesterol, but should not be used in the setting of hypertriglyceridemia (Tikkanen et al., 1978). Use of estrogens has been associated with a significant reduction in CHD mortality in postmenopausal women (Bush et al., 1983; Stampfer et al., 1985).

For patients with elevations in both LDL cholesterol and triglycerides, the drug of choice is niacin. For patients who cannot tolerate this agent, gemfibrozil or lovastatin can be used, as can the combination of resin and niacin or the combination of gemfibrozil and resin.

For patients with hypertriglyceridemia only normal LDL cholesterol levels, there are as yet no clear guidelines for the use of medication. If the patient has fasting triglycerides in excess of 1000 mg/dl while on a restricted diet, use of medication to reduce the risk of pancreatitis is recommended. However, prior to taking this step, the physician should make sure that these patients are not taking estrogens, using alcohol, or have uncontrolled diabetes mellitus. Also caloric and fat restriction and an exercise program are important in these patients. The drug of choice in such patients is generally gemfibrozil because most of these patients have glucose intolerance. In the

Table 5 Lipid-Lowering Medications

	Resins	Niacin	Gemfibrozil	Lovastatin	Probucol
Patient acceptance and compliance	Often poor	Often poor	Generally excellent	Generally excellent	Generally excellent
Side-effects	Constipation, bloating, decreased absorption of certain medicines	Flushing, itching, gastritis hepatotoxicity, hyperuricemia, hyperglycemia	Myositis, hepatotoxicity, GI side effects, coumadin interaction	Hepatotoxicity, myositis, headaches, weight gain, insomnia	GI side effects
Usual dose	8–10 g p.o. BID	1 g p.o. BID with food	600 mg p.o. BID	20 mg p.o. BID	500 mg p.o. BID
LDL reduction	10–20%	10–20%	0–15%	25–35%	10–15%
Triglyceride reduction	a	40%	35%	20%	0%
HDL increase	5%	15–20%	5–15%	5–10%	b
CHD risk reduction	Yes	Yes	Yes	No	No
	19%	20%	34%		
documented	7yr	5yr	5yr		
Long-term safety documented	Yes	Yes	Yes	No	No

a May increase triglycerides.
b Lowers HDL cholesterol 15–25%; both resins and niacins should be started at low doses and gradually increased.

absence of glucose intolerance, niacin can be tried. In patients in whom these agents are not effective or if additional triglyceride reduction is needed, fish oil capsules (1 g) at a dose of 3–5 capsules twice daily are effective in lowering triglycerides.

In patients with moderate hypertriglyceridemia, especially in the setting of HDL deficiency, lifestyle changes including weight reduction and an exercise program are very helpful, as are cessation of beta blockers. If such patients have CHD the use of either niacin, gemfibrozil, or reductase inhibitors should be considered to normalize their lipid levels. The goals of therapy in CHD patients are not only to get their LDL cholesterol below 130 mg/dl but to reduce their triglycerides to less than 200 mg/dl and to increase their HDL cholesterol to over 40 mg/dl. Some authorities advocate lowering LDL cholesterol to less than 100 mg/dl if CHD is present. In the absence of heart disease, only lifestyle modification (diet and exercise) can currently be recommended in patients with hypertriglyceridemia and/or HDL deficiency. An overview of lipid lowering drugs is provided in Table 5, as well as below.

A. Cholestyramine and Colestipol

Cholestyramine and colestipol are anion exchange resins which bind bile acids, increase conversion of liver cholesterol to bile acids, and upregulate LDL receptors in liver, increasing LDL catabolism and decreasing plasma LDL by about 20% (Shepherd et al., 1980). Cholestyramine is bulkier than colestipol, but has flavor. Both resins need to be thoroughly mixed with liquid. Side effects include bloating and constipation, elevation of triglycerides, and interference with the absoirption of digoxin, tetracycline, d-thyroxine, phenylbutazone, and coumadin (give drugs 1 hour before or 4 hours after resin). Cholestyramine (4-g scoops) or colestipol (5-g scoops) can be started at one scoop twice per day and gradually increased to two scoops twice per day (the scoops are half the price of the packets) or two scoops three times daily. Constipation may require treatment. Cholestyramine use has been shown to reduce CHD risk prospectively by 19% over 7 years in middle-aged asymptomatic hypercholesterolemic men (Lipid Research, 1984a, b; Gordon et al., 1988).

B. Niacin

Niacin decreases VLDL (by 40%) and LDL production (by 20%) and raises HDL cholesterol values (by 20%). Niacin should be started at 100 mg p.o. BID with meals and gradually increased to 1 g p.o. BID or TID with meals. Side effects include flushing, gastric irritation, and elevations of uric acid, glucose, and liver enzymes in some patients. Niacin should not be used in patients with liver disease, a history of an ulcer, or in diabetic patients not on insulin. Long-acting niacin causes less flushing but more GI side effects than regular niacin. One aspirin daily will minimize flushing and can be used initially. Niacin should be discontinued if liver enzymes increase to over twice the upper normal limit. Niacin has been shown to reduce the recurrence of myocardial infarction by 20% after a 5-year period of administration in men with CHD. The use of niacin was also associated with an 11% reduction in all cause mortality 10 years after cessation of niacin (Coronary Drug Project, 1975; Canner et al., 1986).

C. Gemfibrozil

Gemfibrozil is given at a dose of 600 mg p.o. BID and is generally well tolerated. The drug is very effective in lowering triglycerides (by 35%) by decreasing production and enhancing breakdown of VLDL. The drug usually lowers LDL cholesterol levels 10–15% and increases HDL 5–15%. Rarely patients may have gastrointestinal symptoms or muscle cramps (elevated CPK, 1%). The drug should not be used in patients with renal insufficiency, and it is also known to potentiate the action of coumadin. The drug may raise LDL levels in some hypertriglyceridemic patients. Gemfibrozil has been found to reduce CHD prospectively by 34% over 5 years in middle-aged asymptomatic hypercholesterolemic men (Frick et al., 1987; Manninen et al., 1988).

D. Lovastatin and Pravastatin

Lovastatin and pravastatin are started at 20 mg/day and can be increased to a maximal dose of 40 mg p.o. BID. These drugs are generally well tolerated, but may occasionally cause liver enzyme elevation, CPK elevation with myalgias and myositis, stomach upset, headaches, decreased sleep duration or mild insomnia, blurred vision, skin rash, and weight gain. Possible differences in the side effect profile of these agents is currently being explored. The drugs inhibit HMG CoA reductase, the rate-limiting enzyme in cholesterol biosynthesis, causing upregulation of LDL receptors, enhancing LDL catabolism, and decreasing plasma LDL 30–45% (Lovastatin Study Group, 1986). These agents also decrease VLDL and LDC by decreasing production and may increase HDL. Long-term safety and efficacy in CHD risk reduction have not been established.

E. Probucol

Probucol is an antioxidant given at a dose of 500 mg p.c. BID and is a second-line drug in lowering LDL 10–15%, which can be used in familial hypercholesterolemia for increasing nonreceptor LDL catabolism. It may cause gastrointestinal side effects. The drug also lowers HDL cholesterol 15–25%. Long-term safety and efficacy in CHD risk reduction have not been established.

F. Combination Therapy

Niacin and resin together are effective, as are resin and gemfibrozil, and lovastatin with resin. Gemfibrozil and lovastatin can be used, but myositis incidence is approximately 7%. Niacin and lovastatin are also effective, but the incidence of significant liver enzyme elevation is >10%. Gemfibrozil with either fish oil capsules or niacin can be used to lower triglycerides.

V. CONCLUSION

Dietary treatments with reduced saturated fat and cholesterol content remain the cornerstone of therapy for elevated LDL cholesterol values. Such diets have been shown to reduce CHD risk by 20% or more in normolipidemic, hypercholesterolemic, and CHD subjects (Dayton et al., 1969; Leren, 1970; Hjermann et al., 1981). In patients with established CHD, aggressive management not only to lower LDL cholesterol but to raise HDL cholesterol levels is warranted based on studies that indicate that when this is achieved there is decreased progression and some regression of existing coronary atherosclerosis (Blankenhorn et al., 1987). Newer, more effective agents for the treatment of lipid disorders (HMG CoA reductase inhibitors) have recently become available. If these agents are shown to be safe in long-term studies and decrease CHD risk, then they will become the agents of choice for LDL reduction. More information is urgently needed with regard to the dietary and drug management of patients with familial dyslipidemia, hypoalphalipoproteinemia, and lipoprotein (a) excess.

REFERENCES

Anderson, C. M., Townley, R. R. W., and Freeman, J. P. (1961). Unusual causes of steatorrhea in infancy and childhood. *Med. J. Aust.* **11**:617.

Assmann, G., Schulte, H., Funke, H., von Eckardstein, A., and Seedorf, U. (1989). The prospective cardiovascular Munster (PROCAM) Study: Identification of high risk individuals for myocardial infarction and the role of high density lipoprotein. In *High Density Lipoproteins, Reverse Cholesterol Transport, and Coronary Heart Disease*. Edited by N. Miller. Princeton, Excerpta Medica, pp. 46–59.

Barbirak, S. P., and Brunzell, J. P. (1989). A subset of patients with familial combined hyperlipidemia have abnormal lipoprotein lipase. *Circulation* II **79A** (abstract).

Bassen, F. A., and Kornzweig, A. L. (1950). Malformation of the erythrocytes in a case of atypical retinitis pigmentosa. *Blood* **5**:381.

Beil, V., Grundy, S. M., Crouse, J. R., and Zech, L. (1982) Triglyceride and cholesterol metabolism in primary hypertriglyceridemia. *Arteriosclerosis* **2**:44.

Berg, K. (1963). A new serum type system in man—The Lp system. *Acta Pathol. Microbiol. Scand.* **59**:369.

Berg, K., Dahlen, G., and Borreson, A. L. (1979). Lp(a) phenotypes, other lipoprotein parameters and a family history of coronary heart disease in middle-aged males. *Clin. Genet.* **16**:347.

Berger, G. M. B., Brown, G., Henderson, H. E., and Bonnici, F. (1983). Apolipoprotein B detected in the plasma of a patient with homozygous hypobetalipoproteinemia: Implications for aetiology. *J. Med. Genet.* **20**:189.

Bjorkem, I., and Skrede, S. (1989). Familial diseases with storage of sterols other than cholesterol: Cerebrotendinous xanthomatosis and phytosterolemia In *Metabolic Basis of Inherited Disease*. Edited by C. R. Scriver, A. L. Beaudet, W. S. Sly, and D. Valle. New York, McGraw-Hill, pp. 1283–1304.

Blankenhorn, D. M., Nessim, S. A., Johnson, R. L., Sanmarco, M. E., Azen, S. P., and Cashin-Hemphill, L. (1987) Beneficial effects of combined colestipol-niacin therapy on coronary atherosclerosis and coronary venous bypass grafts. *JAMA* **257**:3233–3240.

Breckenridge, W. C., Little, J. A., Steiner, G., Chow, A., and Poapst, A. (1978). Hypertriglyceridemia associated with a deficiency of apolipoprotein C-II. *N. Engl. J. Med.* **298**:1265–1273.

Brunzell, J. D. (1989). Familial lipoprotein lipase deficiency, and other causes of chylomicronemia syndrome In *The Metabolic Basis of Inherited Disease*. Sixth edition. Edited by C. R. Scriver, A. L. Beaudet, W. S. Sly, and D. Valle. New York, McGraw-Hill, pp. 1165–1180.

Brunzell, J. D., Albers, J. J., Chait, A., Grundy, S. M., Groszek, E., and McDonald, G. B. (1983). Plasma lipoproteins in familial combined hyperlipidemia and monogenic familial hypertriglyceridemia. *J. Lipid Res.* **24**:147–155.

Brunzell, J. D., Schrott, H. G., Motulsky, A. G., and Bierman, E. L. (1976). Myocardial infarction in the familial forms of hypertriglyceridemia. *Metabolism* **25**:313.

Bush, T. L., Cowan, L. D., Barrett, C. E., Criqui, M. H., Karon, J. M., Wallace, R. B., Tyroler, H. A., and Rifkind, B. M. (1983). Estrogen use and all-cause mortality. Preliminary results from the Lipid Research Clinics program followup. *JAMA* **249**:903–911.

Canner, P. L., Berge, K. G., Wenger, N. K., Stamler, J., Friedman, L., Prineas, R. J., and Friedewald, W. (1986). Fifteen-year mortality in Coronary Drug Project patients: Long-term benefit with niacin. *J. Am. Coll. Cardiol.* **8**:1245–1255.

Castelli, W., Doyle, J. T., Gordon, T., et al. (1977). HDL cholesterol and other lipids in coronary heart disease: the Cooperative Lipoprotein Phenotyping Study. *Circulation* **55**:767–772.

Chait, A., Albers, J. J., and Brunzell, J. D. (1980). Very low density lipoprotein overproduction in genetic forms of hypertriglyceridemia. *Eur. J. Clin. Invest.* **10**:17–22.

Chait, A., Foster, D., Albers, J. J., and Brunzell, J. D. (1981). Familial hyper-cholesterolemia vs. familial combined hyperlipidmia: low density lipoprotein apo-lipoprotein-B kinetics. *Arteriosclerosis* **1**:82.

Cladaras, C., Hadzopoulou-Cladaras, M., Felber, B. K., Pavlakis, G., and Zannis, V. I. (1987). The molecular basis of a familial apo E deficiency. An acceptor splice site mutation in the third intron of the deficient apo E gene. *J. Biol. Chem.* **262**:2310.

Collins, D. R., Knott, T. J., Pease, R. J., Powell, L. M., Wallis, S. C., Robertson, S., Pullinger, C. R., Milne, R. W., Marcel, Y. L., Humphries, S. E., Talmud, P. J., Lloyd, J. K., Miller, N. E., Muller, D., and Scott, J. (1988). Truncated variants of apolipoprotein B cause hypobetalipoproteinema. *Nucleic Acids Res.* **16**:8361.

The coronary drug project research group. (1975). Clofibrate and niacin in coronary heart disease. *JAMA* **231**:360–381.

Cottrill, C., Glueck, C. J., Leuba, V., Millet, F., Puppione, D. and Brown, W. V. (1974). Familial homozygous hypobetalipoproteinemia. *Metabolism* **23**:779.

Dahlen, G. H., Guyton, J. R., Attar, M., Farmer, J. A., Kautz, J. A., and Gotto, A. M., Jr. (1986). Association of levels of lipoprotein Lp(a), plasma lipids, and other lipoproteins with coronary artery disease documented by angiography. *Circulation,* **59**:199.

Dahlen, G. H., Guyton, J. R., Attar, M., Farmer, J. A., Kautz, J. A., and Gotto, A. M. (1986). Association of levels of Lp(a), plasma lipids, and other lipoproteins with coronary artery disease documented by angiography. *Circulation* **74**: 758–765.

Dayton, S., Pearce, M. L., and Hasimoto, S. A. (1969). A controlled clinical trial of a diet high in unsaturated fat in preventing complications of atherosclerosis. *Circulation* **40** (Suppl. 2): 1–63.

The Expert Panel. (1988). Report of the National Cholesterol Education Program Expert Panel on detection, evaluation, and treatment of high blood cholesterol in adults. *Arch. Intern. Med.* **148**:36–69.

Fager, G., Berglund, G., Bondjers, F., et al. (1983). Effects of antihypertensive therapy on serum lipoproteins: treatment with metoprolol, propranolol, and hyd-rochlorothiazide. *Artery* **11**:283–296.

Fless, G. M., Rolih, C. A., and Scanu, A. M. (1984). Heterogeneity of human plasma lipoprotein (a): Isolation and characterization of the lipoprotein subspecies and their apoproteins. *J. Biol. Chem.* **259:**11470.

Fredrickson, D. S., Altrocchi, P. H., Avioli, L. V., Goodman, D. S., and Goodman, H. C. (1961). Tangier disease—combined clinical staff conference a the National Institutes of Health. *Ann. Intern. Med.* **55:**1016.

Fredrickson, D. S., Levy, R. I., and Lees, R. S. (1967). Fat transport in lipoproteins—an integrated approach to mechanisms and disorders. *N. Engl. J. Med.* **276:**34, 94, 148, 214, 273.

Frick, M. H., Elo, O., Haapa, K., Heinonen, O. P., Heinsalmi, P., Helo, P., Huttunen, J. K., Kaitaniemi, P., Koskinen, P., Manninen, V., Maenpaa, H., Malkonen, M., Mantari, M., Norola, S., Pasternak, A., Pikkaranen, J., Romo, M., Sjomblom, T., and Nikkila, E. A. (1987). Helsinki Heart Study: Primary prevention trial with gemfibrozil in middle-aged men with dyslipidemia. *N. Engl. J. Med.* **317:**1237–1245.

Friedewald, W. T., Levy, R. I., and Fredrickson, D. S. (1972). Estimation of low density lipoprotein cholesterol in plasma, without use of the preparative ultracentrifuge. *Clin. Chem.* **18:**499–502.

Gavish, D., Azrolan, N., and Breslow, J. L. (1989). Plasma Lp(a) concentration is inversely correlated with the ratio of the kringle IV/kringle V encoding domains in the apo(a) gene. *J. Clin. Invest.* **84:**2021–2027.

Genest, J. J., Jr., Martin-Munley, S., McNamara, J. R., Salem, D. N., and Schaefer, E. J. (1989). Frequency of genetic dyslipidemia in patients with premature coronary artery disease. *Circulation* **9:**701A.

Genest, J., Sniderman, A., Cianflone, K., et al. (1986). Hyperapobetalipoproteinemia. Plasma lipoprotein response to oral fat load. *Arteriosclerosis* **6:**297–304.

Ghiselli, G., Schaefer, E. J., Gascon, P., and Brewer, H. B., Jr. (1981). Type III hyperlipoproteinemia associated with apolipoprotein E deficiency. *Science* **214:**1249.

Goldstein, J. L., and Brown, M. S. (1989). Familial hypercholesterolemia. In *The Metabolic Basis of Inherited Disease.* Edited by C. R. Scriver, A. L. Beaudet, W. S. Sly, and D. Valle. New York, McGraw-Hill, p. 1215.

Goldstein, J. L., Schrott, H. G., Hazzard, W. R., Bierman, E. L., and Motulsky, A. G. (1973). Hyperlipidemia in coronary heart disease. II. Genetic analysis of lipid levels in 176 families and delineation of a new inherited disorder, combined hyperlipidemia. *J. Clin. Invest.* **52:**1544–1568.

Gordon, D. J., Knoke, J., Probstfield, J. L., et al. (1988). High-density lipoprotein cholesterol and coronary heart disease in hypercholesterolemic men. The Lipid Research Clinics Coronary Primary Prevention Trial. *Circulation* **2:**29–37.

Gotto, A. M., Levy, R. I., John, K., and Fredrickson, D. S. (1971). On the nature of the protein defect in abetalipoproteinemia. *N. Engl. J. Med.* **284:**813.

Greenberg, B. H., Blackwelder, W. C., and Levy, R. I. (1977). Primary type V hyperlipoproteinemia. A descriptive study in 32 families. *Ann. Intern. Med.* **87:**526.

Gurakar, A., Hoeg, J. M., Kostner, G., Papadopoulos, N. M., and Brewer, H. B., Jr. (1985). Levels of lipoprotein Lp(a) decline with neomycin and niacin treatment. *Atherosclerosis* **57**:293.

Hajjar, K. A., Gavish, D., Breslow, J. L., and Nachman, R. L. (1989). Lipoprotein (a) modulation of endothelial cell surface fibrinolysis and its potential role in atherosclerosis. *Nature* **339**:303–305.

Hashim, S. A., and VanItallic, T. B. (1965). Cholestyramine resin therapy for hypercholesterolemia. *JAMA* **192**:289–293.

Hazzard, W. R., Goldstein, J. L., Schrott, H. G., Motulsky, A. G., and Bierman, E. L. (1973). Evaluation of lipoprotein phenotypes of 156 genetically defined survivors of myocardial infarction. *J. Clin. Invest.* **52**:1544.

Hazzard, W. R., O'Donnell, T. F., and Lee, Y. L. (1975). Broad-beta disease (type III hyper-lipoproteinemia) in a large kindred. Evidence for a monogenic mechanism. *Ann. Intern. Med.* **92**:141.

Hegele, R. A., and Angel, A. (1985). Arrest of neuropathy and myopathy in abetalipoproteinemia with high dose vitamin E therapy. *Can. Med. Assoc. J.* **12**: 41.

Hjermann, I., Velve-Byre, K., Holme, I., and Leren, P. (1981). Effect of diet and smoking intervention on the incidence of coronary heart disease. *Lancet* **2**:1303–1309.

Illingworth, D. R., (1984). Mevinolin plus colestipol in therapy for severe heterozygous familial hypercholesterolemia. *Ann. Intern. Med.* **101**:598–604.

Innerarity, T. L., Weisgraber, K. H., Arnold, K. S., et al. (1987). Familial defective apolipoprotein B-100: low density lipoproteins with abnormal receptor binding. *Proc. Natl. Acad. Sci. USA* **84**:6919–6925.

Janus, E. D., Nicoll, A. M., Turner, P. R., Magill, P., and Lewis, B. (1980). Kinetic bases of the primary hyperlipidemias: studies of apolipoprotein B turnover in genetically defined subjects. *Eur. J. Clin. Invest.* **10**:161–172.

Kane, J. P., and Havel, R. J. (1989). Disorders of the biogenesis and secretion of lipoproteins containing the B apolipoproteins In *The Metabolic Basis of Inherited Disease*. Sixth edition. Edited by C. R. Scriver, A. L. Beaudet, W. S. Sly, and D. Valle. New York, McGraw-Hill pp. 1145–1155.

Kane, J. P., Malloy, M. J., Tur, P., Phillips, N. R., Freedman, D. D., Williams, M. L., Rowe, J. S., and Howel, R. J. (1981). Normalization of low density lipoprotein levels in heterozygous familial hypercholesterolemia with a combined drug regimen. *N. Engl. J. Med.* **304**:251–258.

Kannel, W. P., Castelli, W. P., and Gordon, T. (1979). Cholesterol in the prediction of atherosclerotic disease: new perspectives based on the Framingham Study. *Ann. Intern. Med.* **90**:85–91.

Kannel, W. B., Neaton, J. D., Wentworth, D., et al. (1986). Overall and CHD mortality rates in relation to major risk factors in 325, 348 men screened for MRFIT. *Am. Heart J.* **112**:825–836.

Karathanasis, S. K., and Haddad, I. (1987). DNA inversion within the apolipoprotein

A-I/C-III/A-IV encoding gene cluster of certain patients with premature atherosclerosis. *Proc. Natl. Acad. Sci. USA* **84**:7198–7202.

Kayden, H. J., and Traber, M. G. (1986) Clinical, nutritional, and biochemical consequences of apolipoprotein B deficiency. *Adv. Exp. Med. Biol.* **201**:67.

Kesaniemi, Y. A., and Grundy, S. M. (1983). Overproduction of low density lipoproteins associated with coronary heart disease. *Arteriosclerosis* **3**:40.

Kissebah, A. H., Alfarsi, S., and Adams, P. W. (1981). Integrated regulation of very low density lipoprotein triglyceride and apolipoprotein B kinetics in man: Normolipidemic subjects, familial hypertriglyceridemia, and familial combined hyperlipidemia. *Metabolism* **30**:856–868.

Krauss, R. M., Levy, R. I., and Fredrickson, D. S. (1974). Selective measurement of two lipase activities in postheparin plasma from normal subjects and patients with hyperlipoproteinemia. *J. Clin. Invest.* **54**:1107.

Lackner, K. J., Monge, J. C., Gregg, R. E., Hoeg, J. M., Triche, T. J., Law, S. W., and Brewer, H. B., Jr. (1986). Analysis of the apolipoprotein B gene and messenger ribonucleic acid in abetalipoproteinemia. *J. Clin. Invest.* **78**:1701.

Langer, T., Strober, W., and Levy, R. I. (1972). The metabolism of low density lipoprotein in type II hyperlipoproteinemia. *J. Clin. Invest.* **51**:1528–1536.

Le, A. N., and Ginzberg, H. N. (1988). Heterogeneity of apolipoprotein A-I turnover with reduced concentrations of plasma high density lipoprotein cholesterol. *Metabolism* **37**:614–617.

Leren, P. (1970). The Oslo Diet Heart Study: eleven year report. *Lancet* **42**:935–942.

Levy, E., Marcel, Y., Deckelbaum, R. J., Milne, R., LePage, G., Seidman, E., Bendayan, M., and Roy, C. C., (1987). Intestinal apoB synthesis, lipids, and lipoproteins in chylomicron retention disease. *J. Lipid. Res.* **28**:1263.

Levy, R. I., Fredrickson, D. S., Stone, N. G., Bilheimer, D. W., Grown, W. V., Glueck, C. J., Gotto, A. M., Jr., Herbert, P. N., Kwiterovich, P. O., Langer, T., LaRosa, J., Lux, S. E., Rider, A. K., Shulman, R. S., and Sloan, H. R. (1973). Cholestyramine in type II hyperlipoproteinemia: a double bind trial. *Ann. Intern. Med.* **79**:51–59.

Levy, R. I., Langer, T., Gotto, A. M., and Fredrickson, D. S. (1970). Familial hypobetalipoproteinemia, a defect in lipoprotein synthesis. *Clin. Res.* **18**:539.

The Lipid Research Clinics Population Studies Data Book. Vol 1. *The Prevalence Study.* (1980). Washington D. C., Department of Health and Human Services, Public Health Service, National Institutes of Health Publication No. 80-1527, pp. 28–81.

Lipid Research Clinics Program. (1984a). The Lipid Research Clinics Coronary Primary Prevention Trial results: I. Reduction in the incidence of coronary heart disease. *JAMA* **251**:351–364.

Lipid Research Clinics Program. (1984b). The Lipid Research Clinics Coronary Primary Prevention Trial results: II. The relationship of reduction in incidence of coronary heart disease to cholesterol lowering. *JAMA* **251**:365–374.

Loscalzo, J., Weinfeld, M., Fless, G. M., and Scanu, A. M. (1990). Lipoprotein (a), fibrin binding and plasminogen activation. *Arteriosclerosis* **10**:240–245.

Lovastatin Study Group II. (1986). Therapeutic response to lovastatin (mevinolin) in nonfamilial hypercholesterolemia. A multicenter trial. *JAMA* **256**:2829–2834.

Mabuchi, H., Sakari, T., Sakai, Y., Yoshimura, A., Watanabe, A., Wakisugi, T., Koizumi, J., Takeda, R., Reduction of serum cholesterol in heterozygous patients with familial hypercholesterolemia: Additive effects of compactin and cholestyramine. *N. Engl. J. Med.* **308**:609–614.

Malloy, M. J., Kane, J. P., Hardman, D. A., Hamilton, R. L., and Dalal, K. (1981). Normotriglyceridemia abetalipoproteinemia. Absence of the B-100 apoprotein. *J. Clin. Invest.* **67**:1441.

Manninen, V., Elo, O., Frick, M. H., Haapa, K., Heinonen, O. P., Heinsalmi, P., Helo, P., Huttunen, J. K., Kaitaniemi, P., Koskinen, P., Maenpaa, H., Malkonen, M., Mantari, M., Norola, S., Pasternak, A., Pikkaranen, J., Romo, M., Sjomblom, T., and Nikkila, E. (1988). Lipid alterations and decline in the incidence of coronary heart disease in the Helsinki Heart Study. *JAMA* **260**:641–651.

McLean, J. W., Tomlinson, J. E., Kuang, W-J., Eaton, D. L., Chen, E. Y., Fless, G. M., Scanu, A. M., and Lawn, R. M. (1987). cDNA sequence of human apolipoprotein (a) is homologous to plasminogen. *Nature* **330**:132.

McNamara, J. R., Cohn, J. S., Wilson, P. W. F., and Schaefer, E. J. (1990). Calculated values for low density lipoprotein cholesterol in the assessment of lipid abnormalities and coronary disease risk. *Clin. Chem.* **36**:36–42.

McNamara, J. R., and Schaefer, E. J. (1987). Automated enzymatic standardized lipid analyses for plasma and lipoprotein fractions. *Clin. Chim. Acta* **166**:1–8.

Miller, N. E., Forde, O. H., and Thelle, D. S. (1977). The Tromso Heart Study: High density lipoprotein and coronary heart disease: A prospective case control study. *Lancet* **55**:767–772.

Morganroth, J., Levy, R. I., and Fredrickson, D. S. (1975). The biochemical, clinical and genetic features of type III hyperlipoproteinemia. *Ann. Intern. Med.* **82**:158.

Muller, D. P. R., Lloyd, J. K., and Bird, A. C. (1977). Long-term management of abetalipoproteinemia. *Arch. Dis. Child.* **52**:209.

Muller, D. P. R., Lloyd, J. K., and Wolff, O. H. (1983). Vitamin E and neurological function. *Lancet* **1**:225.

Norum, R. A., Forte, T. M., Alaupovic, P., and Ginsberg, H. N. (1986). Clinical syndrome and lipid metabolism in hereditary dificiency of apolipoproteins A-I and C-III, variant I. *Adv. Exp. Med. Biol.* **201**:137–149.

Norum, K. R., Gjone, E., and Glomset, J. A. (1989). Familial lecithin : cholesterol acyltransferase deficiency including fish eye disease. In *Metabolic Basis of Inherited Disease*. Edited by C. R. Scriver, A. L. Beaudet, W. S. Sly, and D. Valle. New York, McGraw-Hill, pp. 1181–1194.

Norum, R. A., Lakier, J. B., Goldstein, S., et al. (1982). Familial deficiency of apolipoproteins A-I and C-III and precocious coronary artery disease. *N. Engl. J. Med.* **306**:1513–1519.

Ordovas, J. M., Cassidy, D. K., Civeira, F., Bisgaier, C. L., and Schaefer, E. J. (1989). Familial apolipoprotein A-I, C-III, and A-IV deficiency with marked high density lipoprotein deficiency and premature atherosclerosis due to a deletion of the apolipoprotein A-I, C-III, and A-IV gene complex. *J. Biol. Chem.* **264:**16339–16342.

Ordovas, J. M., Peterson, J. P., Santaniello, P., Cohn, J., Wilson, P. W. F., and Schaefer, E. J. (1987). Enzyme linked immunosorbent assay for human plasma apolipoprotein B. *J. Lipid Res.* **28:**1216–1224.

Rall, S. C., Jr., Weisgraber, K. H., Innerarity, T. L., Mahley, R. W., and Assmann, G. (1983). Identical structural and receptor binding defects in apolipoprotein E2 in hypo-, normo-, and hypercholesterolemic dysbetalipoproteinemia. *J. Clin. Invest.* **71:**1023.

Ross, R. S., Gregg, R. E., Law, S. W., Monge, J. C., Grant, S. M., Higuchi, K., Triche, T. J., Jefferson, J., and Brewer, H. B. Jr. (1988). Homozygous hypobetahpoproteinemia: A disease distinct from abetalipoproteinemia at the molecular level. *J. Clin. Invest.* **81:**590.

Saku, K., Gartside, P. S., Hynd, B. A., and Kashyap, M. L. (1985). Mechanism of action of gemfibrozil on lipoprotein metabolism. *J. Clin. Invest.* **75:**1702–1712.

Schaefer, E. J. (discussant). (1983). Dietary and drug treatment, in type III hyperlipoproteinemia: Diagnosis, molecular defects, pathology, and treatment. H. B. Brewer, Jr. (moderator). *Ann. Intern. Med.* **98** (part 1):633.

Schaefer, E. J., Anderson, D. W., Zech, L. A., Lindgren, F. T., Bronzert, T. B., Rubalacaba, E. A., and Brewer, H. B., Jr. (1981). Metabolism of high density lipoprotein subfractions and constituents in Tangier disease following the infusion of high density lipoproteins. *J. Lipid Res.* **22:**217.

Schaefer, E. J., Blum, C. B., Levy, R. I., Jenkins, L. L., Alaupovic, P., Foster, D. M., and Brewer, H. B., Jr. (1978). Metabolism of high density apolipoproteins in Tangier disease. *N. Engl. J. Med.* **299:**905.

Schaefer, E. J., Gregg, R. E., Ghiselli, G., Forte, T. M., Ordovas, J. M., Zech, L. A., and Brewer, H. B., Jr. (1986). Familial apolipoprotein E deficiency. *J. Clin. Invest.* **78:**1026.

Schaefer, E. J., Heaton, W. H., Wetzel, M. G., and Brewer, H. B., Jr. (1982). Plasma apolipoprotein A-I absence associated with a marked reduction of high density lipoproteins and premature coronary artery disease. *Arteriosclerosis* **2:**16–26.

Schaefer, E. J., and Levy, R. I. (1985). Pathogenesis and management of lipoprotein disorders. *N. Engl. J. Med.* **312:**1300–1310.

Schaefer, E. J., and Ordovas, J. M. (1986). Metabolism of the apolipoproteins A-I, A-II, and A-IV. In *Methods in Enzymology, Plasma Lipoproteins.* Part B: *Characterization, Cell Biology and Metabolism.* Edited by J. Segrest and J. Albers. Academic Press.

Schaefer, E. J., Ordovas, J. M., Law, S., Ghiselli, G., Kashyap, M. L., Srivastava, L. S., Heaton, W. H., Albers, J. J., Connor, W. E., Lemeshev, Y., Segrest, J., Brewer, H. B., Jr. (1985). Familial apolipoprotein A-I and C-III deficiency, variant II. *J. Lipid Res.* **26:**1089–1101.

Schaefer, E. J., Zech, L. A., Schwartz, D. E., and Brewer, H. B., Jr. (1980).

Coronary heart disease prevalence and other clinical feature in familial high density lipoprotein deficiency (Tangier disease). *Ann. Intern. Med.* **93**:261.

Schmitz, G., Assmann, G., Robeneck, H., and Brennhausen, B. (1985). Tangier disease: A disorder of intracellular membrane traffic. *Proc. Natl. Acad. Sci.* **82**:6305–6308.

Schmitz, G., and Lackner, K. (1989). *High Density Lipoprotein Deficiency with Xanthomas: A Defect in apo A-I Synthesis.* Edited by G. Crepaldi, A. M. Gotto, E. Manzato, and G. Baggio. Amsterdam, Excerpta Medica, p. 399.

Seed, M., Hoppicher, F., Reaveley, D., McCarthy, S., Thompson, G. R., Boerwinkle, G., and Utermann, G. (1990). Relation of serum lipoprotein (a) concentration and apolipoprotein (a) phenotype to coronary heart disease in patients with familial hypercholesterolemia *N. Engl. J. Med.* **322**:1494–1499.

Shepherd, J., Packard, C. J., Bicker, S., Lawrie, T. D. V., and Morgan, H. G. (1980). Cholestyramine promotes receptor mediated low density lipoprotein catabolism. *N. Engl. J. Med.* **302**:1219–1224.

Sigurdsson, G., Nicoll, A., and Lewis, B. (1970). The metabolism of very low density lipoproteins in hyperlipidemia: studies of apolipoprotein B kinetics in man. *Eur. J. Clin. Invest.* **6**:167–177.

Sniderman, A. D., Teng, B., Genest, J., Cianflone, K., Wacholder, S., and Kwiterovich, P. O., Jr. (1985). Familial aggregation and early expression of hyperapobetalipoproteinemia. *Am. J. Cardiol.* **55**:291–295.

Sniderman, A. D., Wolfson, C., Teng, B., Franklin, F. A., Bachorik, P. S., and Kwiterovich, P. O., Jr. (1982). Association of hyperapobetalipoproteinemia with endogenous hypertriglyceridemia and atherosclerosis. *Ann. Intern. Med.* **97**:833–839.

Sprecher, D. S., Schaefer, E. J., Kent, K. M., Roberts, W. C., and Brewer, H. B., Jr. (1984). Cardiovascular features of homozygous familial hypercholesterolemia. *Am. J. Cardiol.* **54**:20–30.

Stampfer, M. J., Willett, W. C., Colditz, G. A., Rosner, B., Speizer, F. E., and Hennekens, C. H. (1985). A prospective study of postmenopausal estrogen use and coronary heart disease. *N. Engl. J. Med.* **313**:1044–1049.

Steinberg, D., Grundy, S. M., Mok, H. I., Turner, J. D., Weinstein, D. B., Brown, W. V., and Albers, J. J., (1979). Metabolic studies in an unusual case of asymptomatic familial hypobetalipoproteinemia and fasting chylomicroemia. *J. Clin. Invest.* **64**:292.

Stone, N. J., Levy, R. I., Fredrickson, D. S., and Verter, J. (1974). Coronary artery disease in 116 kindreds with familial type II hyperlipoproteinemia. *Circulation* **49**:476–485.

Teng, B., Thompson, G. R., Sniderman, A. D., Forte, T. M., Krauss, R. M., and Kwiterovich, P. O., Jr. (1983). Composition and distribution of low density lipoprotein fractions in hyperapobetalipoproteinemia, normolipidemia, and familial hypercholesterolemia. *Proc. Natl. Acad. Sci. USA* **80**:6662–6666.

Third, J. L. H. C., Montag, J., Flynn, M., Freidel, J., Laskarzewski, P., and Glueck,

C. J. (1984). Primary and familial hypoalphalipoproteinemia. *Metabolism* **33**:136–146.

Thompson, G. R., Miller, J. P., and Breslow, J. L. (1985). Improved survival of patients with homozygous familial hypercholesterolemia treated with plasma exchange. *Br. Med. J.* **291**:1671–1678.

Tikkanen, M. J., Nikkila, E. A., and Vartianen. (1978). Natural estrogen use as an effective treatment for type II hyperlipoproteinemia. *Lancet* **2**:490–495.

U.S. Department of Health and Human Services, National Institutes of Health. (1990). Recommendations for improving cholesterol measurement. Publication No. 90-2964, 1–63.

Utermann, G., Haas, J., Steinmetz, A., and Paetzold, R. (1984). Apolipoprotein A-I Gressen (Pro 143-Arg). A mutant that is defective in activating LCAT. *Eur. J. Biochem.* **144**:326–331.

Utermann, G., Manzel, H. J., Kraft, H. G., Duba, H. C., Kemmler, H. G., and Seitz, C. (1987). Lp(a) glycoprotein phenotypes: inheritance and relation to Lp(a) lipoprotein concentrations in plasma. *J. Clin. Invest.* **80**:458–465.

Utermann, G., Pruin, N., and Steinmetz, A. (1977). Polymorphism of apolipoprotein E and occurrence of dysbetalipoproteinemia in man. *Nature* **269**:604.

Vega, G. L., and Grundy, S. M. (1986). In vivo evidence for reduced binding of low density lipoproteins to receptors as a cause of primary moderate hypercholesterolemia. *J. Clin. Invest.* **78**:1410–1418.

Vergani, C., and Bettale, A. (1981). Familial hypoalphalipoproteinemia. *Clin. Chem. Acta.* **114**:45–52.

Weisgraber, K. H., Bersot, T. P., Mahley, R. W., Francheschini, G., and Sirtori, C. R. (1980). A-I milano apoprotein. Isolation and characterization of a cysteine-containing variant of the A-I apoprotein from human high density lipoproteins. *J. Clin. Invest.* **66**:901–909.

Weisgraber, K. H., Rall, S. C., Jr. and Mahley, R. W. (1981). Human apolipoprotein E isoprotein subclasses are genetically determined. *Am. J. Hum. Genet.* **33**:11.

Young, S. G., Bertics, S. J., Curtiss, L. K., Dubois, B. W., and Witztum, J. L. (1987). Genetic analysis of a kindred with familial hypobetalipoproteinemia; evidence for two separate gene defects: One associated with an abnormal apolipoprotein B species, apoB-37, and a second associated with low plasma concentrations of apoB-100. *J. Clin. Invest.* **79**:1842.

Young, S. G., Northey, S. T., and McCarthy, B. J. (1988). Low plasma cholesterol levels caused by a short deletion in the apoB gene. *Science* **241**:591.

Young, S. G., Peralta, F. P., Dubois, B. W., Curtiss, L. K., Boyles, J. K., and Witzum, J. L. (1987b). Lipoprotein B37, a naturally occuring lipoprotein containing the amino-terminal portion of apolipoprotein B-100, does not bind to the apolipoprotein B, E (low density lipoprotein) receptor. *J. Biol. Chem.* **262**:16604.

Zannis, V. I., and Breslow, J. L. (1981). Human very low density lipoprotein apolipoprotein E isoform polymorphism is explained by genetic variation and posttranslational modification. *Biochemistry* **20**:1033.

3

Guidelines for the Detection and Treatment of Dyslipoproteinemia in Adults

John C. LaRosa
George Washington University Medical Center
Washington, D.C.

I. INTRODUCTION

The relationship between circulating lipoproteins and atherosclerosis has been a matter of intense interest and controversy for the last half century. A consensus has developed in the past several years that has settled large elements of that controversy. As a result of numerous laboratory, epidemiological, and clinical studies reviewed elsewhere in this volume, it has become clear that elevated circulating levels of low density lipoprotein (LDL) cholesterol are associated with accelerated atherogenesis and that arrest or even reversal of that process can be achieved if LDL cholesterol levels are lowered.

The scientific consensus that has developed as a result of these accumulated data was first reflected in the statements of the U.S. National Institutes of Health (NIH) "consensus panel," convened to review the evidence linking lowering of blood cholesterol to lowering levels of coronary risk (NIH Consensus Conference, 1985). That conference, in turn, led to the establishment by the National Heart, Lung & Blood Institute of the U.S. National

Cholesterol Education Program (NCEP), which involves the participation of the American Heart Association and a host of other medical and scientific public health, business, and consumer organizations. The overall purpose of the NCEP was to provide the medical community and the lay public with guidelines for the management of a number of issues related to the cholesterol/heart disease relationship. The first major product of this program were guidelines developed by an expert panel for the detection, evaluation, and treatment of high blood cholesterol in adults (> 20 yr). These guidelines have become widely known as the Adult Treatment Panel Guidelines (National Cholesterol Education Program, 1988). This chapter will review those guidelines and some of the thinking that went into their formulation, as well as some of the critiques directed at them and similar guidelines developed in Europe (Study Group, European Atherosclerosis Society, 1987).

II. SCREENING FOR LIPID ABNORMALITIES

The Adult Treatment Panel Guidelines recommend that total blood cholesterol be used as an initial screening measurement. They do not recommend universal (public) screening for adults, except as such screening may occur as part of regular physician/patient encounters. Universal screening was not endorsed because of the panel's concern that before such an endorsement, it was necessary that both the medical profession and the public become more sophisticated about the meaning of abnormalities of circulating lipid and lipoprotein fractions and their relationships to the development of coronary heart disease. In addition, the adult treatment panel withheld endorsement of widespread public screening because separate groups, including one addressing the public health aspects of the cholesterol issue and another looking at the impact of these issues on pediatric practice, also should have a role to play in developing screening guidelines.

Nevertheless, because of widespread interest in cholesterol screening, the NCEP has developed some guidelines according to which screenings should be done if they are to be done at all (U.S. Department of Health and Human Services, 1988). These include careful attention to cholesterol measurement methods, to the presence of personnel capable of appropriate "on-the-spot" counseling for those found to have abnormalities, and to the preparation and enlistment of the medical community to accept referrals generated as a result of the screenings.

While the guidelines do not recommend widespread public screening, they do recommend that a cholesterol measurement be incorporated into any appropriate patient–physician encounter. With a properly informed medical community, lifestyle changes can then be addressed and appropriate counseling provided.

The recommendation that total cholesterol be used as a screening measurement was based on its widespread availability, the relatively advanced status of standardization of measurement methods (compared to other lipoprotein fractions), and the lack of requirement for fasting. Most important, total cholesterol is usually a reasonable indicator of the level of circulating LDL cholesterol.

On the other hand, total cholesterol is the sum of cholesterol carried in all lipoprotein fractions, including LDL, high density lipoproteins (HDL), and very low density lipoproteins (VLDL). Of necessity, it is a less precise predictor of coronary risk than either LDL or HDL cholesterol levels. The recommendation to use total cholesterol as a single screening device has been criticized as one that generates undue concern among those with cholesterol elevations due to high HDL levels and inappropriate reassurance among those with low HDL levels and normal total cholesterols.

On balance, however, total cholesterol measurements provide a reasonable screening device that must, of course, be followed, when indicated, with more detailed lipoprotein analysis.

III. SCREENING CUTPOINTS

On the basis of accumulated epidemiological and clinical data, the NCEP guidelines designate "cutpoints" to divide "normal" from "abnormal" cholesterol levels. Inevitably, these guidelines are somewhat arbitrary. They have generated a good deal of (largely fruitless) debate, which would be the case wherever they were set. It is important to note that, unlike those of the previous consensus statement (NIH Consensus Conference, 1985) and in the interest of simplicity and easy applicability, none of the numerical cutpoints or goals are specified by age or gender.

Based on accelerating coronary risk, those with total cholesterols over 240 mg/dl are classified as having "high blood cholesterol" (Table 1) (National Cholesterol Education Program, 1988). This level corresponds to about the 75th percentile of the U.S. adult population.

Those with cholesterols below 200 mg/dl (corresponding to a point slightly below the 50th percentile of the U.S. adult population) are said to have "desirable" cholesterol levels. Those between 230 and 239 are in the "borderline high" range. Those with cholesterol levels less than 200 mg/dl are required to have a repeat measurement only every 5 years. Although general instruction in risk factor reduction, including general information about diet

Table 1 Thresholds and Cutpoint Goals for Management of Hypercholesterolemia

Screening cutpoints		Treatment thresholds	Treatment goals
Total cholesterol	>240 mg/dl ("high")	LDL cholesterol > 160 mg/dl (no risk factors)	LDL cholesterol < 160 mg/dl (no risk factors)
Total cholesterol	200–239 mg/dl ("borderline")	LDL cholesterol > 130 mg/dl (documented CHD or two risk factors)	LDL cholesterol < 130 mg/dl (two or more risk factors)
Total cholesterol	<200 mg/dl ("desirable")		

Source: National Cholesterol Education Program, 1988.

modification, is recommended, no more specific intervention is required. In fact, since the Step 1 American Heart Association Diet is recommended for all adults, the dietary recommendations for these various cholesterol subgroups differ not in content, but in the intensity of the instruction and the frequency of follow-up.

Those with cholesterol levels greater than 240 mg/dl are advised to have a more detailed lipoprotein analysis on a blood sample obtained after a 12-hour fast. This analysis should include repeat total cholesterol as well as total triglycerides, HDL cholesterol (HDL-C), and an "estimated" LDL cholesterol (LDL-C) level. LDL-C is determined by the formula (Friedewald et al., 1972):

$$LDL-C = \text{total cholesterol} - \left[HDL-C + \frac{\text{triglyceride}}{5} \right]$$

This formula is valid as long as all parameters are expressed in mg/dl and triglyceride levels measure less than 400 mg/dl.

Those with cholesterols between 200 and 239 mg/dl without coronary heart disease or other risk factors (Table 2) (National Cholesterol Education Program, 1988) should receive dietary counseling (more intense than the general counseling noted above but not requiring a dietitian) and an annual remeasurement of total cholesterol. If they have documented coronary disease or two or more other risk factors as outlined in Table 1, they require the same lipoprotein analysis as those with total cholesterols over 200 mg/dl. Since male sex is considered to be one risk factor, males need only one other risk

Table 2 Risk Factors Determining Lower LDL Treatment Thresholds and Goals

---

Male sex
Family history of premature CHD (death or myocardial infarction before age 55 in a
    parent or sibling)
Cigarette smoking ($>$10 per day)
Hypertension
HDL cholesterol $<$ 35 mg/dl
Diabetes mellitus
History of CVA or peripheral vascular disease
Obesity ($>$30% over ideal body weight)

Source: National Cholesterol Education Program, 1988.

factor to qualify for additional lipoprotein analysis. This portion of the
guidelines contains a logical inconsistency. One of the risk factors, HDL
cholesterol $<$ 35 mg/dl, is, itself, part of the lipoprotein analysis and,
therefore, unknown until the analysis is performed. In fact, the larger issue of
the role of HDL cholesterol in these guidelines is one that will be revisited
below, where critiques of the guidelines are discussed.

This inconsistency aside, however, these guidelines provide a rational
procedure for utilizing total cholesterol as a method for screening and initially
classifying a patient. Further classification, however, is dependent on the
lipoprotein analysis required of *all* cholesterols over 240 mg/dl and those over
200 mg/dl with documented coronary vascular disease or two risk factors.

IV. SELECTING PATIENTS FOR
CHOLESTEROL-LOWERING THERAPY

Once the patient has been identified as requiring lipoprotein analysis, the
focus of the guidelines shifts from total to LDL cholesterol levels. It is
reasonable to ask why LDL rather than HDL is emphasized. The reasons are
several, and include 1) the broader database relating LDL cholesterol to
coronary risk and LDL lowering to the prevention of that risk, 2) the wider
therapeutic armamentarium, including dietary and drug interventions, which
can be applied to LDL lowering and the database confirming the value of such
intervention, and 3) the better understanding of LDL's role in atherogenesis.
None of this is to say that HDL is unimportant in the prevention of atherosclerosis, or that, as understanding of HDL–atherogenetic relationships become
more precise, future versions of these guidelines will not be revised. In view

of the large and consistent database relating LDL to atherogenesis and its prevention, however, the emphasis placed on LDL in these guidelines is warranted.

As with total cholesterol levels, LDL-C "cutpoints," of necessity somewhat arbitrary, must be selected. Those with LDL-C below the 130 mg/dl range, corresponding in population studies but not in individuals to about 200 mg/dl of total cholesterol, are said to have "desirable" LDL levels. Those with LDL-Cs over 160 mg/dl (corresponding roughly to total cholesterols of 240 mg/dl) have "high risk" levels, and those in the 130–159 mg/dl range "borderline high risk."

Those with LDL-C levels less than 130 mg/dl are given general risk factor and dietary counseling and asked to return within 5 years. This group will contain a large number of individuals whose HDL, not LDL, cholesterol level is responsible for the total cholesterol elevation that necessitated lipoprotein analysis. Those with LDL cholesterol levels in the 130–159 mg/dl range (the borderline high risk range) with no risk factors require more intensive dietary counseling and annual monitoring. The presense of two or more risk factors (Table 2) in these borderline cases or the presence of an LDL cholesterol over 160 mg/dl, regardless of other risk factors, dictates more extensive evaluation and intervention. It should be emphasized that at no point should decisions about classification or therapeutic recommendations be made without at least two repeated measurements of lipid and lipoprotein fractions.

Additional evaluation of patients falling into these high risk categories should include laboratory tests to eliminate secondary causes of LDL elevations, including diabetes, nephrosis, renal failure, hypothyroidism, dysgammaglobulinemia, and obstructive liver disease. The vigor with which the physician will approach therapeutic interventions may also be influenced by the patient's age, sex, and the presence of documented familial lipoprotein abnormalities. In reality, the initial intervention should always be dietary and is usually quite innocuous. Nuances of physician judgment have much more influence when drug therapy is under consideration.

V. SETTING GOALS FOR THERAPY

For those whose LDL cholesterol levels require more than annual monitoring, it is first necessary to decide what the goal of therapeutic intervention should be. In general, it is desirable to maintain LDL cholesterols below 130 mg/dl, corresponding to total cholesterol levels of about 200 mg/dl. This is particularly true for those with two or more risk factors. Without drug intervention, however, such a goal is not practical for many individuals. For those without risk factors and LDL cholesterol levels below 160 mg/dl (corresponding to total cholesterol levels of about 240 mg/dl), this goal is sufficient, particularly if achieving lower levels would require drug therapy.

In general, once an LDL goal has been reached and the relationship to LDL cholesterol is established in an individual patient, total cholesterol levels may be used as a surrogate so that the more expensive lipoprotein profiles, with estimated LDL determinations, need be done only every year or so.

VI. DIETARY INTERVENTION

Details of the scientific rationale and implementation of dietary therapy for hypercholesterolemia are discussed elsewhere in this volume. Table 3 summarizes the composition of the recommended diet for hypercholesterolemia compared to the current composition of the average American diet.

The guidelines recommend that patients requiring dietary intervention be initially instructed in the Step 1 diet by the physician (or, more likely, someone on the physician's staff) without utilizing the services of a registered dietitian. This recommendation is based on the relative scarcity of registered dietitians. There are four physicians for every registered dietitian. Most registered dietitians are employed in institutional settings and are not available (and perhaps not even trained) to see patients referred for lipid disorders. The skepticism and indifference with which many physicians regard dietary intervention is a major factor in the failure of diet to produce convincing cholesterol lowering in many patients. These guidelines were meant to be of practical value. In addition, however, they were meant to stimulate the growth of resources not currently available. It is unlikely that they will reach their full potential without more sophisticated dietary counseling and monitoring than is currently available through many physicians' offices.

Patients who, after repeat LDL testing at 6 weeks and 3 months, have achieved their goal on diet can be followed up every 4 months or so in the first year and semiannually thereafter. If, after 3 months, goal levels of LDL cholesterol have not been reached, referral to a registered dietitian, when possible, and/or intensification of dietary counseling are required.

After an additional 3 months on the more restricted Step 2 diet, failure to achieve LDL-C goals should lead to consideration of drug therapy. As is true of all of these guidelines, this approach to diet should not be regarded as a locke-step approach to therapy. Clearly, some patients with severe genetic abnormalities will be poor dietary responders and will not require 6 months to

Table 3 National Cholesterol Education Program/American Heart Association Recommended Diet

	Estimated current U.S. adult diet (% daily calories)	Step 1	Step 2	Lipoprotein effect	
				LDL	HDL
Total fat	35–40	<30%	<30%	decrease	no change
Saturated	15	<10%	<7%	decrease	no change
Polyunsaturated	7	10%	10%	decrease	decrease
Monounsaturated	16	10%	10%	decrease	no change
Carbohydrate	40	50–60%	50–60%	no change	? decrease
Protein	40	10–20%	10–20%	no change	no change
Cholesterol	500 mg/day	<300 mg/d	<200 mg/d	decrease	? decrease

Current U.S. intake is contrasted with composition of recommended diets. Recommended diets are prescribed in two stages, with the second stage including further limitations in saturated fat and cholesterol intake.
Source: LaRosa, 1988.

demonstrate that. Others with less severe abnormalities may take longer than 6 months to reach LDL-C goals on diet. A patient moving in the right direction with diet should not be rushed to drug intervention.

Above all, the physician and his or her staff must demonstrate their own commitment to and knowledge of the effectiveness and desirabilty of dietary changes.

VII. DRUG INTERVENTION

Individual lipid-lowering agents will not be reviewed here in detail. (That is done in other portions of this volume.) Table 4 (National Cholesterol Education Program, 1988) lists drugs currently considered to be acceptable lipid-lowering agents according to the NCEP guidelines. Bile acid sequestrants (cholestyramine and colestipol) and niacin were, at the time the report was made public, the only drugs that demonstrated both the ability to lower LDL-C and coronary risk. In addition, these drugs were effective LDL-lowering agents and had proven long-term safety records. In the well-known Helsinki Study (Frick et al., 1987), gemfibrozil, although only modestly effective as an LDL-lowering drug, was demonstrated to reduce coronary heart risk, probably related to both LDL reduction and HDL elevation. Its long-term safety, however, is less well established. Other drugs, including lovastatin (the most potent LDL-lowering drug currently available in the United States) and probucol, a unique agent that appears to lower LDL's atherogenic potential to a greater extent than its circulating levels, as yet have not been shown to prevent coronary atherosclerotic sequalae and also do not have the long-term safety record of sequestrants or niacin.

Whichever drug is selected for therapy, however, it is important to note

Table 4 Lipid-Lowering Drugs

Drugs of first choice
bile acid sequestrants (cholestyramine and colestipol)
niacin
New drugs
lovastatin
Other drugs
gemfibrozil
probucol
clofibrate

Source: National Cholesterol Education Program, 1988.

that the LDL criteria for diet and drug intervention differ importantly. The panel that formulated these guidelines had considerable concern for the possibility that long-term drug therapy, particularly with newer agents and unlike diet therapy, might be associated with severe side effects. If that were the case, whatever gains might be achieved from cholesterol lowering might then be compromised by such side effects. The thresholds for drug intervention, therefore, were set 30 mg/dl higher than those for dietary intervention, i.e., LDL cholesterol levels greater than 190 mg/dl if no other risk factors are present and greater than 160 mg/dl if two or more risk factors are present and with greater than 160 mg/dl with two or more risk factors.

Goals of therapy remain the same for both diet and drug therapy. LDL cholesterol should be less than 160 mg/dl or less than 130 mg/dl with and without risk factors, respectively. Drug therapy with any agent should be given 3 months before any other agent is substituted. Combination therapy should, when possible, be arranged with the help of a specialist in lipid disorders. In general, bile acid sequestrants may be combined with other agents without undue concerns about toxicity. Other combinations, however, should be avoided without a specialist's help.

During the evaluation period of a drug regimen, monitoring may occur as often as once a month. Once a regimen has been established, visits more often than three times per year are really necessary. Semiannual visits are, in the opinion of this author, a minimum requirement to maintain good diet and drug adherence.

VIII. CRITIQUES OF THE ADULT TREATMENT PANEL GUIDELINES

These guidelines represent a set of straightforward suggestions that, while not as simple as the panel might have originally hoped, are nevertheless usable with the resources available to most physicians. In general, they appear to have been widely and favorably accepted. They promise to form the cornerstone for a widespread and successful educational program for both practicing physicians and their patients.

The guidelines, however, have engendered some critical commentaries. Some comments have focused on the emphasis on LDL cholesterol as the critical measurement for therapeutic decision making. Emphasis on LDL places heavy reliance on a parameter that is not directly measured but, rather, estimated from direct measurements of total and HDL cholesterol and total triglyceride. It also ignores HDL cholesterol except as part of the LDL calculation and as a risk factor, the latter use limited by the logical inconsistency mentioned above (i.e., low HDL cholesterol serves as an indicator for its own measurement). Failure to include HDL cholesterol as a screening device, moreover, leaves undetected those individuals with total cholesterols under 200 mg/dl but with HDLs low enough (i.e., < 30–35 mg/dl) to put them at increased coronary risk (LaRosa et al, 1986; Abbott et al., 1988).

The focus on LDL cholesterol, moreover, ignores those individuals with triglycerides in the 200–400 mg/dl range who may be carrying atherogenic lipoproteins despite LDL-C levels below the thresholds for diet or drug intervention.

Each of these concerns has validity. On the other hand, the epidemiological and clinical trial database which allows an approximation of thresholds and therapeutic goals for LDL-C levels simply does not exist for HDL-C and triglyceride levels (Grundy et al., 1989). In the final analysis, it is that, more than anything else, which, thus far, has directed the focus of the guidelines away from HDL-C and triglyceride and toward LDL-C levels.

Attempts have been made in similar recommendations promulgated by the European Atherosclerosis Society to incorporate HDL and the triglyceride measurements more fully into the therapeutic decision-making process (Table 5) (Study Group, European Atherosclerosis Society, 1987). Rather than rely on LDL-C determinations, these guidelines create several categories of patients depending on total cholesterol and triglyceride measurements. Cutpoints for total cholesterol are similar to those in U.S. guidelines. While HDL-C levels are not part of the classification mechanism, they are, as in the NCEP Guidelines, regarded as additional risk factors. Recommendations about screening and the progression of testing are less precise than in the NCEP Guidelines. In the opinion of this author, these European guidelines, while of interest, rest on a less secure database. In fact, they reinforce rather than refute the notion that the clinical database justifying aggressive intervention in modest hypertriglyceridemia and/or low HDL-C states is simply insufficient to justify recommendations that can command a wide consensus.

Table 5 European Atherosclerosis Society Lipoprotein Cutpoints

Total cholesterol	> 200–250 mg/dl
Total triglyceride	> 200–500 mg/dl
HDL cholesterol	< 35 mg/dl

Source: Adapted from Study Group, European Atherosclerosis Society, 1987.

IX. SUMMARY

The National Cholesterol Education Program's Adult Treatment Panel Guidelines:

1. Are based on total cholesterol as a nonfasting screening measurement.
2. Focus on LDL cholesterol as a major factor in making therapeutic decisions.
3. Do not address either altered HDL-C or triglyceride levels as therapeutic goals.
4. Provide numerical cutpoints and goals for cholesterol and LDL-C that are neither age nor gender specific.
5. Require higher thresholds for drug intervention than for dietary intervention.
6. Emphasize dietary therapy as the first and foremost therapeutic maneuver.
7. Require that drugs of first choice be those that can be shown to lower both LDL-C and coronary risk and have proven, long-term safety records.
8. Should be regarded as guidelines, not as rigid dictum, requiring considerable physician judgment and latitude for their proper application.

REFERENCES

Abbott, R. D., Wilson, P. W. F., Kannel, W. B., and Castelli, W. P. (1988). High density lipoprotein cholesterol, total cholesterol screening, and myocardial infarction: The Framingham Study. *Arteriosclerosis* **8**:207–211.

Frick, M. H., Elo, Olli, Happa, K., Heinonen, O. P., Heinsalmi, P., Helo, P., Huttunen, J. K., Kaitaniemi, P., Koskinen, P., Manninen, V., Mäenpää, H., Mälkönen, M., Mänttäri, M., Norolo, S., Pasternack, A., Pikkarainen, J., Romo, M., Sjöblom, T., and Nikkilä, E. A. (1987). Helsinki heart study: Primary-prevention trial with gemfibrozil in middle-aged men with dyslipidemia. *New Engl. J. Med.* **317**:1237–1245.

Friedewald, W. T., Levy, R. I., and Frederickson, P. S. (1972). Estimation of the concentration of low-density lipoprotein cholesterol in plasma, without use of preparative ultracentrifuge. *Clin. Chem.* **18**:499–502.

Grundy, S. M., Goodman, D. S., Rifkind, P. M., and Cleeman, J. I. (1989). The place of HDL in cholesterol measurement. *Arch. Intern. Med.* **149**:505–510.

LaRosa, J. C. (1988). Lipoproteins: Their role in atherosclerosis and its prevention (a monograph). Needham Heights, MA, Damon Clinical Laboratories, pp. 1–19.

LaRosa, J. C., Chambless, L. E., Criqui, M. H., Frantz, I. D., Glueck, C. J., Heiss, G., and Morrison, J. A. (1986). Patterns of dyslipoproteinemia in selected North American populations. *Circulation* **73**:I-12–I-29.

National Cholesterol Education Program (1988). Report of the expert panel on detection, evaluation, and treatment of high blood cholesterol in adults. *Arch. Intern. Med.* **148**:36–80.

NIH Consensus Conference. (1985). Lowering blood cholesterol for the prevention of heart disease. *JAMA* **253**:2080–2096.

Study Group, European Atherosclerosis Society. (1987). Strategies for the prevention of coronary heart disease: A policy statement of the European Atherosclerosis Society. *European Heart Journ.* **8**:77–88.

U.S. Department of Health and Human Services: Health Services. (1988). Recommendations regarding public screening for blood cholesterol: Summary of a National Heart, Lung & Blood Institute Workshop, October 1988. NIH Publication No. 89-3045.

4

Clinical Trials of Lipid-Lowering Drugs

Jacques E. Rossouw

National Heart, Lung, and Blood Institute
National Institutes of Health
Bethesda, Maryland

I. INTRODUCTION

Diet remains the cornerstone of the management of high blood cholesterol, not least because of the size of the problem. Fifty-seven percent of North American adults aged 20–70 years have cholesterol levels that are borderline-high (> 200 mg/dl) according to National Cholesterol Education Program cutpoints, and a further 27% have high levels (> 240 mg/dl) (Sempos et al., 1989). Estimates of the proportion of adults who will need immediate follow-up because of a high initial blood cholesterol or because of a borderline-high level and the presence of coronary heart disease (CHD) or two or more risk factors vary from 41% of males (35% of females) (Sempos et al., 1989) to 35% of males (19% of females) (Wilson et al., 1989). These are the individuals who (but only if they do not respond sufficiently well to an adequate trial of diet) may be considered for cholesterol-lowering drug therapy.

The National Cholesterol Education Program has built in a further safeguard to discourage unnecessary and premature drug therapy: the low-density lipoprotein cholesterol must exceed 190 mg/dl if there are no other risk factors or 160 mg/dl if there is CHD or two or more risk factors (one of which may be male sex) before drug therapy is entertained (Expert Panel, 1988). Applied to the Framingham Offspring Study population, the guidelines will yield 16% of males and 10% of females who will qualify for drug therapy if there is no response to diet, compared to only 7% of males (4% of females) if diet results in a 10% reduction in serum cholesterol (Wilson et al., 1989). Since a 10% reduction in serum cholesterol by diet is feasible, particularly in a motivated high risk group, assiduous application of diet therapy should result in only a small minority (4–7%) of the adult population, and only about 20% of the individuals who need immediate follow-up after initial screening, who would eventually qualify for drug therapy.

Further reasons for drug therapy to take second place to diet are the cost of drugs and their adverse effects. Fortunately most of the common side effects, while a nuisance, are not serious, and those of a more serious nature are uncommon. In reviewing the clinical trials of cholesterol lowering, any benefit in terms of a reduction in MI needs to be balanced against the risk of serious adverse effects and the possible discomforts consequent upon taking drugs.

The trials to be reviewed in this chapter had as their primary endpoint a reduction in MI (or stabilization/regression of angiographic lesions), rather than modification of blood lipids only. They are important as evidence for proving the cholesterol hypothesis, and they provide a rationale for the treatment of lipid disorders. There would be little incentive to treat the biochemical disorder if it could not be shown that such treatment reduces the severity and occurrence of disease endpoints. Some 25 randomized cholesterol-lowering clinical trials have been reported; however, many were far too small or were of too short a duration to yield meaningful results, used drugs now known to be toxic (estrogen, thyroxin), or had other design faults. This review will focus on a select group of eight drug trials (and mention four diet trials), which had MI as the primary endpoint, and on three angiographic studies. The clinical trials of MI reduction were selected on uniform criteria of size (at least 100 in each group), random allocation to treatment group, duration at least 3 years, and no co-intervention on other risk factors. The angiographic studies were selected on similar criteria, except that 30 subjects in each group, a 2-year intervention, and a double-blind design were required.

The selected trials will be described briefly, highlighting particular lessons that can be learned from each. Thereafter they will be analyzed in aggregate, including a "meta-analysis." Such a meta-analysis provides a statistical power the individual trials cannot provide, and thereby allows certain questions to be explored: Does lowering cholesterol reduce the risk of MI? Is the benefit extended to fatal as well as nonfatal MI, and to persons with preexisting CHD? Is overall mortality reduced? Are there risks attached to cholesterol lowering? How do the different classes of drugs compare to each other, and to diet, in respect of efficacy and risk? Finally, some of the implications of the clinical trial results for clinical practice and for public health policy will be reviewed.

II. CLINICAL TRIALS

A. Lipid Research Clinics Coronary Primary Prevention Trial (LRC-CPPT)

Reported in 1984 (Lipid Research Clinics Program, 1984a), this was a large, carefully designed and executed primary prevention trial of cholesterol-lowering drug therapy. Men aged 35–59 with primary hypercholesterolemia (Type IIA) were prescribed either 24 g/day of cholestyramine resin ($n = 1906$) or placebo ($n = 1900$) for an average period of 7.4 years. In addition, both groups were put on a moderate lipid-lowering diet. The diet reduced serum cholesterol by about 4%, as envisaged in the design. The net fall in serum cholesterol on cholestyramine relative to placebo over the study period was 9%, and that of low density lipoprotein cholesterol was 13%. The net fall in serum cholesterol was less than the expected 25% on which the sample size calculations were based (Lipid Research Clinics Program, 1979). This decreased the power of the study; nevertheless, at the end of 7.4 years there was a significant 17% difference for the primary endpoint of definite nonfatal plus fatal MI (155 in the cholestyramine group vs. 187 in the placebo group, one-tailed $p < 0.05$) (Table 1). This favorable result is validated by the internal consistency of the study: other relatively frequent endpoints such as new positive exercise tests, angina, and coronary bypass surgery decreased by 25%, 18%, and 17%, respectively. Parenthetically, over 20% of placebo participants developed one or more of the secondary cardiovascular endpoints, so that decreases of the order of 17–25% in these endpoints are of considerable clinical importance. (Note that the method of calculation of percent change used throughout may result in small inconsistencies compared to published figures. Percent change is expressed as $(a - b)/b \times 100$, where a is the rate in treated group, and b is the rate in control group.)

The variation in compliance and in response of serum lipids allowed a clear and significant ($p < 0.001$) dose-response relationship between cholesterol reduction and reduction in MI to be demonstrated. The one-third of participants who reduced their low-density lipoprotein cholesterol levels by more

Table 1 Myocardial Infarctions and Deaths in Drug Trials of Cholesterol Lowering

Trial[a]	Number randomized		Number of myocardial infarctions						Number of deaths					
			Nonfatal		Fatal		All		Cardio-vascular		Noncardio-vascular		All	
LRC (cholestyramine)	1906	1900	130	158*	30	38	155	187*	37	47	31	24	68	71
Helsinki (gemfibrozil)	2051	2031	45	71*	11	13	56	84*	22	23	23	19	45	42
WHO (clofibrate)	5331	5296	131	174*	36	34	167	208*	68	62	94	65	162	127*
CDP (clofibrate)	1103	2789	144	386	195	535	309	839	241	633	29	54	281	709
CDP (niacin)	1119	2789	114	386**	203	535	287	839*	238	633	30	54	273	709
Newcastle (clofibrate)	244	253	30	46	25	44*	52	81**	n/a		n/a		n/a	
Edinburgh (clofibrate)	350	367	25	41	34	35	54	72	n/a		n/a		43	47
Stockholm (clofibrate + niacin)	279	276	35	50	47	73**	72	100*	54	75*	7	7	61	82*
Sum of Observed-Expected Events Σ(O-E)			−106***		−45**		−135***		−30*		+32**		−1	

[a]Trials selected on size (at least 100 in each group), duration (at least 3 years), random assignment to treatment group and no confounding co-intervention on other risk factors. Trials using drugs now known to be toxic (thyroxin, estrogens) were excluded. LRC = Lipid Research Clinics, WHO = World Health Organization, CDP = Coronary Drug Project, n/a = not available. $*p < 0.05$, $**p < 0.01$, $***p < 0.001$ represent significances of differences between treated and control groups, as reported by the investigators, or as calculated by chi-square where not reported. The meta-analysis of all trials combined was performed as described by Mantel and Haenszel (1959) and applied by Yusuf et al. (1985). Σ(O-E) is the sum of the differences between the number of events expected (E) in each of the treated groups if there were no treatment effects, and the numbers actually observed (O). If treated and control groups are equal in size, Σ(O-E) is about one half of actual difference in events.

than 25% had a 64% reduction in MI risk (Lipid Research Clinics Program, 1984b). For serum cholesterol, a dose-response relationship of a 2% reduction in MI for every 1% reduction was obtained.

Although there were 10 fewer deaths due to cardiovascular disease in the cholestyramine group, this group had 7 more noncardiovascular deaths than the placebo group, so that the all-cause mortality was almost identical (68 vs. 71). The only noncardiovascular cause of death that appeared to be unduly frequent in the cholestyramine group was accidents and violence (11 vs. 4, not significant). Detailed analyses of these cases did not suggest any relation to either CHD or cholesterol lowering. Cancer deaths were equally frequent in the two groups.

Gastrointestinal side effects were common: in the first year 68% of the cholestyramine patients (vs. 43% of the placebo patients) complained of (one or more) constipation, heartburn, abdominal pain, belching, bloating, gas, or nausea. Side effects were generally not severe, could be dealt with by standard clinical means, and decreased with time.

The LRC-CCPT is of particular importance because, unlike the other studies to be discussed, it was a predominantly cholesterol-lowering study. Participants were selected for hypercholesterolemia, and those with hypertriglyceridemia were excluded. The effect of the drug used is for practical purposes limited to lowering total and low density lipoprotein cholesterol. The small increases in high density lipoprotein cholesterol and triglycerides observed accounted for a reduction in CHD risk of 2% and 0%, respectively (Lipid Research Clinics Program, 1984b). It thus provides strong support for the causal role of serum cholesterol for CHD, and for the treatment of high blood cholesterol. Rightly, it has had a decisive impact on clinical practice and on public health recommendations. Both the Consensus Conference Statement on Lowering Blood Cholesterol to Prevent Heart Disease (1985) and the Adult Treatment Panel Report of the National Cholesterol Education Program (Expert Committee, 1988) were influenced by the findings from this study.

B. Helsinki Heart Study

The Helsinki study, like the LRC-CPPT, was a large, multicenter, double-blind, placebo-controlled primary intervention study (Frick et al., 1987). It included 2051 men aged 40–55 in the active drug group and 2031 in the placebo group. All participants were placed on a lipid-lowering diet. It differed from the LRC-CPPT in several respects: the drug used was the fibric acid derivative gemfibrozil (at a total daily dose of 1200 mg), and selection procedures allowed a mixture of hyperlipoproteinemic phenotypes to be recruited (63% were Type IIA, 28% Type IIB, and 9% Type IV). Mean low density lipoprotein cholesterol levels at baseline were lower, and triglycerides higher, than in the LRC-CPPT.

Gemfibrozil brought about net reductions in total cholesterol of 10%, in low density lipoprotein cholesterol of 11%, in triglycerides of 35%, and increased high-density lipoprotein cholesterol by 11%. The most marked reductions in low-density lipoprotein cholesterol were seen in the Type IIA subgroup, with the Type IIB subgroup intermediate, and a small increase in the Type V subgroup (Manninen et al., 1988). Triglycerides responded most in the Type IIB and V subgroups, while the high density lipoprotein cholesterol response was about equal in all subgroups. After 5 years of intervention, the number of MIs was 35% lower on gemfibrozil treatment than on placebo (56 vs. 84, $p < 0.02$). In multivariate regression analyses of the entire gemfibrozil-treated group, changes in both low and high density lipoprotein cholesterol appeared to contribute to reduction in myocardial infarction incidence, though the association appeared stronger for high density lipoprotein cholesterol.

Cardiovascular mortality was equal in the two groups (22 vs. 23), mainly because a nonsignificant excess of hemorrhagic stroke in the gemfibrozil group (5 vs. 1) counterbalanced the reduction in CHD deaths (14 vs. 19). As in the LRC-CPPT, there was a nonsignificant excess of deaths from accidents and violence in the active treatment group (10 vs. 4). Cancer deaths were equal (11 in each group). Total deaths were 45 on gemfibrozil, 42 on placebo (not significant).

Upper gastrointestinal side effects were most common, with 11% of gemfibrozil and 7% of placebo patients complaining of moderate-to-severe symptoms in the first year, decreasing to 2% and 1% in subsequent years. Operations for gallstones were somewhat more frequent on gemfibrozil (18) than on placebo (12), although this was not statistically significant. The greater number of abdominal operations in the gemfibrozil group was significant (81 vs. 54, $p < 0.02$).

The Helsinki study confirmed that the effects of the fibric acid derivative are predominantly on triglycerides, and that they also raise high density lipoprotein cholesterol levels. Their effect on low density lipoprotein cholesterol varied according to the underlying lipoprotein phenotype, paradoxically being most marked in Type IIA and progressively less marked or even inverse in situations where triglycerides were raised, and yet the greatest benefit in terms of reduction in MI appeared to be in the latter situations (Types IIB and V). These observations raise the possibility that, in certain subgroups of patients, a reduction in triglycerides and an increase in high density lipoprotein cholesterol is as important as is a reduction in low density lipoprotein in others (the latter was exemplified by the Type IIA patients in the LRC-CPPT). Although triglycerides did not appear to contribute to myocardial infarction reduction in multivariate analysis, in view of the inverse metabolic relationship between triglycerides and high density lipoprotein cholesterol, this finding does not exclude a role for triglycerides. The larger variance of triglycerides compared to high density lipoprotein cholesterol would, if they were both entered into a multivariate analysis, favor high density lipoprotein cholesterol displacing a real effect of triglycerides (Austin, 1989). Triglycerides and high density lipoprotein cholesterol may thus represent different sides of the same coin.

C. The World Health Organization Cooperative Trial on Primary Prevention of Ischemic Heart Disease Using Clofibrate to Lower Serum Cholesterol (WHO Study)

This is the largest primary cholesterol-lowering intervention study ever undertaken, and its results would have ranked among the most important if serious design faults had not complicated their interpretation. Most pertinently, the design does not allow the in-trial results to be presented on an intent-to-treat basis, and the out-of-trial follow-up mortality data are incomplete. As a result of these various problems, the reliable results are those relating to nonfatal myocardial infarctions (after nonfatal infarct participants were withdrawn from further participation in the trial); however, for the sake of completeness, fatal MIs and other causes of death will be discussed. Limited follow-up data (up to one year after withdrawal) are included in these analyses.

The WHO Study randomized 5331 men aged 30–59 into in the upper third of the cholesterol distribution into an active treatment group receiving 1.6 g of clofibrate daily, and 5296 men into the placebo group (Committee of Principal Investigators, 1978). The study was double-blind and lasted 5.3 years. The net reduction of serum cholesterol was 8%, and the reduction in MI was 20% (167 in clofibrate and 207 in placebo group, $p < 0.05$, all the reduction being accounted for by nonfatal myocardial infarctions).

Total deaths (162 on clofibrate, 127 on placebo) and noncardiovascular deaths (94 on clofibrate, 65 on placebo) were significantly more frequent in the clofibrate group, while there was no difference in cardiovascular deaths (68 vs. 62). However, for the reasons mentioned earlier, mortality data from the in-trial period of this study is not reliable. This judgment is strengthened by the diffuse nature of the causes of death; no particular cause predominated, in spite of the large differences in total deaths. Such a pattern is difficult to reconcile with drug toxicity. Nevertheless, the group of causes of death relating to "liver, gallbladder and intestines" deserve mention, as in-trial cholecystectomies were significantly more frequent on clofibrate, and deaths from this group of diseases were higher. This excess of deaths persisted over the total 13-year follow-up (Committee of Principal Investigators, 1980, 1984). These findings are consistent with the known propensity for clofibrate to increase gallstone formation. Fatalities from neoplasms were somewhat more frequent in the clofibrate group during the trial (58 vs. 42, not significant), but not over the entire follow-up (206 vs. 197).

Because withdrawals for nonfatal MI occurred less frequently in the clofibrate group (131 vs. 174), the clofibrate group had a smaller overall number of withdrawals (477 vs. 501). However, withdrawals for reasons other than MI were more frequent in the clofibrate group (346 on clofibrate, 327 on placebo). Gallstone operations, diabetes, weight gain, indigestion, diarrhea, and impotence were significantly more frequent on clofibrate, while hypertension was less frequent.

The large apparent difference in noncardiovascular mortality has distracted attention from the fact that the trial, flawed though it may be, did succeed in its primary objective—that of demonstrating that cholesterol lowering reduces MI. However, rather than this positive finding leading to increased enthusiasm for cholesterol management, the negative (and possibly misleading) findings in regard to mortality have dominated thinking and have retarded acceptance of the value of such management.

D. The Coronary Drug Project (CDP)

The CDP was designed to explore the efficacy and safety of lipid-lowering drugs in patients with existing coronary heart disease, i.e., in the setting of secondary prevention. Men aged 30–64 with at least one documented previous MI were recruited in 53 centers (Coronary Drug Project Research Group, 1975). Unlike the primary prevention studies, they were unselected in regard to serum cholesterol level. Originally they were randomized into 5 treatment groups and a placebo group; however, the two estrogen groups and the dextro-thyroxine group were discontinued early on because of an unacceptably high incidence of toxic effects. The clofibrate and niacin active treatment groups completed the planned 6 years of the double-blind placebo-controlled trial.

Clofibrate

Clofibrate was given at a total daily dose of 1.8 g to 1103 men. Compared to the 2789 men in the placebo group, clofibrate reduced serum cholesterol by 6% and triglycerides by 22%. Nonfatal plus fatal MI decreased by 7% (309 in clofibrate group vs. 839 in placebo group, not significant). Small decreases in cardiovascular mortality and increases in noncardiovascular mortality were not significant, and there was no change in total mortality.

Clofibrate was well tolerated by the participants, as demonstrated by a nonadherance rate of only 4.7%, similar to the 5.1% on placebo. However, higher proportions of patients on clofibrate complained of loss of libido or impotence, of breast enlargement or tenderness, and of increased appetite. They also gained more weight and manifested more gallbladder disease, hepatomegaly, intermittent claudication, angina, arrhythmia, and pulmonary embolism, and were more often prescribed digitalis and anticoagulants. Laboratory monitoring showed that clofibrate lowers bilirubin and hematocrit slightly, decreases alkaline phosphatase substantially, and increases blood urea nitrogen and potassium slightly.

Overall, this large and well-conducted study failed to provide evidence in favor of using clofibrate in unselected patients with CHD. The small decrease in serum cholesterol meant that it did not provide an adequate test of the cholesterol hypothesis. The correspondingly small decreases in MI morbidity and mortality were offset by increases in other cardiovascular and noncardiovascular endpoints. Some of these may be significant by chance (since a large number of variables were examined), but others such as gallstones are clearly related to the drug's known actions. In the 15-year follow-up of the CDP participants, there was no excess total mortality in the clofibrate group (57.8% mortality vs. 58.2% in the placebo group) (Canner et al., 1986). This finding is in contrast to that of the WHO study, where there was still a 11% (nonsignificant) excess mortality in the clofibrate group at 13 years follow-up (Committee of Prinicpal Investigators, 1984). The CDP was, of course, a secondary rather than a primary prevention study, and this may offer a partial explanation for the divergent findings since cardiovascular deaths formed a much larger proportion of deaths in the CDP. Like the WHO Study, the decision to do the follow-up was a post hoc one, however, the exhaustive nature and cross-referencing of vital status ascertainment in the CDP engenders more confidence in the reliablity of its findings.

Niacin

The 1119 patients who received a total of 3 g niacin per day experienced a net decrease (compared to the 2789 on placebo) in serum cholesterol of 10% and in triglycerides of 26%. At the end of 6 years MI had decreased by 15% (287 on niacin vs. 839 on placebo, $p < 0.05$). Other cardiovascular endpoints also tended to decrease, significantly so for stroke and new angina, except that there was a significant excess of cardiac arrhythmias. Noncardiovascular deaths increased slightly, and cardiovascular and total deaths decreased slightly and nonsignificantly, so that there was no difference in all-cause deaths.

Niacin was not nearly as well tolerated as was clofibrate. Nonadherence was 15.5% compared to 5.1% on placebo. Cutaneous adverse effects were almost universal in the form of flushing (92%), itching, urticaria, or other rashes, and there was an increased incidence of icthyosis, hyperpigmentation, and acanthosis nigricans on clinical examination. Upper gastrointestinal tract symptoms (nausea, pain, loss of appetite) were also fairly common. Although the mean serum uric acid increased very little, the proportion that had abnormal levels (43.5% on niacin vs. 19.6% on placebo), developed acute gout (6.4% vs. 4.3%), or were prescribed gout medication (11.4% vs. 6.1%) was considerably higher on niacin. There were slight decreases of blood urea nitrogen, potassium, and white blood cell count, and slight increases of alkaline phosphatase and plasma glucose. Though the proportion with abnormal fasting or stimulated plasma glucose levels increased, there was no increase in frank diabetes.

In spite of its relatively poor tolerance, niacin was a more effective lipid-lowering agent than clofibrate. The investigators suggested that it could be used cautiously in secondary prevention. They expressed concern about arrhythmias, gastrointestinal problems, and abnormal chemistry findings and the lack of decrease in total mortality. The major contribution of the CDP came some years later, when the 15-year follow-up did show a 10% reduction in total mortality (mortality 52.2% in niacin group vs. 58.2% in the placebo group, $p < 0.0004$), and thereby provided the first firm evidence that an early reduction in CHD morbidity and mortality may over a longer period translate into a reduced total mortality (Canner et al., 1986). Most of the benefit came from a reduced CHD mortality; however, small reductions also occurred in other causes of death. Importantly, median survival was 1.63 years longer in the niacin group than the placebo group.

E. The Newcastle and Edinburgh Trials of Clofibrate in the Treatment of Ischemic Heart Disease

Both these secondary prevention trials were unusual, in that they included patients with angina as well as those with MI, and a small proportion of females as well as males. Participants were unselected in regard to lipid levels, except that those with serum cholesterol levels exceeding 400 mg/dl or with xanthomata were excluded in Newcastle. Participants were aged less than 65 years in Newcastle and 40–69 years in Edinburgh (Group of Physicians of the Newcastle upon Tyne Region, 1971; Research Committee of the Scottish Society of Physicians, 1971). Both trials were double-blind placebo-controlled studies of rather small size: there were 244 participants on clofibrate and 253 on placebo in the Newcastle trial, and 350 on clofibrate and 367 on placebo in the Edinburgh trial. Patients on anticoagulants were equally distributed among the clofibrate and placebo groups. The dose of clofibrate was 1.5–2.0 g per day, and duration was 5 years in Newcastle and 6 years in Edinburgh.

The serum cholesterol levels in Newcastle fell by 10% compared to controls, and in Edinburgh by 15%. Significantly fewer (−33%) MIs occurred in the clofibrate compared to the placebo group in Newcastle (52 vs. 81, $p <$ 0.01). In Edinburgh the 21% reduction in MIs was not significant (54 vs. 72). In both studies the subgroups who had angina at entry had significantly fewer sudden deaths on treatment than the controls, and there were more such patients in Newcastle than in Edinburgh, possibly accounting for the more favorable results in regard to all myocardial events in the Newcastle trial. Only the Edinburgh trial reported all-cause mortality: 43 deaths in the drug group vs. 47 in the placebo group (not significant).

The incidence of side effects necessitating withdrawal was low (3%) on clofibrate and only marginally in excess of the rate (2%) on placebo. Gastrointestinal side effects predominated, clinical myositis was not seen, but one case of reversible alopecia was noted.

The reports of these early studies created some interest at the time of their publication because both concluded that the beneficial effects in regard to MI were relatively independent of the initial level of serum cholesterol and of the response to treatment. If true, this would suggest a nonlipid mode of action for clofibrate. However, these studies were far too small to allow for meaningful conclusions to be drawn from such subgroup analyses, so that they could not test this hypothesis. Also, in the much larger WHO clofibrate primary prevention trial, benefit was more marked in those with highest levels of serum cholesterol at baseline and in those who had the greatest fall on treatment.

F. The Stockholm Ischemic Heart Disease Secondary Prevention Study

This trial was a small, randomized (but not blinded) comparison of a combination of clofibrate (2 g/day) plus niacin (3 g/day) with no treatment, in consecutive survivors of MI below 70 years of age (Carlson and Rosenhammer, 1988). There were 279 participants in the active treatment group and 279 in the control group. One fifth were females, but these were not analyzed separately. The treatment period was 5 years.

The net change in serum cholesterol was 13% in the actively treated group, while serum triglycerides declined by 19%. Myocardial infarctions decreased by 28% (72 in the treated group, 100 in the control group, $p < 0.05$). Unique among the trials, in-trial all-cause mortality was also significantly lower in the treated group (61 vs. 82, $p < 0.05$). Six percent of the treated group withdrew because of the side effects.

Subgroup analyses seemed to indicate that individuals who had elevated triglycerides, and those who showed the greatest decline in triglycerides, had the greatest reductions in MI. No such relationships were noted for serum cholesterol. The findings might suggest that the role of triglycerides in the etiology of MI needs to be reassessed. While provocative, the subgroup analyses are not sufficient to make the case, due to the small numbers in each of the subgroups.

III. ANALYSES OF THE COMBINED CLINICAL TRIALS

Meta-analysis allows the results of trials to be examined in aggregate (Yusuf et al., 1985). Many clinical trials are too small to yield statistically meaningful results individually; however, they can contribute information when combined with the results of the larger studies. Such a meta-analysis can provide a more stable estimate of the effectiveness of a treatment than can even the largest study on its own. The eight drug trials discussed above were subjected to meta-analysis, as were four diet trials (Research Committee to the Medical Research Council, 1965, 1968; Dayton et al., 1969; Leren, 1970). The diet trials were selected using the same criteria as the drug trials and were included for purposes of comparison. In addition to the meta-analysis, the percentage reductions in serum cholesterol and MI (weighted for study size) were calculated.

The efficacy of drug treatment in reducing the primary endpoint of MI is shown in Table 1. Significantly fewer MIs (nonfatal, fatal, and all) were observed in the treatment groups than would be expected to occur if treatment was without effect, i.e., treatment was effective in reducing the MI rate. Treatment appeared to be successful in secondary as well as primary prevention studies (Fig. 1). For all MIs, the mean 9% reductions in serum cholesterol obtained produced reductions of 21% in primary, and 15% in secondary prevention trials (i.e., about 2% reduction in MI rate for every 1% reduction

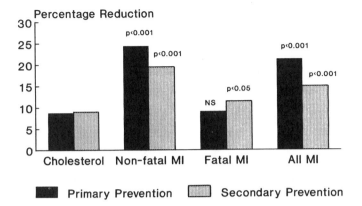

Figure 1 Mean percentage reductions in serum cholesterol and nonfatal, fatal, and all myocardial infarcts (MI) in three primary and five secondary prevention drug trials of cholesterol lowering. Details of trials are given in text. Means are weighted for number of all MIs in each trial, so that the larger trials have more influence on the overall mean. The significance of the reductions in the treated groups versus the control groups were obtained by meta-analysis (Yusuf at al., 1985).

in serum cholesterol). Reductions in nonfatal MIs (24% and 20%) were somewhat higher than the reductions in fatal MIs (9% and 11%). Given the short duration of the trials in relation to the evolution of coronary atherosclerosis, it would be expected that less severe manifestations would respond first.

The success of treatment appears to depend primarily on the degree of cholesterol lowering obtained, rather than the method used. The ratio of 2:1 appears to apply whether the method used was diet or a variety of drugs (Fig. 2). Gemfibrozil may be an exception, since its ratio is better than 3:1; however, this finding should be interpreted with caution since it depends on one study only.

These positive findings in respect of the primary study endpoint of MI have to be tempered by another finding from the meta-analysis: though cardiovascular deaths are significantly reduced, the reduction is balanced by a significant increase in noncardiovascular deaths, so that all deaths are unaltered (Table 1). The reasons for the increase in noncardiovascular deaths are not known. The extent of the increase shown on the table may be exaggerated, since the largest contribution was made by one study (the WHO trial), which may well have overestimated deaths in the treated group. Nevertheless, the

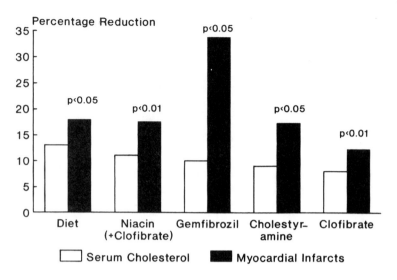

Figure 2 Mean percentage reductions in serum cholesterol and in myocardial infarcts in diet trials (Research Committee to the Medical Research Council, 1965; Research Committee to the Medical Research Council, 1968; Dayton et al., 1969; Leren, 1970), trials using niacin (Coronary Drug Project Research Group, 1975; Carlson and Rosenhammer, 1988), gemfibrozil (Frick et al., 1987), cholestyramine (Lipid Research Clinics Program, 1984), and clofibrate (Group of Physicians of the Newcastle upon Tyne Region, 1971; Research Committee of the Scottish Society of Physicians, 1971; Coronary Drug Project Research Group, 1975). Calculations were performed as in Figure 1.

trend towards an increase in noncardiovascular deaths was also present in the remaining studies.

The causes of excess noncardiovascular death varied in different studies (accidents and violence in some, no predominant cause in most), so that it is difficult to attribute the excess noncardiovascular mortality to cholesterol lowering per se. Importantly, only the WHO trial suggested an excess of cancer (58 vs. 42) among the drug trials, and only one diet trial (Dayton et al., 1970) suggested an excess (7 vs. 2); the excess was not significant in either of these trials. It is possible that some deaths were due to the drugs used, though with the exception of gallbladder disease in the case of the fibrates, there are no plausible mechanisms for such an effect. The lowered cardiovascular mortality may have allowed a competing cause of death to intervene (Rose and Shipley, 1990), and finally chance may be operating. More data from a number of clinical trials currently in progress should shed some light on these questions. In the interim, it is of interest to note that there is a trend towards decreased all-cause mortality under two disparate sets of conditions: diet treatment and treatment of patients with existing CHD.

The lack of decrease in all-cause mortality should not distract attention from the main finding of the clinical trials—that cardiac morbidity and mortality is decreased. The large and significant decrease in nonfatal MI remains as a net gain from treatment. In itself, this is a worthwhile goal, since the number of persons with nonfatal CHD far exceeds that of CHD deaths in any one year; also, the direct costs (e.g., outpatient medical treatment, hospitalizations, surgical procedures) of nonfatal CHD far exceed those of fatal disease.

The benefit of treatment also has to be weighed against the side effects of treatment. In the case of some drugs such as cholestyramine and niacin, side effects were common. For cholestyramine, side effects were generally not of a severe nature and were largely confined to the gastrointestinal tract. For niacin, cardiac arrythmias and gout were worrisome (but relatively infrequent) during the Coronary Drug Project, and so was gout during the Stockholm study, while cutaneous side effects were almost universal. The fibrates as a group had a low incidence of side effects, but clofibrate also had the lowest efficacy in respect of lowering cholesterol. The results of diet therapy were as good as those of drugs, and diet would of course have the lowest rate of side effects.

IV. ANGIOGRAPHIC STUDIES

Studies using coronary angiographic endpoints are of interest because they allow direct visualization of the response of the atheromatous lesion to therapy, and thus allow for testing of the hypothesis that cholesterol lowering will arrest lesion growth or induce its regression. Also, because of the quantitative nature of the angiographic endpoint and because the investigator does not have to wait for a clinical event to occur, the numbers of participants needed are smaller than in clinical trials. Three recent randomized, double-blind angiographic studies are of particular interest: the NHLBI Type II Coronary Intervention Study, the Cholesterol-Lowering Atherosclerosis Study, and the Familial Atherosclerosis Treatment Study.

A. NHLBI Type II Coronary Intervention Study

The trial selected patients aged 21–55 years (81% males, 19% females) with elevated low density lipoprotein cholesterol levels (Type II hyperlipoproteinemia) and angiographic evidence of coronary artery disease (Brensike et al., 1984). The mean levels of serum cholesterol of the patients was very high at 323 mg/dl. After one month of diet, 59 patients were randomized to receive 24 g of cholestyramine daily and 57 to receive placebo for 5 years. During the trial period, serum cholesterol levels were 11% lower, low density lipoprotein cholesterol 19% lower, and high density lipoprotein cholesterol 5% higher on cholestryramine than on placebo. The trial failed to show a significant result for the primary endpoint; the same small proportion (7%) of the cholestyramine and control groups showed apparent regression. However, fewer patients on cholestyramine showed lesion progression (32% vs. 49%, one-sided $p < 0.05$), and stabilization (no change, or mixed progression and regression) tended to be more common on cholestyramine (61% vs. 44%).

Safety monitoring showed a rise in alkaline phosphatase and in serum iron-binding capacity, and a drop in carotene levels in the cholestyramine group. Clinical side effects were surprisingly infrequent, most commonly gas (7%) and leg cramps (6%).

This study provided some evidence that it is possible to slow progression in patients with Type II hyperlipoproteinemia, but it was not able to demonstrate regression. The failure to show regression is not surprising in view of the still-high level of serum cholesterol while on drug treatment (256 mg/dl).

B. Cholesterol-Lowering Atherosclerosis Study (CLAS)

CLAS enrolled nonsmoking men aged 40–59 who had previously undergone coronary artery bypass grafting and who had demonstrated good compliance and good response in serum cholesterol to the study medications (Blankenhorn et al., 1987). Participants were thus a more favorable group to intervene on than those in the NHLBI study. Unlike the NHLBI patients, the CLAS patients were unselected in regard to baseline lipids, and they had lower mean serum cholesterol levels (246 mg/dl in drug group, 243 mg/dl in placebo group) and a wide range of levels (185–350 mg/dl). Patients were randomly allocated to groups (94 in each group) receiving either colestipol 30 g/day plus niacin 3–12 g/day, or placebos. All patients were placed on a cholesterol-lowering diet.

During the 2 years of the study, the mean serum cholesterol in the drug group was 22% lower, low density lipoprotein cholesterol 39% lower, and high density lipoprotein cholesterol 37% higher than in the placebo group. At the end of the study, 39% of the drug group patients showed progression against 61% of placebo group, stabilization occurred in 45% against 37%, and regression in 16% against 2% (difference in proportions showing regression significant, $p < 0.002$). Both native vessels and the grafts benefited by treatment, and the global change score (derived from a blinded assessment of lesion severity in pre- and posttreatment angiograms) was significantly better for the drug group ($p < 0.001$).

As may be expected from the doses of drugs used in this study, side effects were common. Flushing occurred in 91% of treated patients, warm skin in 69%, itching in 60%, rash in 37%, tingling in 26%, dry skin in 15%, constipation in 31%, nausea in 23%, stomach discomfort in 23%, heartburn in 20%. Diffuse abdominal pain, sore throat, and vomiting were also more common in the drug group. The niacin-induced cutaneous effects tended to persist, but the gastrointestinal symptoms abated with time. The only clinical event more common in the drug group was gouty arthritis (5%), ascribed to the known uricemic effect of niacin.

CLAS confirmed that drug treatment can slow the progression of coronary artery disease, and in addition suggested that regression is possible. The degree of lipid lowering obtained in this study was much greater than in the NHLBI study. It may be that the mean levels of serum cholesterol (180 mg/dl) and low density lipoprotein cholesterol (97 mg/dl) achieved in CLAS represent the kind of levels needed to obtain regression. Additionally, the drug-induced elevation of mean high density lipoprotein cholesterol (from 45 mg/dl to 61 mg/dl) may have been important.

C. Familial Atherosclerosis Treatment Studies (FATS)

To be eligible for this trial, men aged less than 62 years had to have a family history of premature coronary disease, elevated apolipoprotein B levels, and angiographic coronary artery disease, but not have undergone coronary artery bypass grafting (Brown et al., 1989). Two types of combination therapy were assessed: colestipol (30 g/day) plus niacin (4 g/day) ($n = 36$), and colestipol plus lovastatin (40 mg/day) ($n = 38$). The control group ($n = 46$) received placebo (and in some cases, colestipol). All patients were placed on a cholesterol-lowering diet. The trial duration was 2.5 years. In the controls, modest decreases in low density lipoprotein cholesterol (7%) and increases in high density lipoprotein cholesterol (+5%) were observed, percent stenosis increased by 2.1%, progression was observed in 46% of patients and regression in 11%. In the colestipol plus niacin group, low density lipoprotein cholesterol decreased by 32%, high-density cholesterol increased by 43%, mean stenosis decreased by 0.9 percentage points ($p < 0.005$ compared to controls), progression was found in 25%, and regression in 39% ($p < 0.006$). In the colestipol plus lovastatin group, the low density lipoprotein cholesterol decreased by 46%, the high density lipoprotein cholesterol increased by 15%, mean stenosis decreased by 0.7 percentage points ($p < 0.02$), progression was found in 21%, and regression in 32%. The investigators conclude that favorable changes in lesion severity were mediated by change in both low and high density lipoprotein cholesterol levels.

Together with the CLAS results, FATS confirms that regression is indeed possible, provided that the lipid abnormality is aggressively treated. Combination drug thereapy will often be needed to achieve the kind of response necessary.

V. IMPLICATIONS

The clinical trials and angiographic studies of cholesterol lowering have been of decisive importance in persuading scientific and public opinion that elevated serum cholesterol is a causal element in the chain of events leading to CHD, and that treatment by diet and drugs is effective in lowering the risk of CHD. The correctness of these opinions is well illustrated by the analyses of the combined trials, which show that the clinical event rate can be lowered by 20% if cholesterol levels are lowered by 10%. Furthermore, the angiographic studies are increasingly demonstrating that actual regression of established coronary lesions is feasible.

The studies reviewed also provide information about the efficacy and safety of diet and of individual drugs, useful in making appropriate therapeutic choices. Diet is as effective as most of the established drugs in lowering serum cholesterol and in decreasing the myocardial infarction rate. Its freedom from side effects underlines the importance of committed and intensive diet therapy as the cornerstone of treatment. The resins cholestyramine and colestipol are effective in lowering the clinical event rate in patients with high blood cholesterol and can arrest or slow the progression of established coronary artery disease. They do have bothersome gastrointestinal side effects, but appear to be free of serious side effects. In view of their proven efficacy in regard to CHD, the resins must remain drugs of first choice for the treatment of high blood cholesterol. The newer HMG CoA reductase inhibitors are more effective than the resins at lowering serum cholesterol, but have yet to be shown to alter the clinical event rate. In combination with colestipol, lovastatin has achieved regression of coronary atherosclerosis in one recent study (Brown et al., 1989), so that the outcomes of further angiographic studies and of primary and secondary prevention trials using HMG CoA reductase inhibitors alone and in combination will be of some interest.

Niacin is difficult to evaluate, since it appears to be both effective and toxic. In the one study where it was used as monotherapy (the Coronary Drug Project), it did produce a significant 15% reduction in myocardial infarctions, but was also associated with serious toxicity (e.g., gout, arrythmias) and with annoying cutaneous symptoms. When used in combination with resins or with clofibrate, it was effective in reducing myocardial infarction and in inducing regression. Also, niacin featured in both studies which have thus far demonstrated a reduction in all-cause mortality (the CDP 15-year follow-up and the Stockholm study). Therefore, until a drug of demonstrably superior efficacy and lower side effects is available, niacin must retain a place in the treatment of both high blood cholesterol and triglycerides. It would appear to be particularly useful when used in combination with resins or HMG CoA reductase inhibitors.

The fibrates are generally poor at lowering serum cholesterol, being more effective at lowering triglycerides. Nevertheless, an extensive clinical trial experience of the oldest member of the fibrate family, clofibrate, has been accumulated and indicates that CHD is lowered to a degree commensurate with the modest cholesterol lowering achieved. In combination with niacin, clofibrate reduced cardiovascular and all-cause mortality in the Stockholm study. Toxicity appears to be low (if the results from the WHO study are discounted), except for an increase in gallstone-related complications. Newer fibrates may be better choices, since they are somewhat better at lowering serum cholesterol, and gemfibrozil has been successful in lowering MI rates, particularly in patients with elevated triglycerides (Frick et al., 1987).

The value of combined therapy was underscored especially by the angiographic studies. While monotherapy lowers serum cholesterol sufficiently to reduce the incidence of clinical events, combined therapy appears to be necessary to achieve the degree of cholesterol lowering needed to induce regression of atheromatous lesions. Also, combined therapy allows more facets of dyslipidemia to be corrected. Thus, the positive results of the combination of colestipol with niacin in CLAS and FATS, and of colestipol and lovastatin in FATS, may well be due not only to the marked degree of cholesterol lowering obtained, but also to the simultaneous improvement in high density lipoprotein and triglyceride levels. The Helsinki study provides further support for the idea that improvement in these lipid fractions are advantageous, though final judgment will have to await a trial specifically designed to test the hypothesis.

From the public health point of view, the trials encourage wide application of the principles of a cholesterol-lowering diet, since it will be effective in lowering serum cholesterol and of CHD, is safe, and, most importantly, will reduce the number requiring intensive medical treatment. In the clinical setting also, the number of patients requiring drug therapy can be lowered by effective diet therapy. Misconceptions about the efficacy of diet may on occasion have led to the token institution of a "trial of diet therapy," rather than a whole-hearted commitment on the part of doctor and patient alike. The choice of drugs, when needed, will be predicated to some extent by the type of lipid disorder: resins or niacin (or, likely in the near future, HMG CoA reductase inhibitors) for isolated high serum cholesterol; niacin or gemfibrozil (or possibly, HMG CoA reductase inhibitors) for mixed hyperlipidemias. The primary purpose of treatment remains the reduction of total and low density lipoprotein cholesterol; however, the possibility of an additional benefit from improving other aspects of the lipid profile at the same time should not be ignored. In many instances combinations of drugs will be needed to achieve optimal lowering of serum cholesterol or to treat all elements of the disorder. It would be particularly appropriate to institute such intensive diet and combination drug therapy in patients with existing CHD, in view of their high risk of reinfarction if left untreated.

REFERENCES

Austin, M. (1989). Plasma triglyceride as a risk factor for coronary heart disease. The epidemiologic evidence and beyond. *Am. J. Epidemiol.* **129**:249–259.

Blankenhon, D. H., Nessim, S. A., Johnson, R. L., Sanmarco, M. E., Azen, S. P., and Cashin-Hemphill, L. (1987). Beneficial effects of combined colestipol-niacin therapy on coronary atherosclerosis and coronary venous bypass grafts. *J.A.M.A.* **257**:3233–3244.

Brensike, J. F., Levy, R. I., Kelsey, S. F., Passamani, E. R., Richardson, J. M., Loh, I. K., Stone, M. J., Aldrich, R. F., Battaglini, J. W., Moriarty, D. J., Fisher, M. R., Friedman, L., Friedewald, W., Detre, K. M., and Epstein, S. E. (1984). Effects of therapy with cholestyramine on progression of coronary arteriosclerosis: results of the NHLBI Type II Coronary Intervention Study. *Circulation* **69**:313–324.

Brown, B. G., Albers, J. J., Fisher, L. D., Schaefer, S. M., Lin, J-T., Kaplan, C., Zhao, X-Q., Bisson, B. D., Fitzpatrick, V. F., and Dodge, H. T. (1990). Regression of coronary artery disease as a result of intensive lipid-lowering therapy in men with high levels of apolipoprotein B. *N. Engl. J. Med.* **323**:1289–1298.

Canner, P. L., Berge, K. H., Wenger, N. K., Stamler, J., Fiedman, L., Prineas, R. J., and Friedewald, W. (1986). Fifteen year mortality in Coronary Drug Project patients: long-term benefit with niacin. *J. Am. Coll. Cardiol.* **8**:1245–1255.

Carlson, L. A., and Rosenhammer, G. (1988). Reduction in mortality in the Stockholm Ischaemic Heart Disease Secondary Prevention Study by combined treatment with clofibrate and nicotinic acid. *Acta Med. Scand.* **223**:405–418.

Committee of Principal Investigators. (1978). A cooperative trial in the primary prevention of ischaemic heart disease using clofibrate. *Br. Heart J.* **40**:1069–1118.

Committee of Prinicpal Investigators. (1980). W.H.O. coooperative trial on primary prevention of ischaemic heart disease with clofibrate to lower serum cholesterol: Mortality follow-up. *Lancet* **2**:279–385.

Committee of Principal Investigators. (1984). W.H.O. cooperative trial on primary prevention of ischaemic heart disease with clofibrate to lower serum cholesterol: Final mortality follow-up. *Lancet* **2**:600–604.

Consensus Conference Statement on Lowering Blood Cholesterol to Prevent Heart Disease. (1985). *J.A.M.A.* **253**:2080–2086.

Coronary Drug Project Research Group. (1975). Clofibrate and niacin in coronary heart disease. *J.A.M.A.* **231**:360–381.

Dayton, S., Pearce, M. L., Hashimoto, S., Dixon, W. J., and Tomiyasu, U. (1969). A controlled clinical trial of a diet high in unsaturated fat in preventing complications of atherosclerosis. *Circulation* **40** (Supplement 2):1–63.

Expert Panel. (1988). Report of the National Cholesterol Education Program expert panel on detection, evaluation, and treatment of high blood cholesterol in adults. *Arch. Intern. Med.* **148**:36–69.

Frick, M. H., Elo, O., Haapa, K., Heinonen, O. P., Heinsalmi, P., Helo, P., Huttunen, J., Kaitaniemi, P., Koskinen, P., Manninen, V., Mäenpää, H., Mälkönen, M., Mänttäri, M., Norola, S., Pasternack, A., Pikkarainen, J., Romo, M., and Nikkilä, E. A. (1987). Helsinki Heart Study: Primary-prevention trial with gemfibrozil in middle-aged men with dyslipidemia. Safety of treatment, changes in risk factors, and incidence of coronary heart disease. *N. Engl. J. Med.* **317**:1237–1245.

Group of Physicians of the Newcastle upon Tyne Region. (1971). Trial of clofibrate in the treatment of ischaemic heart disease. *Br. Med. J.* **4**:767–75.

Leren, P. (1970). The Oslo Diet-Heart Study. Eleven-year report. *Circulation* **42**:935–942.

Lipid Research Clinics Program. (1979). The Coronary Primary Prevention Trial: Design and implementation. *J. Chron. Dis.* **32**:609–631.

Lipid Research Clinics Program. (1984a). The Lipid Research Clinics Coronary Primary Prevention Trial results. I. Reduction in incidence of coronary heart disease. *J.A.M.A.* **251**:351–364.

Lipid Research Clinics Program. (1984b). The Lipid Research Clinics Coronary Primary Prevention Trial results. II. The relationship of reduction in incidence of coronary heart disease to cholesterol lowering. *J.A.M.A.* **251**:365–374.

Manninen, V., Elo, O., Frick, M. H., Haapa, K., Heinonen, O. P., Heinsalmi, P., Helo, P., Huttunen, J., Kaitaniemi, P., Koskinen, P., Mäenpää, H., Mälkönen, M., Mänttäri, M., Norola, S., Pasternack, A., Pikkarainen, J., Romo, M., Sjöblom, T., and Nikkilä, E. A. (1988). Lipid alterations and decline in the incidence of coronary heart disease in the Helsinki Heart Study. *J.A.M.A.* **260**:641–651.

Mantel, N., and Haenzel, W. (1959). Statistical aspects of the analysis of data from retropective studies of disease. *J. Natl. Cancer Inst.* **22**:719–748.

Research Committee of the Scottish Society of Physicians. (1971). Iscaemic heart disease: A secondary prevention trial using clofibrate. *Br. Med. J.* **4:**775–784.

Research Committee to the Medical Research Council. (1965). Low-fat diet in myocardial infarction—a controlled trial. *Lancet* **2:**501–504.

Research Committee to the Medical Research Council. (1986). Controlled trial of soya-bean oil in myocardial infarction. *Lancet* **2:**693–700.

Rose, G., and Shipley, M. (1990). Effects of coronary risk reduction on the pattern of mortality. *Lancet* **335:**275–277.

Sempos, C., Fulwood, R., Haines, C., Carroll, M., Anda, R., Williamson, D. F., Remington, P., and Cleeman, J. (1989). The prevalence of high blood cholesterol levels among adults in the United States. *J.A.M.A.* **262:**45–52.

Wilson, W. F., Christiansen, J. C., Anderson, K. M., and Kannel, W. B. (1989). Impact of national guidelines for cholesterol risk factor screening. The Framingham Offspring Study. *J.A.M.A.* **262:**41–44.

Yusuf, S., Peto, R., Collins, R., and Sleight, P. (1985). Beta blockade during and after myocardial infarction: An overview of randomized trials. *Progr. Cardiovasc. Dis.* **27:**355–371.

5

Bile Acid Sequestrants

Donald B. Hunninghake

Heart Disease Prevention Clinic
University of Minnesota
Minneapolis, Minnesota

There are two bile acid sequestrants, cholestyramine and colestipol, available for clinical use. The bile acid sequestrants (resins) were defined as drugs of first choice for lowering low density lipoprotein cholesterol (LDL-C) in the National Cholesterol Education Program Adult Treatment Panel report (Expert Panel, 1988). This recommendation was based upon their efficacy in lowering LDL-C, long-term safety data, and evidence for reduction in risk of coronary heart disease (CHD). However, limited acceptance of the use of this class of drugs by both health professionals and patients has occurred because of gastrointestinal side effects and lack of palatability. The frequency of these problems is generally overestimated. This chapter will provide the rationale for the appropriate use of the resins.

I. EFFECT ON CORONARY HEART DISEASE

The major study that documented association of lowering of total and LDL-cholesterol with a reduction in CHD risk was the Lipid Research Clinics Coronary Primary Prevention Trial (Lipid Research Clinics Program, 1984a,b). This was a randomized, double-blind trial of 3806 middle-aged men who were asymptomatic for CHD and with LDL-C levels above 175 mg/dl after diet. The patients were randomized to receive either placebo or cholestyramine 24 g per day. The cholestyramine group had greater mean reductions in total and LDL-C of 8.5% and 12.6%, respectively, than those observed in the placebo group. At the end of an average of 7.4 years of follow-up, there was a statistically significant 19% reduction in the primary endpoint for the study, fatal and nonfatal myocardial infarction. The total number of definite fatal and nonfatal myocardial infarctions in the placebo group was 187 and in the cholestyramine group 155 ($p < 0.05$). The clinical significance of this 19% reduction in the primary endpoint for this study has been questioned by some. However, it is important to recognize that there were similar or greater reductions in the frequency of all other manifestations of CHD including positive exercise test, angina pectoris, and coronary artery bypass surgery. The total number of coronary events in the placebo group was 1036 compared to 831 in the cholestyramine group, and the total numbers of cardiovascular events were 1159 and 943, respectively.

Additionally, the bile-acid sequestrants have been used in three major angiographic studies to determine their effect on the rate of progression and/or regression of CHD. The NHLBI type II study used only cholestyramine, and the results suggested that the cholestyramine group had a reduced rate of progression (Brensinke et al., 1984). The Cholesterol Lowering Atherosclerosis Study (CLAS), which used a combination of colestipol and nicotinic acid, showed a reduced rate of progression in the drug-treated group compared to the placebo group and also noted regression after 2 years in 16% of the patients (Blankenhorn et al., 1987). The recently completed Familial Atherosclerosis Treatment Study (FATS) had two active treatment groups consisting of colestipol plus either nicotinic acid or lovastatin. Regression and reduced rate of progression and fewer clinical endpoints were reported in the two treatment groups as compared to the control (Brown et al., 1989). Finally, in an uncontrolled trial with colestipol, which should be interpreted as inconclusive, it was reported that CHD mortality was decreased (Dorr et al., 1978).

II. LONG-TERM SAFETY

Cholestyramine has been used clinically since the 1960s, and no major adverse effects have been reported. However, the only large, long-term trial with a bile-acid sequestrant has been the LRC-CPPT. No significant major adverse effects were noted in this trial (Lipid Research Clinics Program, 1984a). Three suspect areas have occasionally been discussed. One relates to the fact that there were 4 traumatic deaths (accident, homicide, suicide) in the placebo group compared to 11 in the cholestyramine group. This difference was not statistically significant, and it appears that this was a chance observation. The second observation was that there were 6 cases of cancer of the oral cavity–pharynx in the cholestyramine group compared to none in the placebo group. Again, the observed frequency in the two groups was not statistically different and was compatible with that expected in the population. Furthermore, the total number of malignancies was 57 in both the placebo and cholestyramine groups with 15 and 16 malignant deaths, respectively. There were 30 hospitalizations for gallstones and other gallbladder and biliary tract disease in the placebo group and 38 in the cholestyramine group (not significant). An additional 6-year follow-up of patients in the LRC-CPPT has been completed, and these results should be available soon. The resins are administered as the chloride salts, and rare cases of hyperchloremia acidosis have been observed.

III. MECHANISM OF ACTION

Both cholestyramine and colestipol are highly charged compounds which are not absorbed from the gastrointestinal tract. The lack of systemic effect would predict that this class of drugs would not have systemic toxicity, should not require special monitoring for adverse effects, and could be considered for use in special populations such as children. Cholesterol-lowering drugs are not recommended during pregnancy, but the resins can be safely administered until the pregnancy is confirmed without adverse effects on the fetus.

The mechanism of action of the resins is dependent upon their highly charged nature and lack of absorption from the gut. Approximately 97% of the bile acids undergo an enterohepatic recirculation with only a small percentage being excreted in the feces. The resins are administered as either the chloride or hydrochloride salts. The chloride ion is exchanged for the negatively charged bile acid. The net effect is that both cholestyramine and colestipol bind the bile acids in the gut, interrupt their normal enterohepatic recirculation, and increase fecal bile acid excretion (Moore et al., 1968). This increases the conversion of cholesterol to bile acids in the liver by the enzyme 7-alpha dehydrogenase. Thus hepatic cholesterol content is decreased, and this is the stimulus for upregulation or increased number of LDL receptors. The increased number of receptors increases the uptake of LDL from the plasma and increases the rate of catabolism of LDL, which is the desired clinical effect. The preceding mechanisms appear to be the major reason for the observed decrease in plasma LDL-C, but other mechanisms such as smaller, denser than normal LDL particles depleted of cholesterol esters have been described (Witztum et al., 1979). The mechanism for this observation is not clear.

The decrease in hepatic cholesterol levels can produce an increase in hepatic cholesterol synthesis due to an increase in the enzyme HMG-CoA reductase, which regulates cholesterol synthesis (Grundy et al., 1971). However, the increase in conversion of cholesterol to bile acids is greater than the increase in cholesterol synthesis, and the net effect is a reduction in plasma total and LDL cholesterol. This increase in hepatic cholesterol synthesis does limit the total amount of lowering that can be obtained with resin therapy alone, but also explains the additive or synergistic effects of combining a resin with an agent that inhibits cholesterol synthesis (HMG-CoA reductase inhibitor). The mechanism of action of the resins differs from all currently available hypolipidemic agents, and thus the resins can be used in combination with all currently available classes of hypolipidemic agents for lowering LDL-C.

The resins can not only bind bile acids in the gut, but can also bind other negatively charged (anionic) drugs administered simultaneously. There is also some evidence that there may be some nonspecific adsorption of other drugs to the resins. Thus if resins are administered simultaneously with other drugs, there may be a decrease in the absorption of these drugs. Specific drug interactions will be described later.

IV. CLINICAL USE OF BILE ACID SEQUESTERING AGENTS

A. Lipid and Lipoprotein Effects

The resins are primarily effective in lowering total and LDL cholesterol. They also produce modest increases in HDL-C and either have no effect or cause a variable increase (frequently transitory) in serum triglyceride levels. A summary of the effect of resins on the serum lipid and lipoprotein levels with commonly administered dosages of the resins is illustrated in Table 1.

Table 1 Effect of Resins on Serum Lipid and Lipoprotein Levels

Lipid/Lipoprotein	Change
Total C	12–25% decrease
LDL-C	15–30% decrease
HDL-C	3–7% increase
Triglycerides	No effect or increase

The reductions in total and LDL-C are dose dependent (Angelin and Einarsson, 1981; Hunninghake et al., 1981; Illingworth, 1987). The reported LDL-C response in clinical trials has been variable, and this may be related to factors such as compliance, dietary restriction, and patient selection for study. Many clinical trials have demonstrated much greater reductions in LDL-C with smaller doses of resin (2–3 packets per day) than were observed in the LRC-CPPT. Although not confirmed by multiple trials, there is a perception that greater percent reductions in LDL-C are obtained with small doses of resins in patients with modest elevations of LDL-C as compared to those with more severe elevations.

It should be emphasized that the dose response for many drugs, including the resins, is not a linear response. This means that there is a relatively greater response with the initial smaller doses of drug (e.g., a 15% decrease with two scoops or packets of resin), and then each increment in dose produces a progressively smaller additional percent lowering of LDL-C.

A typical response in three patients with varying LDL-C levels after maximum diet therapy who were treated with different doses of resins is indicated in Table 2. It is assumed that the same percent reduction in LDL-C will be obtained no matter what the LDL-C levels after maximum dietary therapy, although the percent reduction may be greater in patients with lower LDL-C levels. These data indicate that one might expect to achieve the minimum NCEP target LDL-C goal of <130 mg/dl in a patient with an LDL-C of 160 mg/dl and two major risk factors with two to three packets of resin per day. Similar doses of resin would also be required to achieve the minimum NCEP target goal of an LDL-C level of <160 mg/dl in a patient with an LDL-C of 190 mg/dl without two major risk factors. As will be

Table 2 Typical LDL-C Responses in Patients with Varying Levels of LDL-C after Administration of Resin Therapy

Resin dosage (packets/day)	Expected mean % reduction in LDL-C	LDL-C levels (mg/dl) after maximum diet		
		160	190	225
2	15	136	162	192
3	20	128	152	180
4	24	122	144	171
6	30	112	133	157

discussed later, most patients tolerate two to three packets of resin per day without significant gastrointestinal complaints. In contrast, a patient with heterozygous familial hypercholesterolemia and an LDL-C level of 225 mg/dl may not achieve target LDL-C levels with maximum doses of resin, and the expected frequency of gastrointestinal side effects would be high. Unfortunately, many of the attitudes and beliefs of physicians regarding the use of resin therapy were derived in the era before the current guidelines for management of high blood cholesterol were developed. At that time, the only patients who were usually treated with drugs were those with familial hypercholesterolemia who usually received maximal doses of resin (six packets). Most patients will manifest significant gastrointestinal side effects when the maximal dose of resin is used.

The resins also produce increases in HDL, which generally range from 3 to 5%, although larger increases are occasionally reported. This increase in HDL has also been shown to contribute to the reduced CHD risk associated with the administration of the resins (Gordon et al., 1989). The exact mechanism for the increase in HDL has not been established, but it appears that there is an increased synthesis of apolipoprotein A-1, one of the major apolipoproteins in HDL. There is also recent evidence that the resins may increase the formation of HDL particles that contain only apoA-1, and this type of particle appears to be better correlated with cholesterol efflux from cells (Puchois et al., 1987).

The resins can either have no effect or may increase triglyceride levels; sometimes the increase is only transient. In patients who have increased LDL levels, modest increases in triglyceride levels (generally 10–25%) are seen if these patients also have triglyceride levels >300 mg/dl or occasionally when levels exceed 250 mg/dl. This is not a contraindication to the use of resins, but other drugs such as nicotinic acid are preferable. The resins are contraindicated in patients who have phenotypes characterized by increased cholesterol and triglyceride levels, but without increased LDL levels. These would include types III, IV, and V hyperlipoproteinemias. Administration of a resin to these patients will cause a dramatic increase in both cholesterol and triglyceride levels. In the patients with high VLDL or VLDL and chylomicrons levels, the increase in triglycerides may be so great as to significantly increase the risk of pancreatitis.

B. Time and Frequency of Administration

The frequency and time of administration of the resins are important both for compliance and maximizing the lipid-lowering effects. Twice-daily administration is as effective as more frequent administration of the same total daily dose (Blum et al., 1976). Compliance is frequently better with twice-daily administration as many patients have difficulty taking medication at noon. A few patients will have difficulty taking more than one packet of resin per dose; in these situations more frequent schedules may be indicated. Studies have also indicated that single-dose administration with the evening meal may be as effective as twice-daily administration (Hunninghake et al., 1979). A single morning dose is less effective. Resins should also be administered within an hour of the evening meal to achieve the maximal effect (Peters and Hunninghake, 1985). A very popular dosage regimen in our clinic is a single daily dose of two packets of resin shortly before the evening meal. This regimen also eliminates many of the problems regarding timing of administration of the resins to avoid altering the absorption of other drugs.

C. Side Effects

Since the resins are nonabsorbable drugs, the side effects are limited to gastrointestinal complaints and palatability concerns. Upper gastrointestinal complaints include belching or bloating, gas, heartburn, nausea and vomiting, and abdominal pain; lower gastrointestinal complaints are primarily constipation, and rarely diarrhea with high doses.

Problems with palatability can frequently be decreased by appropriate selection of the vehicle for preparation. An unsweetened juice to provide a different flavor and use of a heavier juice such as a tomato juice or pulpy orange juice may help to disguise the gritty consistency. Belching or bloating is frequently related to rapid ingestion of the resin as well as large amounts of air. Nausea and vomiting can also be related to dislike of taste and consistency. Gas and heartburn can also occur, and symptomatic treatment with antacids may be necessary. Patients with hiatus hernia or who consume large amounts of alcohol are especially susceptible to these symptoms.

Constipation is the more frequent lower gastrointestinal complaint. Constipation is variously defined by individuals as decreased frequency of bowel movements or increased consistency of the stool. In the case of resin administration it is usually increased consistency of the stool. In many patients there will only be a temporary increase in the consistency of the stool, which reverts back to its normal consistency in a short period of time. If constipation persists, it can frequently be alleviated by increased fluid and fiber. In addition to alleviating the constipation, increased intake of various soluble fiber such as oat bran or psyllium may not only decrease the degree of constipation, but also enhance the cholesterol-lowering effect because these compounds have independent cholesterol-lowering properties (Bell et al., 1989). However, controlled trials that document an additive effect of soluble fiber such as psyllium, when added to a resin, have not been reported. Many patients will also report improvement in their bowel habits with regular bowel movements of normal consistency following administration of resin. Diarrhea is rarely a problem, but is more likely to occur with the higher doses of resin.

D. Use in Children

The National Cholesterol Education Program is currently developing guidelines for the treatment of children with high blood cholesterol levels, including indications for drug therapy. Some clinicians treat children with a positive family history of premature CHD and/or markedly elevated total and LDL-C levels with cholesterol-lowering drugs. If drug therapy is considered, many believe that the resins are the only class of drugs that can safely be administered to children because of their safety record and lack of systemic effect. Limited studies in children indicate that the resins are not associated with any special form of toxicity and that growth and development proceed normally (Stein, 1989).

V. EFFECT ON ABSORPTION OF DRUGS AND NUTRIENTS

Resins are highly charged compounds which are not absorbed from the gut, and thus they can alter the absorption of other drugs by direct binding, adsorption or interference with the enterohepatic recirculation. Certain vitamins and nutrients require bile acids for their absorption.

There are a limited number of clinical studies to evaluate the effect of the resins on the absorption of other drugs. Many of these studies have only tested single doses of resin and thus may not truly measure the effects of chronic resin administration. Significant interaction between the resins and the following classes of drugs have been reported (Hunninghake, 1986).

Cardiac glycosides—The absorption of digitoxin, which has a large binding affinity for the resin and an extensive enterohepatic recirculation, is decreased by the resins. Digoxin does not have these properties and is much less likely to be affected.

Coumarin anticoagulants—Siginificant decreases in the absorption of both warfarin and phenprocoumon (not used in the United States) have been documented. The prothrombin time can be used to monitor for a clinical interaction.

Diuretics—Chlorothiazide and hydrochlorothiazide have been studied, but one would expect other thiazide diuretics and chlorthalidone to be affected.

When cholestyramine is administered simultaneously with hydrochlorothiazide, the absption of the latter is decreased by 85%. There will probably always be a modest (25%) decrease in absorption of diuretics even with maximum differences in time of administration of resin and diuretics.

Beta-blockers—The effects on the absorption of propranolol have been studied, but it is likely that other drugs in this class would be affected. Some estimate of the potential interaction can be obtained by monitoring pulse rate.

Thyroid hormone—The absorption of exogenously administered thyroid hormone is decreased, but there is no interference with endogenous hormone.

For all the drugs listed above, the interference with absorption can be minimized by separating the time of administration of resin from other drugs by at least 4 hours and preferably 6 hours. There is some evidence that cholestyramine decreases the absorption of other drugs more than colestipol, but this has not been carefully documented. Since the effect of the resins on the absorption of most drugs used clinically has not been tested, the routine recommendation is to administer other drugs either 1 hour before or 4 hours after the resin, although the absorption of many drugs is probably not altered by the administration of resins.

Because of the gastrointestinal complaints that can accompany the use of resins, antacids and H_2-histamine antagonists are occasionally used for symptomatic relief. These two classes of drugs can alter the absorption or metabolism of a variety of drugs. The resins are also given in combination with other hypolipidemic agents. Although there are occasional reports of some decreased bioavailability of these drugs, there are no reports which document a diminution in the lipid-lowering effects when combination therapy is administered simultaneously as compared to separating the time of administration of the hypolipidemic agents.

The resins do not interfere with the absorption of fat-soluble vitamins in adults unless there is an associated severe disturbance in bile acid metabolism due to either severe hepatic or small bowel disease. There have been isolated reports of a decrease in the absorption of vitamin B_{12}, folic acid, and iron in adult patients receiving resin therapy, but one should also always look for other causes. Children should be monitored more carefully for potential changes in vitamin and nutrient levels; they may be more sensitive to the changes in absorption produced by the resins, or their diets may be inadequate and their absolute requirements increased (West and Lloyd, 1973).

VI. COMPLIANCE

It is important for health professionals to have an objective viewpoint on the incidence of side effects with different doses of the resins. The beliefs and attitudes of health professionals are conveyed to the patient by both verbal and nonverbal communication. Both the advantages and disadvantages of the use of resins should be explained. Some patients are much more likely to tolerate the nuisances of resin therapy if they understand the nonabsorbable nature of the resins and long-term safety information plus the reduced number of visits and laboratory tests that are required with the resins as compared to other drugs. The patients' first experience with the resin may determine whether they will continue the drug. Since therapy will generally be for a lifetime and it is not an emergency, it is important to initiate therapy slowly and with small doses. Adequate instruction of the patient regarding administration of the resins is essential for good compliance. An approach that we have used (written instructions will simplify and are recommended) is as follows.

Initiate therapy with one scoop of resin within an hour of the evening meal. The initial goal is to determine the best method for administering the resin: volume, temperature, and type of fluid. If water is unsatisfactory, unsweetened juices are used to improve flavor. Heavier juices such as a pulpy orange juice or tomato juice are better for complaints related to the gritty consistency. I personally believe that use of elaborate methods for preparation (blenders, sauces, etc.) frequently conveys a negative message and should usually be avoided.

The titration period follows. The dose is increased to two packets per day (either twice daily or both in the evening). The effect on the lipoproteins is then measured and the dosage is increased as necessary. In my clinic, the most commonly administered total daily dose is two to three scoops per day. Most patients tolerate this dose without significant side effects, and approximately 60–65% of the maximum LDL-C lowering effect is obtained. In most patients it is prudent not to exceed a total daily dose of four scoops per day. There is only a small additional decrease in LDL-C that can be obtained, but the frequency of side effects increases dramatically. Occasional patients may be adequately controlled with one scoop per day.

A. Preparations and Cost

One should be aware of the cost of the resins at various pharmacies in the community. There can be significant variations. The resins are generally cheaper when provided in bulk containers as compared to individual packets.

Comparable unit dosages of active drug of cholestyramine and colestipol are 4 g and 5 g, respectively. The following preparations are available:

Cholestyramine

Questran—5 g of additives per dose. Available both as packets and bulk cans.
Questran-Light—1 g of additives per dose. Available both in packets and bulk cans.
Cholybar—Bar form only. Additional calories and additives are dependent upon the flavor.

Colestipol

Colestid—No additional additives. Available in both packets and bulk cans.

Some patients will have a preference for one of the above preparations, and if one preparation is disliked it is advisable to try another. It does require additional visit time, but we frequently give patients several sample packets of the above, allow them to test the different preparations, and select the prefered one. One can either give multiple prescriptions at the time of the visit or call the pharmacy later. Rare patients have developed allergic reactions to the dyes that were present in Questran in the past, but there has been some reformulation. If there is a question of an allergic response, colestipol should be tried because there are no additional additives.

VII. WHO SHOULD RECEIVE RESINS

Resins can be considered for use in any patient whose LDL-C level has not been adequately controlled with diet. Their long-term safety record and the reduced number of visits and laboratory tests that are required are desirable features. Negatives aspects are related to the palatability and gastrointestinal complaints which are more likely with higher doses.

Resins are ideal drugs for:

Primary prevention
Safety-conscious individuals
Women of child-bearing potential
Children (if indicated)
Modest increases in LDL-C where low-dose resin therapy is indicated
In combination therapy for patients with familial hypercholesterolemia or where aggressive lowering of LDL-C is indicated because of presence of CHD

Resins must be used cautiously in patients who:

Have constipation, hemorrhoids, hiatus hernia, or multiple gastrointestinal complaints

Are receiving multiple other drugs with multiple dosing schedules

Resins are contraindicated:

Lipoprotein phenotypes without significant elevation of LDL-C, i.e., types III, IV, and V phenotypes

VIII. SUMMARY

The bile acid sequestrants (resins) produce dose-dependent reductions in low-density lipoprotein cholesterol (LDL-C). The reduction in LDL-C and use of less than maximal doses of resins produce most of the LDL-C lowering effect, but significantly reduce the frequency of side effects. Side effects are also dose-dependent. The resins have also been shown to reduce the risk of CHD and to be safe for long-term administration. The resins are ideal drugs for primary prevention, especially as single drug therapy for individuals with modest elevations of LDL-C. The resins can also be used effectively in combination with other drugs for lower LDL-C.

REFERENCES

Angelin, B., and Einarsson, K. (1981). Cholestyramine in type IIa hyperlipoproteinemia. *Atherosclerosis* **38**:33–38.

Bell, L. P., Hectorne, K., Reynolds, H., Balm, T. K., and Hunninghake, D. B. (1989). Cholesterol-lowering effects of psyllium hydrophilic mucilloid. *JAMA* **261**:3419–3423.

Blankenhorn, D. M., Nessim, S. A., Johnson, R. L., Sanmarco, M. E., Azen, S. P., and Cashin-Hemphill, L. (1987). Beneficial effects of combined colestipol-niacin therapy on coronary atherosclerosis and coronary venous bypass grafts. *JAMA* **257**:3233–3240.

Blum, C. B., Havlik, R. J., and Morganroth, J. (1976). Cholestyramine: An effective twice daily dosage regimen. *Ann. Intern. Med.* **85**:287–289.

Brensike, J. F., Levy, R. I., Kelsey, S. F., Passamani, E. R., Richardson, J. M., Loh, I. K., Stone, N. J., Aldrich, R. F., Battaglini, J. W., Moriarty, D. J., Fisher, M. R., Friedman, L., Friedewald, W., Detre, K. M., and Epstein, S. E. (1984). Effects of therapy with cholestyramine on progression of coronary arteriosclerosis: results of the NHLBI Type II Coronary Intervention Study. *Circulation* **69**:313–324.

Brown, G., Albers, J. L., Fisher, L. D., Schaeffer, S. M., Lin, J. T., Kaplan, C., Zhao, X. Q., Bisson, B. D., Fitzpatrick, V. F. and Dodge, H. T. (1990). Regression of coronary artery disease as a result of intensive lipid-lowering therapy in men with high levels of apolipoprotein B. *N. Engl. J. Med.* **323**:1289–1298.

Brown, B. G., Lin, J. T., Schaefer, S. M., Kaplan, C. A., Dodge, H. T., and Albers, J. J. (1989). Niacin or lovastatin, combined with colestipol, regress coronary atherosclerosis and prevent clinical events in men with elevated apolipoprotein B. *Circulation* **80**(Suppl. II):II-266 (abstract).

Dorr, A. E., Gundersen, K., Schneider, J. C. Jr., Spencer, T. W., and Martin, W. B. (1978). Colestipol hydrochloride in hypercholesterolemic patients—effect on serum cholesterol and mortality. *J. Chron. Dis.* **31**:5–14.

The Expert Panel. (1988). Report of the National Cholesterol Education Program Expert Panel on detection, evaluation, and treatment of high blood cholesterol in adults. *Arch. Intern. Med.* **148**:36–69.

Gordon, D. J., Probstfield, J. L., Garrison, R. J., Neaton, J. D., Castelli, W. P., Knoke, J. D., Jacobs, D. R. Jr., Bangdiwala, S., and Tyroler, A. (1989). High-density lipoprotein cholesterol and cardiovascular disease: Four prospective American studies. *Circulation* **79**:8–15.

Grundy, S. M., Ahrens, E. H., Jr., and Salen, G. (1971). Interruption of the enterohepatic circulation of bile acids in man: Comparative effects of cholestyramine and ileal exclusion on cholesterol metabolism. *J. Lab. Clin. Med.* **78**:94–121.

Hunninghake, D. B., Peterson, F., Swenson, M., Kurtz, K., and Bell, C. (1979). Efficacy of once versus twice-a-day dosage of cholestyramine in type IIa hyperlipoproteinemia. *Pharmacologist* **21**:176 (abstract).

Hunninghake, D. B., Probstfield, J. L., Crow, L. O., and Isaacson, S. -O. (1981). Effect of colestipol and clofibrate on plasma lipid and lipoproteins in type IIa hyperlipoproteinemia. *Metabolism* **30**:605–609.

Hunninghake, D. B. (1986). Resin therapy. Adverse effects and their management. In *Pharmacological Control of Hyperlipidemia*. Edited by J. Fears. Barcelona, J. R. Prous Science Publishers, S. A., pp. 67–89.

Illingworth, D. R. (1987). Lipid-lowering drugs: An overview of indication and optimum therapeutic use. *Drugs* **33**:259–279.

Lipid Research Clinics Program (1984a). The Lipid Research Clinics Coronary Primary Prevention Trial results: I. Reduction in the incidence of coronary heart disease. *JAMA* **251**:351–364.

Lipid Research Clinics Program (1984b). The Lipid Research Clinics Coronary Primary Prevention Trial results: II. The relationship of reduction in incidence of coronary heart disease to cholesterol lowering. *JAMA* **251**:365–374.

Moore, R. B., Crane, C. A., and Frantz, I. D., Jr. (1986). Effect of cholestyramine on the fecal excretion of intravenously administered cholesterol-4-^{14}C and its degradation products in a hypercholesterolemic patient. *J. Clin. Invest.* **47**:1664–1671.

Peters, J. R., and Hunninghake, D. B. (1985). Effect of time of administration of cholestyramine on plasma lipids and lipoproteins. *Artery* **13**:1–6.

Puchois, P., Kandoussi, A., Fievet, P., Fourrier, J. L., Bertrand, M., Koren, E., and Fruchart, J. C. (1987). Apolipoprotein A-I containing lipoproteins in coronary artery disease. *Atherosclerosis* **68**:35–40.

Stein, E. A. (1989). Treatment of familial hypercholesterolemia with drugs in children. *Arteriosclerosis* **9**(Suppl. I):I-145–I-151.

West, R. J., and Lloyd, J. K. (1973). *Arch. Dis. Child* **48**:370–373.

Witztum, J. L., Schonfeld, G., Wiedman, S. W., Giese, W. E., and Dillingham, M. A. (1979). Bile sequestrant therapy alters the composition of low density and high density lipoproteins. *Metabolism* **28**:221–229.

6

Fibric Acid Derivatives

D. Roger Illingworth
Oregon Health Sciences University
Portland, Oregon

I. INTRODUCTION

The development of hypolipidemic drugs can be traced back to the synthesis of *p*-chlorophenoxyisobutyric acid (CPIB) by Thorp and his colleagues at ICI in 1947 (Thorp, 1962). The ester form of CPIB (clofibrate) was introduced as a hypolipidemic agent in the United Kingdom in 1962 and was approved by the FDA for prescription use in the United States in 1967. Clofibrate was the most widely prescribed hypolipidemic drug in the early 1970s, but its use has decreased progressively since 1978 (Wysowski et al., 1990). This decrease was precipitated by the results of the World Health Organization (WHO) co-operative trial of clofibrate, published in 1978 (Committee of Principal Investigators, 1978), which demonstrated that despite a 9% reduction in blood cholesterol levels (compared to placebo), the sum of all cardiovascular events including cardiac mortality was not significantly reduced and that, overall, total mortality was higher in the clofibrate treated patient. This increase in total mortality was not due to any single cause, although death from cancers of the gastrointestinal tract were higher as were the number of deaths related to cholecystectomy. Although a follow-up study of the participants in the WHO trial (Committee of Principal Investigators, 1984) failed to show any persistent increase in mortality in the patients treated with clofibrate, the use of clofibrate as a hypolipidemic drug has continued to diminish (Wysowki et al., 1990).

The potential for clofibrate to cause gallstone formation in many patients (Coronary Drug Project Research Group, 1977) coupled with the inability of this drug to significantly reduce the plasma concentration of low density lipoproteins (LDL) has stimulated interest in the development of other fibric acid derivatives which display a more favorable benefit to risk ratio when used in the long-term treatment of hyperlipidemia. With the exception of gemfibrozil, a nonhalogenated phenoxypentanoic acid which is structurally distinct from clofibrate, all of the other second-generation fibrates (e.g., bezafibrate, fenofibrate, ciprofibrate, beclafibrate, etofibrate, and clinofibrate) are structurally related to clofibrate. The structures of clofibrate, bezafibrate, fenofibrate, ciprofibrate, and gemfibrozil are shown in Figure 1. Despite structural differences, gemfibrozil has been classed with other fibrates and will be discussed in this context in the present review.

Gemfibrozil was first marketed in the United States in 1982, and its use has shown a progressive increase; at the present time it is the second most widely prescribed hypolipidemic drug in this country (Wysowki et al., 1990). Gemfibrozil was utilized as the lipid-lowering drug in the Helsinki Heart Study (Frick et al., 1987; Manninen et al., 1988), a primary prevention trial in 4081 middle-aged men with primary dyslipidemia who recieved either placebo or gemfibrozil. Over the 5-year period of treatment, gemfibrozil therapy reduced plasma concentrations of total and LDL cholesterol by 10 and 11%, reduced triglycerides by 35%, and increased HDL cholesterol by 11%; these changes were associated with a 34% decrease in cardiovascular endpoints but no changes in total mortality. In contrast to the WHO trial, gemfibrozil therapy was not associated with an increased incidence of gastrointestinal malignancies, nor was there a significant increase in the number of operations for gallstones. Subgroup analysis on the basis of lipoprotein phenotypes has disclosed that the largest decrease in cardiovascular events occurred in those patients with increased plasma concentrations of very low density lipoproteins (VLDL), those with combined increases in VLDL and LDL, and in those patients whose initial HDL cholesterol concentrations were below 0.9 mM/liter (35 mg/dl) (Manninen et al., 1988).

At the present time (1990), clofibrate and gemfibrozil are the only two drugs in the fibric acid class to be approved for prescription use in the United States or Canada. Clinical trials have, however, been conducted with several

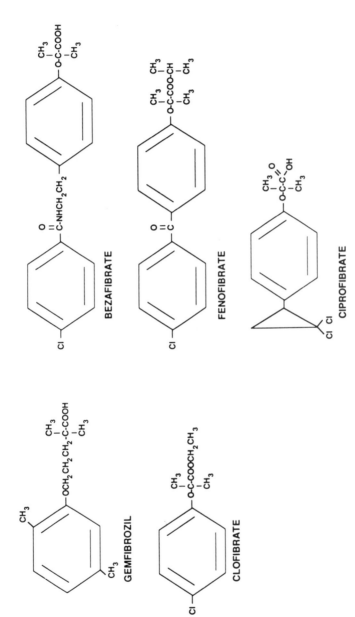

Figure 1 Chemical structures of the most widely available fibric acid derivatives.

of the second-generation fibrate drugs in North America and Europe, and it is anticipated that some of these drugs will be approved by the FDA in the foreseeable future. Although their current availability differs from country to country, fenofibrate, bezafibrate, and ciprofibrate have been approved by regulatory authorities in a number of European and Middle Eastern countries, and bezafibrate has been approved in New Zealand. Fenofibrate appears to be the most widely available of the second-generation fibrates and has been approved for prescription use in France for the last 10 years. To date, however, no primary or secondary prevention trials have utilized fenofibrate, bezafibrate, or ciprofibrate, and the potential ability of these drugs to reduce cardiovascular morbidity and mortality remains unproven.

II. CLINICAL PHARMACOLOGY OF FIBRATE DRUGS

Absorption of all of the fibrate drugs exceeds 90% following oral administration with a meal in humans but is less efficient when given without food. Peak plasma concentrations are attained 2–4 hours after administration of single doses (Monk and Todd, 1987; Todd and Ward, 1988; Balfour and Heel, 1990). In the case of clofibrate and fenofibrate, hydrolysis by tissue and plasma esterases to clofibric acid and fenofibric acid occurs rapidly, and these are the principal active metabolites in humans. As a class, the fibrate drugs are extensively protein bound, and more than 95% of the concentrations of these drugs in plasma are bound to albumin. The plasma half-lives of the fibrates, however, differ quite widely, with clofibrate having the slowest rate of elimination. Reported plasma half-lives are 13–25 hours for clofibric acid (Gugler and Hartlapp, 1978), 19–26 hours for fenofibrate (Balfour and Heel, 1990), 7.6 hours for gemfibrozil (Todd and Ward, 1988), and approximately 2 hours for bezafibrate (Monk and Todd, 1987). The extensive protein binding of fibrate drugs renders these agents virtually nondialyzable from plasma. Tissue distribution studies in animals have indicated that drug concentrations that exceed those found in plasma occur in the liver, kidney, and intestine, whereas concentrations in other tissues are below those found in plasma. Data on the placental transfer of fibrate drugs as well as their ability to be secreted into human milk is incomplete, but, on the basis of data in monkeys, gemfibrozil is transferred across the placenta (Todd and Ward, 1988); this indicates that fibrate drugs, as a class, should not be given to women during pregnancy or lactation.

The high binding affinity of fibrate drugs to serum albumin suggests that these agents may potentially displace other albumin-bound drugs, particularly warfarin. Prolongation of the prothrombin time has been observed in patients treated with clofibrate and a twofold increase in the unbound warfarin fraction has been noted in the plasma of patients receiving gemfibrozil (Todd and Ward, 1988). In the absence of data to the contrary, it is prudent to monitor prothrombin times in patients who are receiving warfarin with the recognition that the dose may have to be decreased following concurrent administration of one of the fibrate drugs. However, because the milligram amounts of drug administered are greater for clofibrate and gemfibrozil as compared to fenofibrate, bezafibrate, and ciprofibrate, this tendency to affect warfarin binding may be greater for the former two drugs than with the newer more potent second-generation fibrates (Table 1).

The fibrate drugs all undergo further metabolism and are excreted predominantly as glucuronide conjugates in the urine. The fibrate drugs and their metabolites are not lipophilic and do not, therefore, accumulate in adipose tissue during prolonged therapy. Studies in humans have indicated that 60–90% of orally administered doses of gemfibrozil, fenofibrate, clofibrate, or bezafibrate are excreted in the urine with smaller amounts being present in the feces (Monk and Todd, 1987; Todd and Ward, 1988; Balfour and Heel, 1990). Fecal excretion of fibrates is attributable to biliary excretion, and the drugs undergo some enterohepatic cycling.

Excretion of fenofibrate, bezafibrate, and clofibrate is impaired in patients with renal insufficiency, and these drugs should be used cautiously and at a reduced dose or not used at all in patients with renal insufficiency. The potential of these drugs to accumulate in plasma is illustrated by pharmacokinetic studies after a single oral dose of fenofibrate in patients with renal failure (creatinine clearance 0–45 ccs/minute) in whom the half-life of fenofibrate was 143 hours as compared to a normal half-life of approximately 21 hours (Desager et al., 1982). Excretion of gemfibrozil may be less severely compromised in patients with renal insufficiency than is seen with other fibrates, and, in one study (Evans et al., 1987), the elimination half-life and

Table 1 Recommended Dosage Schedules for Different Fibrates

Drug	Recommended dosage schedule	Total daily dose (mg)
Clofibrate	1 g B. I. D.	2000
Gemfibrozil	600 mg B. I. D.	1200
Bezafibrate[a]	200 mg T. I. D.	600
Fenofibrate	100 mg T. I. D.	300
Ciprofibrate	100–200 mg Q. D.	100–200

[a]A 400-mg sustained release preparation has also been developed for once daily therapy.

clearance of gemfibrozil was not impaired in a group of older patients with renal insufficiency. In contrast, however, plasma concentrations of gemfibrozil metabolites were three to four times higher in anephric patients than in control subjects (Todd and Ward, 1988). More data on the use of gemfibrozil in patients with renal insufficiency is needed. Gemfibrozil may, however, be the preferred fibrate for use in selected patients with renal insufficiency in whom drugs of this class are therapeutically indicated, but, in the opinion of the author, this drug should be used at lower than normal doses and with careful clinical and biochemical monitoring.

Although data on the pharmacokinetics of fibrate drugs in patients with cholestasis is unavailable, this class of drugs has no role in the therapy of hyperlipidemia in patients with hepatic dysfunction.

III. TOXICOLOGY OF FIBRATES

All of the fibrate drugs have been shown to cause hepatomegaly and peroxisome proliferation in rodents, particularly the male rat (Blane, 1987). Hepatic adenomas and hepatocellular carcinomas also develop in rodents given doses of fibrates that are at least 12-fold higher than the recommended therapeutic human doses. Proliferation of peroxisomes has not been seen in dogs or monkeys treated with gemfibrozil (Todd and Ward, 1988), nor have similar changes been observed in liver biopsy studies in human patients treated with clofibrate, fenofibrate, or gemfibrozil (Blane, 1987). Preclinical studies have failed to demonstrate any teratogenic effects of the fibrate drugs in animals, although an embryotoxic effect of fenofibrate was noted at very high doses (360 mg/kg). As discussed previously, the benefit to risk ratio does not normally justify the use of fibrate drugs during pregnancy or lactation in humans.

IV. THE INFLUENCE OF FIBRATES ON LIPID METABOLISM

The influence of fibrate drugs on plasma concentrations of lipids, lipoproteins, and apoproteins has been extensively examined in normal human volunteers and patients with hyperlipidemia, but the precise cellular mechanism(s) responsible for the observed changes have not been fully clarified, particularly at the molecular level. Fibrates have the potential to influence plasma concentrations of all lipoprotein particles, but the effects vary with the different fibrate drugs and are also dependent upon the lipoprotein phenotype and genotype of the patient being treated. In general, however, the predominant influence of fibrate drugs is to reduce the plasma concentrations of triglyceride-rich lipoproteins and, in patients without hypertriglyceridemia, the concentrations of LDL cholesteral and to increase plasma concentrations of HDL cholesterol. What cellular changes in lipid metabolism are responsible for these changes in lipoproteins?

Decreases in the plasma concentrations of triglyceride-rich lipoproteins could result from a reduction in hepatic synthesis, an increased rate of triglyceride hydrolysis in plasma, or by a combination of both of these effects. Clofibrate has been shown to reduce fasting concentrations of free fatty acids in humans and reduces the rate of their release from adipose tissue in response to stimulation with epinephrine (Rifkind, 1966; Kissebah et al., 1974). Hepatic triglyceride synthesis is known to be influenced by the availability of free fatty acids and, in the absence of compensatory increases in hepatic synthesis of fatty acids, these effects would be expected to reduce hepatic triglyceride production. In addition, fibrates appear to reduce the de novo synthesis of fatty acids in the liver by inhibition of acetyl CoA carboxylase, the rate-limiting enzyme in fatty acid synthesis (Kritchevsky et al., 1979). In addition to reducing the availability of free fatty acids for triglyceride synthesis, fibrates also have been reported to increase mitochondrial and peroxisomal fatty acid oxidation (Kloer, 1987). Gemfibrozil and bezafibrate have both been shown to reduce hepatic triglyceride synthesis from radiolabeled oleic acid or glycerol (Kloer, 1987; Todd and Ward, 1988) and, in a rat model of triton-induced hypertriglyceridemia, fenofibrate suppresses the accumulation of triglyceride-rich lipoproteins in plasma by about 60% (Kloer, 1987).

The rate of intravascular catabolism of triglyceride-rich lipoproteins is influenced primarily by the activity of lipoprotein lipase but is also affected by the activities of lipid transfer proteins, hepatic lipase, and by the apoprotein composition of the lipoprotein particles. Lipoprotein lipase is present on the endothelial cells of capillaries in skeletal muscle and adipose tissue, and the activity of this enzyme, particularly in muscle, is increased during therapy with fibrate drugs (Kloer, 1987; Todd and Ward, 1988; Balfour and Heel, 1990). The influence of clofibrate, fenofibrate, and bezafibrate on the activity of post-heparin lipoprotein lipase was examined by Heller and Harvengt (1983) in 10 healthy volunteers given each of these drugs for a period of 8 days. The magnitude of increase in post-heparin lipoprotein lipase activity was highest after administration of clofibrate (102% increase) as compared to an increase of 43% during therapy with bezafibrate and 39% during treatment with fenofibrate. In this study, the activity of hepatic lipase was slightly, but not significantly, increased with all three drugs, and the activity of lecithin cholesterol acyl transferase (LCAT) was increased during treatment with fenofibrate. To what extent fibrate drugs influence lipid transfer activity has not been adequately studied. Table 2 summarizes some of the known effects of fibrate drugs on triglyceride metabolism.

In addition to their influence on triglyceride metabolism, fibrates have also been reported to influence the synthesis and excretion of cholesterol. Clofibrate has been shown to reduce the activity of hepatic 3-hydroxy-3-methyl glutaryl coenzyme A (HMG CoA) reductase (Berndt et al., 1978), but, parenthetically, an increase in hepatic sterol biosynthesis has been observed in rats treated with gemfibrozil (Maxwell et al., 1983). Whether this difference is attributable to different mechanisms of action of these two drugs on cholesterol metabolism is unclear. Studies with fenofibrate have indicated that this drug reduces hepatic synthesis of cholesterol from ^{14}C-labeled acetate, whereas incorporation of [^{14}C]mevalonate into cholesterol was not reduced (Kloer, 1987). The latter results suggest that the reduction in cholesterol synthesis observed with some, but not all, fibrate drugs is due to an effect of these agents on HMG CoA reductase or a step prior to this enzyme. Under in vitro conditions, however, fenofibrate does not inhibit the activity of HMG CoA reductase (Kloer, 1987) and indicates that fenofibrate may influence the synthesis, degradation, or activation of this enzyme rather than acting as a specific competitive inhibitor. Fenofibrate has been reported to reduce the activity of HMG CoA reductase in freshly isolated mononuclear leukocytes from patients treated with this drug (Schneider et al., 1985), but, in contrast to patients treated with lovastatin (Pappu et al., 1989), concentrations of mevalonic acid in the urine are not reduced during therapy with fibrates. The ability of some fibrate drugs to decrease cholesterol synthesis may, however, provide the link between the action of these drugs on intracellular cholesterol

Table 2 The Influence of Fibrate Drugs on Triglyceride Metabolism

Reduced synthesis	Increased catabolism
Inhibition of de novo fatty acid synthesis	Increased activity of lipoprotein lipase in muscle (± adipose tissue)
Reduction of plasma free fatty acid concentrations	Increase in apoprotein CII:CIII ratio favoring an increased activation of lipoprotein lipase
Stimulation of fatty acid oxidation	Increased hepatic uptake of remnant lipoproteins (?)
Inhibition of hepatic triglyceride synthesis from oleic acid and glycerol	

homeostasis and the increased catabolism of low density lipoproteins observed in hypercholesterolemic patients treated with fenofibrate and bezafibrate (discussed below). Some of the reported effects of fibrate drugs on cholesterol metabolism are summarized in Table 3.

V. THE INFLUENCE OF FIBRATE DRUGS ON LIPOPROTEIN COMPOSITION AND METABOLISM

Analysis of the composition of lipoproteins isolated from the plasma of patients with hypertriglyceridemia demonstrates that the triglyceride content of both LDL and HDL is increased, whereas the content of free and esterified cholesterol and phospholipid is reduced (Deckelbaum et al., 1984; Eisenberg et al., 1984). These compositional changes result in decreases of up to 50% in the cholesterol content of LDL and HDL particles and may contribute to an altered metabolism of these lipoproteins. LDL particles isolated from the plasma of patients with hypertriglyceridemia have a higher density and are smaller than those seen in normal subjects. Hypertriglyceridemia also influences the relative proportions of HDL subfractions with a greater reduction in the plasma concentrations of particles isolated in the HDL2 density spectrum; these changes in concentration are associated with triglyceride enrichment in lipoproteins isolated in both the HDL2 and HDL3 density spectrums.

Several investigators have demonstrated that these abnormalities in the composition of both LDL and HDL particles are corrected following therapy with a number of fibrate drugs including bezafibrate (Eisenberg et al., 1984) and gemfibrozil (Manttari et al., 1990). In addition to changes in the lipid composition of lipoproteins, fibrate drugs may also change the apoprotein content, rendering the particles more or less susceptible to hydrolysis by

Table 3 The Influence of Fibrate Drugs on Cholesterol Metabolism

Reduced synthesis	Increased catabolism
Inhibition of cholesterol synthesis (fenofibrate, clofibrate) from isotopic precursors	Increased biliary excretion of cholesterol
Decreased activity of HMG CoA reductase in freshly isolated mononuclear leukocytes	Increase in LCAT activity in plasma
	Increased fractional catabolism of ^{125}I-LDL in hypercholesterolemic patients

lipoprotein lipase or catabolism via receptor-mediated or non–receptor-mediated pathways. Apoprotein CII has been shown to be the apoprotein that activates lipoprotein lipase activity, whereas inhibition of this enzyme has been demonstrated in the presence of increasing concentrations of apoprotein CIII (Posner et al., 1983; Wang et al., 1985). Changes in the relative proportions of these two apoproteins may therefore be one factor that modulates the rate of intravascular catabolism of chylomicron and VLDL particles. Treatment with fenofibrate has been shown to reduce plasma concentrations of apoprotein CIII to a greater extent than those of apoprotein CII and suggests that the triglyceride-rich lipoproteins present in the plasma of patients treated with this drug will be better substrates for hydrolysis by lipoprotein lipase (Franceschini et al., 1985).

From the preceding discussion it is clear that treatment with fibrate drugs markedly changes the composition of all lipoprotein particles and that such changes are likely to influence their subsequent metabolism.

The influence of fibrate drugs on the synthesis and rates of intravascular catabolism of VLDL, LDL, and HDL have been examined by several investigators in patients with primary hypertriglyceridemia as well as in patients with increased plasma concentrations of LDL cholesterol. Kissebah et al. (1976) examined VLDL synthesis from [^{14}C]palmitate in patients with hypertriglyceridemia before and after therapy with gemfibrozil. The synthetic rate for VLDL triglycerides fell by about 50% in response to gemfibrozil therapy, and these changes were accompanied by an increase in the fractional rate of catabolism of VLDL triglycerides. Parallel studies in which the apoprotein B moiety of VLDL was labeled with ^{125}I also showed a reduction in VLDL apoB production and an increase in FCR during gemfibrozil therapy (Kissebah et al., 1976). Kesaniemi and Grundy (1984) examined VLDL triglyceride kinetics in a group of hypertriglyceridemic patients during therapy with clofibrate and then again when the patients were taking gemfibrozil. In agreement with the results of Kessebah et al. (1976), gemfibrozil therapy was associated with a decrease in the synthesis of VLDL triglycerides and an increased rate of VLDL catabolism. In contrast, therapy with clofibrate did not significantly reduce the rate of synthesis of VLDL triglycerides, but such treatment was associated with an increase in the rate of catabolism of VLDL particles. These results indicate that gemfibrozil may have a more potent effect in reducing triglyceride synthesis than does clofibrate but that both drugs enhance the rate of catabolism of triglyceride-rich lipoproteins. Shepherd et al. (1984) observed a threefold increase in the fractional catabolic rate for VLDL apoprotein B in six patients with hypertriglyceridemia during treatment with bezafibrate. Despite a 60% decrease in the plasma concentrations of VLDL and apoprotein B, the rate of synthesis of this apoprotein was not significantly reduced (although it was lower in four of the six patients when they were being treated with bezafibrate). In a more extensive investigation Packard et al. (1986) studied the kinetics of ^{125}I-labled VLDL apoprotein B in patients with type III hyperlipidemia on diet only and then after subsequent treatment with bezafibrate. In agreement with previous studies, an increased rate of VLDL catabolism was again demonstrated, but, in contrast to their earlier work (Shepherd et al., 1984), bezafibrate therapy was also associated with a reduction in the synthesis of VLDL apoprotein B. Table 4 summarizes the influence of fibrate drugs on VLDL metabolism in humans.

Fibrate drugs consistently reduce the plasma concentrations of VLDL, but their effects on both the concentration and metabolism of LDL are strongly influenced by the lipoprotein phenotype and potentially the genotypic etiology of hypercholesterolemia in a given patient. In patients with hypertriglyceridemia and concurrent low or normal concentrations of LDL, the usual response to fibrate therapy is a reduction in VLDL concentrations which is most frequently paralleled by an increase in the concentrations of LDL cholesterol and apoprotein B and, less frequently, by no change or a slight decrease. The response in patients with combined elevations of VLDL and LDL is again heterogeneous, and the uniform decrease in VLDL concentrations is sometimes accompanied by a paradoxical increase in LDL, whereas in other patients LDL concentrations remain stable or decrease. The ability to reduce LDL concentrations in this patient population is most frequently seen in patients treated with more potent second-generation fibrates (e.g., fenofibrate, bezafibrate, and ciprofibrate) as compared to gemfibrozil.

Table 4 The Influence of Fibrates on Very Low Density Lipoprotein Metabolism

Drug	VLDL synthesis	VLDL-FCR	Ref.
Gemfibrozil	↓ Synthesis VLDL TG	↑	Kissebah et al., 1976
Clofibrate	No change VLDL TG	↑	Kesaniemi and Grundy, 1984
Gemfibrozil	↓ VLDL TG	↑	Kesaniemi and Grundy, 1984
Bezafibrate	Nonsignificant decrease in VLDL apoB	↑	Shepherd et al., 1984
Bezafibrate	↓ Synthesis in VLDL apoB (type III hyperlipidemia)	↑	Packard et al., 1986

In patients with primary hypercholesterolemia, in whom triglyceride concentrations are normal, fibrate therapy results in a small decrease in triglycerides, which is usually paralleled by a decrease in the concentrations of LDL cholesterol and apoprotein B. As will be discussed later, the individual fibrates differ in their relative potency to lower LDL concentrations in these patient populations.

Studies on the rates of synthesis and catabolism of low density lipoproteins in patients with different lipoprotein phenotypes have sought to explain the heterogeneous response in LDL concentrations seen during treatment with fibrates. Such studies have provided evidence that the metabolism of LDL in response to fibrate therapy in patients with preexistent hypertriglyceridemia is different from that seen in patients with primary hypercholesterolemia who do not concurrently have hypertriglyceridemia. Kinetic studies of ^{125}I-LDL metabolism in patients with hypertriglyceridemia studied before and after treatment with either gemfibrozil (Vega and Grundy, 1985) or fenofibrate (Shepherd et al., 1985) had demonstrated that the FCR for LDL is high in patients with hypertriglyceridemia and that this is reduced in response to fibrate therapy. In contrast, the rate of synthesis of LDL apoprotein B in these patients either decreased moderately during gemfibrozil therapy (Vega and Grundy, 1985) or remained unchanged in response to treatment with fenofibrate (Shepherd et al., 1985). These kinetic studies indicate that the rise in LDL that commonly occurs in response to fibrate therapy is not due to an increase in LDL production but rather results from a decrease in the rate of LDL catabolism. These results are also consistent with the view that the increased catabolism of VLDL in response to fibrate therapy results in an increase hepatic uptake of VLDL particles, an enhanced delivery of cholesterol to the liver, and a downregulation of hepatic LDL receptors.

Studies on the metabolism of LDL in patients with primary hypercholesterolemia, in whom LDL concentrations decrease to a variable degree in response to fibrate therapy, have indicated that this decrease results primarily from an increased rate of receptor-mediated LDL catabolism. An increased FCR for ^{125}I-LDL has been consistently observed in patients with heterozygous familial hypercholesterolemia treated with either fenofibrate (Malmendier and Delecroix, 1985) or bezafibrate (Stewart et al., 1982); in both of these studies the calculated rates of LDL apoprotein B synthesis increased during fibrate therapy. These results are consistent with the view that therapy with fibrate drugs in patients with primary hypercholesterolemia reduces the intracellular pool of cholesterol in hepatocytes, which in turn triggers an increased expression of high affinity LDL receptors on liver cell membranes and leads to an enhanced rate of catabolism of LDL particles from plasma. To what extent changes in LDL composition, with resultant changes in the surface expression of the receptor binding domain of apoprotein B, may influence the observed changes in LDL catabolism is unclear.

Decreases in the plasma concentration of triglyceride-rich lipoproteins that occur in patients with hypertriglyceridemia during therapy with fibrate drugs are commonly accompanied by an increase in the concentrations of both HDL cholesterol and apoproteins AI and AII. These changes appear to be due to an increase in the rate of synthesis of apoprotein AI and AII rather than reduced rates of catabolism (Malmendier and Delecroix, 1985; Saku et al., 1985).

VI. THE HYPOLIPIDEMIC EFFECTS OF FIBRATE DRUGS

A. Effects in Patients with Primary Hypercholesterolemia

The hypolipidemic effects of fibrate drugs in patients with primary hypercholesterolemia have been evaluated in a number of controlled clinical trials in which active drug therapy has been compared to either placebo or another hypolipidemic drug. These studies have indicated that the different fibrate drugs vary in their ability to reduce plasma concentrations of LDL cholesterol and apoprotein B and that, in general, the second-generation fibrate drugs exert a greater LDL-lowering effect than occurs with clofibrate or gemfibrozil. Table 5 summarizes representative studies on the comparative efficacy of different fibrate drugs to decrease LDL cholesterol concentrations in patients with heterozygous familial hypercholesterolemia.

The ability of fibrates to reduce LDL cholesterol concentrations appears to be similar in patients with heterozygous familial hypercholesterolemia as compared to patients with less well-characterized causes of primary hypercholesterolemia (Brown, 1989; Balfour and Heal, 1990). In contrast to their different efficacies in reducing concentrations of LDL cholesterol in patients with primary hypercholesterolemia, the different fibrate drugs exert similar effects on the concentrations of plasma triglycerides and HDL cholesterol. In patients with initial triglyceride concentrations below 1.7 mM/liter (150 mg/dl) decreases of 24, 30, 31, 32, and 42% have been observed during treatment with clofibrate, ciprofibrate, fenofibrate, bezafibrate, and gemfibrozil, respectively (Hunninghake and Meinertz, 1987; Peters, 1986). In this same population, increases in the plasma concentrations of HDL cholesterol of 1, 6, 14, 15, and 7%, respectively, were observed during treatment with clofibrate, fenofibrate, ciprofibrate, bezafibrate, and gemfibrozil (Hunninghake and Meinertz, 1987; Peters, 1986). In those studies where apoproteins have been measured, decreases in LDL cholesterol concentrations have been

Table 5 Comparative Efficacy of Fibric Acid Derivatives in Decreasing LDL Cholesterol Concentrations in Patients with Heterozygous Familial Hypercholesterolemia

Drug	Dose (g/day)	Initial LDL cholesterol (mM/L)[a]	No. of patients studied	% Decrease in LDL cholesterol	Ref.
Clofibrate	2	7.4	10	4.6	Levy et al., 1972
Gemfibrozil	1.2	8.0	9	9.6	Meinertz, 1986
Bezafibrate	0.6	8.1	12	28	Eisenberg et al., 1987
Bezafibrate	0.6	6.8	18	18.3	Curtis et al., 1988
Ciprofibrate	0.1	7.6	10	24	Illingworth et al., 1982
Ciprofibrate	0.1	8.7	20	19.5	Rouffy et al., 1985
Ciprofibrate	0.2	8.7	20	27	Rouffy et al., 1985
Fenofibrate	0.3	8.0	9	24	Weisweiler et al., 1985
Fenofibrate	0.3	8.0	21	25	Rouffy et al., 1985
Fenofibrate	0.4	8.0	21	31	Rouffy et al., 1985

[a]To convert mM/liter cholesterol to mg/dl, multiply by 38.6.

paralleled by smaller reductions in the concentrations of apoprotein B, by a decrease in apoprotein E, and by increases in apoprotein AI and AII (Goldberg et al., 1987; Balfour and Heel, 1990).

B. Effects of Fibrates in Patients with Combined Hyperlipidemia

The influence of fibrate drugs on the concentrations of plasma lipoproteins in patients with combined hyperlipidemia in which concentrations of VLDL and LDL are increased (phenotypic type IIB hyperlipidemia) is variable, but the ability of these drugs to reduce LDL concentrations is less than that seen in patients with primary hypercholesterolemia in whom triglyceride concentrations are normal. All of the fibrate drugs are effective in reducing triglyceride concentrations in patients with combined hyperlipidemia and the magnitude of increase in HDL is usually greater than that seen in patients with primary hypercholesterolemia. Table 6 summarizes representative studies in which the influence of gemfibrozil, clofibrate, fenofibrate, bezafibrate, and ciprofibrate on plasma lipid and lipoprotein concentrations have been examined in patients with combined hyperlipidemia. In these studies, plasma concentrations of LDL cholesterol were greater than 5 mMol/liter, and during fibrate therapy these either did not change in response to gemfibrozil or clofibrate or decreased during treatment with fenofibrate, bezafibrate, or ciprofibrate. However, even with the more potent second-generation fibrate drugs, the magnitude of response in LDL cholesterol in individual patients with combined hyperlipidemia varies widely; in eight patients studied by Eisenberg et al. (in whom the mean concentration of LDL cholesterol decreased by 23.4%), the individual response varied between a 2.4% increase and a 62.4% decrease. Shepherd and Packard (1986) have proposed that LDL cholesterol concentrations are most likely to rise in those patients with hypertriglyceridemia in whom LDL cholesterol concentrations are initially below 3.9 mM/liter (150 mg/dl).

The ability of fibrate drugs to accelerate the catabolism of VLDL particles in plasma suggests that these drugs should be extremely effective in the therapy of patients with type III hyperlipidemia in whom VLDL and chylomicron remnant particles accumulate in plasma (Mahley and Angelin, 1984). Although uncommon, patients with type III hyperlipidemia are at substantially increased risk for the premature development of both coronary and peripheral vascular disease and frequently develop characteristic palmar and tuberous xanthomas which regress in response to effective hypolipidemic therapy. Fibrate drugs are extremely effective in the therapy of those patients with type III hyperlipidemia who remain significantly hyperlipidemic following the correction of secondary factors and maximal dietary therapy. Table 7 summarizes changes in lipid and lipoprotein concentrations from studies in which patients with type III hyperlipidemia have been treated with gemfibrozil (Houlston et al., 1988), clofibrate (Illingworth and O'Malley, 1990), bezafibrate (Klosiewicz-Latoszek et al., 1987), and fenofibrate (Fruchart et al., 1987). All of the drugs substantially reduced plasma concentrations of cholesterol and triglyceride and, when measured, dramatically reduced the concentrations of VLDL-remnant particles. In contrast to the greater efficacy of the second-generation fibrates (bezafibrate, fenofibrate, and ciprofibrate) as compared to clofibrate and gemfibrozil to reduce concentrations of LDL

Table 6 Influence of Different Fibrate Drugs on Lipid and Lipoprotein Concentrations in Patients with Combined Hyperlipidemia

	Gemfibrozil[a] (1200 mg/day)	Clofibrate[b] (2000 mg/day)	Fenofibrate[b] (300–400 mg/day)	Bezafibrate[b] (400–600 mg/day)	Ciprofibrate[b] (100–200 mg/day)
Initial lipid conc. (mM/liter)					
Plasma cholesterol	8.43	7.80	8.44	8.47	8.67
Plasma triglycerides	3.31	3.05	3.17	3.40	3.00
LDL cholesterol	5.92	5.18	5.62	5.67	6.30
HDL cholesterol	0.98	1.04	1.19	1.24	1.35
Percent change with therapy					
Total cholesterol	−11	−10	−21	−19	−19
LDL cholesterol	−3	−4	−20	−17	−21
HDL cholesterol	+26	+18	+10	+10	−2
Triglycerides	−54	−37	−46	−48	−37

[a]From East et al., 1988.
[b]Adapted from Hunninghake and Peters, 1987.

Table 7   Hypolipidemic Effects of Fibrate Drugs in Patients with Type III Hyperlipidemia

	Gemfibrozil[a] (n = 13)	Clofibrate[b] (n = 12)	Bezafibrate[c] (n = 9)	Fenofibrate[d] (n = 9)
Initial lipid conc. (mM/liter)				
Plasma cholesterol	12.6	13.0	8.5	9.3
Plasma triglycerides	10.2	8.9	5.2	5.5
VLDL cholesterol	NR	7.8	NR	NR
LDL cholesterol	NR	3.6	3.5	3.1
HDL cholesterol	1.1	0.91	0.97	0.83
Percent change with therapy				
Total cholesterol	−40	−40	−20	−38
VLDL cholesterol	NR	−61	NR	NR
LDL cholesterol	NR	−0.7	+19	−7
HDL cholesterol	+45	+31	−2	+25
Triglycerides	−70	−52	−50	−56

NR, not reported; *n*, number of patients.
[a]From Houlston et al., 1988.
[b]From Illingworth and O'Malley, 1990.
[c]From Klosiewicz-Latoszek et al., 1987.
[d]From Fruchart et al., 1987.

cholesterol in patients with combined hyperlipidemia, all of the fibrate drugs (with the possible exception of bezafibrate) appear to be equally effective in the treatment of patients with type III hyperlipidemia. At the present time, no studies directly comparing different fibrate drugs in the treatment of patients with type III hyperlipidemia have been reported, but in the opinion of the author clofibrate remains a first choice drug.

In addition to substantially reducing plasma concentrations of cholesterol and triglyceride, Fruchart et al., (1987) reported substantial changes in apoprotein concentrations in nine patients with type III hyperlipidemia during treatment with fenofibrate. Plasma concentrations of apoproteins AI and AII rose by 11 and 15%, respectively, whereas concentrations of apoproteins B, CII, CIII, and E fell by 31, 21, 48, and 62%, respectively. Among individual lipoprotein particles, the greatest change occurred in those containing apoprotein E and B and is consistent with a decrease in the absolute number of VLDL remnant particles in plasma in response to fenofibrate therapy.

C. The Effects of Fibrates in Moderate Hypertriglyceridemia

Treatment of patients with moderate hypertriglyceridemia (plasma triglycerides 3.4–11.3 mM/liter [300–1000 mg/dl] in which plasma concentrations of VLDL are increased but in which chylomicronemia is not present with lipid-lowering drugs remains controversial but is most appropriate in patients with familial combined hyperlipidemia, patients with early onset atherosclerosis, and diabetics. Patients with moderate hypertriglyceridemia frequently have low levels of HDL cholesterol, and therapy aimed at reducing VLDL levels usually results in a corresponding increase in the levels of HDL cholesterol. The Helsinki Heart Trial included patients with primary hypercholesterolemia (phenotypic type IIA), combined hyperlipidemia (phenotypic type IIB), and moderate hypertriglyceridemia (type IV phenotype), and in these patients treatment with gemfibrozil was associated with the largest decrease in cardiovascular morbidity and mortality in those patients with the type IIB and type IV phenotypes (Manninen et al. 1988).

For selected adult patients who remain hypertriglyceridemic despite maximal dietary therapy and appropriate correction of potentially exacerbating secondary factors and in whom the decision to use lipid-lowering drugs is made, fibrates represent an appropriate alternative to nicotinic acid. Fibrates may be particularly useful in patients with mild hyperglycemia or hyperuricemia in whom these metabolic abnormalities would be exacerbated by therapy with nicotinic acid. As previously discussed, abnormalities in the composition of LDL and HDL are invariably present in patients with hypertriglyceridemia, and reduction in the concentrations of VLDL particles is associated with a correction of the triglyceride-enrichment of both LDL and HDL (Manttari et al. 1990). Results from representative studies in which the effects of clofibrate, gemfibrozil, fenofibrate, bezafibrate, and ciprofibrate on plasma lipid and lipoprotein concentrations have been examined in patients with moderate hypertriglyceridemia are presented in Table 8. All of the drugs reduce the concentrations of plasma triglycerides and increase the concentrations of HDL cholesterol but also result in increases in the plasma concentrations of LDL cholesterol. In some patients this rise may be of sufficient magnitude to warrant addition of a second drug, whose primary role is to reduce plasma concentrations of LDL cholesterol (East et al., 1988).

D. The Effects of Fibrates in Patients with Severe Hypertriglyceridemia

The goals of lipid-lowering therapy in patients with severe hypertriglyceridemia (plasma triglycerides > 11.3 mM/liter [1000 mg/dl]) associated with

Table 8 Influence of Fibrate Drugs on Plasma Lipids and Lipoproteins in Patients with Moderate Hypertriglyceridemia (Type IV Phenotype)

	Gemfibrozil[a] ($n = 8$)	Clofibrate[b] ($n = 16$)	Fenofibrate[c] ($n = 88$)	Bezafibrate[c] ($n = 70$)	Ciprofibrate[c] ($n = 502$)
Initial lipid conc. (mM/liter)					
Plasma cholesterol	6.75	6.89	7.41	6.48	6.58
Plasma triglycerides	4.30	4.90	7.06	5.80	4.20
LDL cholesterol	3.78	3.79	3.73	3.86	4.17
HDL cholesterol	0.80	0.93	0.93	0.80	1.11
Percent change with therapy					
Total cholesterol	+7	-8	-20	-0	-10
LDL cholesterol	+29	+10	+4	+5	-14
HDL cholesterol	+26	+19	+21	+30	+12
Triglycerides	-40	-53	-59	-51	-37

n, number of patients.
[a]From East et al., 1988.
[b]Rabkin et al. 1988.
[c]Adapted from Hunninghake and Peters, 1987.

combined elevations in VLDL and chylomicron particles are to reduce the sequellae of chylomicronemia (hepatosplenomegaly, abdominal pain, eruptive xanthomas, and potentially pancreatitis) and, second, to reduce the long-term risk of atherosclerosis. In the opinion of the author, drug therapy is indicated for patients in whom triglycerides remain above 11.3 mM/liter on dietary therapy and after correction of potentially exacerbating secondary factors. Gemfibrozil (Leaf et al., 1989), clofibrate (Nye et al., 1980), fenofibrate (Goldberg et al., 1989), and bezafibrate (Saku et al., 1989) have all been shown to be effective in the treatment of type V hyperlipidemia, but the comparative efficacy of these drugs in patients with severe hypertriglyceridemia has not been thoroughly evaluated. Nye et al. (1980) compared the hypolipidemic effects of clofibrate and gemfibrozil in a heterogeneous group of 33 men with varying degrees of hypertriglyceridemia and observed greater reductions in plasma triglycerides during treatment with gemfibrozil. Saku et al. (1989) treated eight patients with type V hyperlipidemia (baseline triglycerides 19.8 mM/liter [1755 mg/dl] with a slow-release preparation of bezafibrate (400 mg daily); plasma triglycerides decreased by 61% after 2 months on therapy and were 51% below baseline after 4 months. Total cholesterol concentrations fell by 19%, whereas concentrations of both LDL and HDL rose. Goldberg et al. (1989) observed a 54% decrease in total plasma triglycerides in a heterogeneous group of patients with moderate to severe hypertriglyceridemia (baseline triglycerides 5.6–16.9 mM/liter [500–1500 mg/dl] treated with 300 mg/day of fenofibrate. In a recent study from our laboratory (Leaf et al., 1989), the hypolipidemic effects of gemfibrozil were assessed in a double-blind placebo-controlled crossover trial in 13 patients with type V hyperlipidemia. Chylomicrons were eliminated from the plasma in 12 of 13 patients during treatment with gemfibrozil, and, overall, plasma triglyceride concentrations decreased by 74%. Figure 2 illustrates the changes in plasma triglycerides in the 13 individual patients who participated in this study when they were receiving either placebo or gemfibrozil. Overall gemfibrozil therapy was associated with a 99% decrease in the concentrations of chylomicron cholesterol and triglyceride, a 68% decrease in VLDL cholesterol, and a 38% increase in the concentration of HDL cholesterol. Concentration of LDL cholesterol rose from an initially low value of 1.8 mM/liter to 3.08 mM/liter, a 68% increase. In the author's opinion gemfibrozil is the fibrate of choice for patients with type V hyperlipidemia and appears to exert a greater inhibitory effect on triglyceride synthesis than is seen with the other fibrates (Table 4).

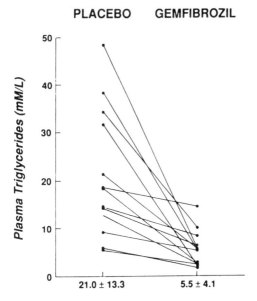

PLACEBO   GEMFIBROZIL

Figure 2 Changes in plasma triglyceride concentrations in 13 patients with type V hyperlipidemia during treatment with placebo or gemfibrozil (600 mg twice daily). (Adapted from Leaf et al., 1989).

E. The Influence of Fibrates in Patients with Hypoalphalipoproteinemia

The ability of fibrate drugs to increase plasma concentrations of HDL cholesterol and apoprotein AI and AII in patients who concurrently have hypertriglyceridemia has been well documented (Monk and Todd, 1987; Todd and Ward, 1988; Balfour and Heel, 1990). The Helsinki Heart Study demonstrated that treatment with gemfibrozil was most beneficial in decreasing cardiovascular morbidity and mortality in those patients whose initial concentrations of HDL cholesterol were less than 0.9 mM/liter (35 mg/dl) and who concurrently had hypertriglyceridemia or combined hyperlipidemia. Despite convincing evidence that low levels of HDL cholesterol, even in the absence of significant hypercholesterolemia or hypertriglyceridemia, are associated with an increased risk of premature atherosclerosis (Grundy et al., 1989), the potential benefit to be derived from pharmaceutical therapy aimed at raising plasma concentrations of HDL cholesterol in these patients is unknown.

In recent studies Vega and Grundy (1989) compared the lipid-modifying effects of gemfibrozil and lovastatin in 22 patients with hypoalphalipoprotein-emia (HDL cholesterol concentrations < 0.91 mg/dl) who had neither con-current hypercholesterolemia (total cholesterol < 5.2 mM/liter) or hypertrig-lyceridemia (plasma triglycerides < 2.2 mM/liter). Concentrations of total cholesterol and triglycerides fell from 5.12 to 4.76 mM/liter and from 2.11 to 1.33 mM/liter, respectively, on gemfibrozil, and these changes were accom-panied by a decrease in VLDL cholesterol (from 1.01 to 0.65 mM/liter) a slight but not significant decrease in LDL cholesterol (3.31 to 3.23 mM/liter), and a 9% rise in HDL cholesterol (from 0.78 mM/liter at baseline to 0.85 mM/liter on gemfibrozil). Lovastatin was more effective in reducing con-centrations of LDL cholesterol and resulted in a 12% increase in HDL cholesterol. However, with both drugs plasma concentrations of HDL cholesterol remained below 0.91 mM/liter, and neither drug significantly increased plasma concentrations of apoproteins AI or AII. The authors con-cluded that gemfibrozil is not effective in raising HDL cholesterol con-centrations in normolipidemic patients with isolated hypoalphalipoproteine-mia, and the potential benefits of treatment with fibrate drugs in this patient population are unproven.

F. The Effects of Fibrates on Lp(a)

Increased plasma concentrations of lipoprotein (a) (Lp(a)) have been shown to be a strong risk factor for the premature development of atherosclerosis, particularly in patients with concurrent hypercholesterolemia (Seed et al., 1990). Studies to examine the influence of fibrate drugs on plasma con-centrations of Lp(a) are incomplete, but, on the basis of available data, neither clofibrate (Albers et al. 1975) nor a more potent second-generation fibrate, bezafibrate (Kostner, 1988), reduces plasma concentrations of Lp(a). Further studies, particularly in patients with high levels of Lp(a) treated with fibrates, are, however, necessary before this data can be considered definitive.

G. Hypolipidemic Effects of Fibrates in Secondary Hyperlipidemia

Hyperlipidemia due to increased plasma concentrations of any of the major lipoproteins (LDL, VLDL remnants, and chylomicrons), often in association with abnormalities in HDL, may be attributable to genetic and environmental factors, secondary causes, or a combination of both. Identification and treatment of the primary abnormality responsible for secondary hyperlipidemia may result in complete reversal of the lipid abnormality (e.g., treatment of hypothyroidism), but in other cases the underlying primary cause is not amenable to correction and the secondary hyperlipidemia persists. Diet and drug therapy aimed at reducing the long-term complications of hyperlipidemia is appropriate in some patients with persistent secondary causes of hyperlipidemia, particularly those with diabetes, and potentially in patients with hyperlipidemia associated with the nephrotic syndrome, chronic renal failure, or the hyperlipidemia that frequently occurs following renal or cardiac transplantation.

Hyperlipidemia, particularly hypertriglyceridemia and concurrent low concentrations of HDL cholesterol, is commonly seen in patients with diabetes mellitus (particularly type II diabetes), and these patients are at unusually high risk for the premature development of atherosclerosis (Garg and Grundy, 1990). Available data indicates that the effects of gemfibrozil (Todd and Ward, 1988), clofibrate (Kobayashi et al., 1988), bezafibrate (Monk and Todd, 1987), and fenofibrate (Balfour and Heel, 1990) to reduce concentrations of triglyceride-rich lipoproteins and increase HDL cholesterol levels are similar in patients with diabetes as compared to nondiabetic subjects. One potential advantage of fibrate drugs when used as hypotriglyceridemic agents in diabetes is that these agents may improve glucose tolerance and may also exert a slight uricosuric effect. These effects are in contrast to nicotinic acid, which has the opposite effects on blood glucose and serum concentrations of uric acid.

Hypertriglyceridemia is commonly seen in patients with chronic renal failure and uremia, and in these patients an acquired deficiency of lipoprotein lipase appears to contribute to the lipid disorder. With the possible exception of gemfibrozil (Evans et al., 1987) renal excretion of fibrate drugs is impaired in parallel with a reduction in creatinine clearance and use of fibrate drugs in patients with uremia is associated with an increased risk of myopathy (Digiulio et al., 1977). Unless facilities to monitor drug concentrations of fibrate drugs are available, these drugs cannot be recommended for use in patients with hypertriglyceridemia who concurrently have chronic renal failure.

Severe hyperlipidemia with plasma cholesterol concentrations of between 10 and 15 mM/liter, often in association with mild hypertriglyceridemia, is commonly seen in patients with the nephrotic syndrome in whom rates of synthesis of VLDL and LDL apoprotein B are increased (Vega and Grundy, 1988). Studies in the 1970s indicated that the use of clofibrate, whose active metabolites are highly protein bound, in patients with the nephrotic syndrome was associated with an increased risk of myopathy and potentially rhabdomyolysis (Bridgeman et al., 1972), and for this reason clofibrate is contradicated in patients with hyperlipidemia and the nephrotic syndrome or in patients with secondary hyperlipidemia associated with hypoalbuminemia (e.g., a protein-losing enteropathy). In the absence of data to the contrary, the use of second-generation fibrate drugs (e.g., bezafibrate or fenofibrate) in patients with hyperlipidemia and nephrosis should be regarded as investigational and use of these agents cannot be recommended. In a recent report Groggel et al. (1989) evaluated the efficacy of gemfibrozil (600 mg twice daily) in 11 adult patients with the nephrotic syndrome, all of whom had serum creatinine concentrations of below 3 mg/dl. When compared to placebo, treatment therapy with gemfibrozil lowered total cholesterol concentrations from 9.64 to 8.19 mM/liter (-15.1%) and triglycerides from 3.48 to 1.72 mM/liter (-50.7%). Concentrations of LDL cholesterol decreased 12.5%, and HDL cholesterol levels rose 17.8%. However, despite the ability of gemfibrozil to lower concentrations of total and LDL cholesterol in these patients, mean LDL cholesterol concentrations on therapy with gemfibrozil remained elevated (6.17 mM/liter). The authors concluded that monotherapy with gemfibrozil was inadequate for optimal control of hyperlipidemia in this patient population but in a subset of patients observed additional lipid lowering when gemfibrozil was combined with colestipol. No drug-related side effects were observed in this study, and renal function remained stable. Although gemfibrozil may be useful in the therapy of selected patients with the nephrotic syndrome in whom hypertriglyceridemia is the predominant lipid abnormality, lovastatin (Vega and Grundy, 1988; Golper et al., 1989) or simvastatin (Rabelink et al., 1988) both appear to be more effective in reducing LDL cholesterol concentrations in this patient population.

VII. THE USE OF FIBRATES IN CHILDREN WITH HYPERLIPIDEMIA

Limited data is available concerning the efficacy of fibrate drugs in the therapy of hyperlipidemia in children, and no data concerning their long term safety in this population is available. Steinmetz et al. (1981) treated 17 hypercholesterolemic children with fenofibrate at a dose of 5 mg/kg per day for a period of 3 months and observed decreases of 22 and 39%, respectively, in the plasma concentrations of cholesterol and triglyceride. In a double-blind placebo-controlled crossover study, Wheeler et al. (1985) evaluated the hypolipidemic effects of bezafibrate (10–20 mg/kg/day) in 14 children aged 4–15 with heterozygous familial hypercholesterolemia who received active drug for a period of 3 months. Treatment with bezafibrate was well tolerated and reduced total plasma cholesterol and triglyceride concentrations by 16 and

33%, respectively. In the opinion of the author the benefit-to-risk ratio does not justify the use of fibrate drugs in the treatment of children with heterozygous familial hypercholesterolemia, and their use should be restricted to the rare pediatric patient with severe hypertriglyceridemia or type III hyperlipidemia (Lindner and Illingworth, 1988) in whom the benefit from therapy is felt to outweigh concerns over unproven long-term safety.

VIII. FIBRATES IN COMBINATION DRUG THERAPY FOR HYPERLIPIDEMIA

The potential usefulness of fibrates in combination therapy with other hypolipidemic drugs has been evaluated in a number of studies in patients with primary hypercholesterolemia or combined hyperlipidemia. Although combination therapy with a second-generation fibrate and a bile acid seques-trant may be useful in patients with heterozygous familial hypercholesterol-emia (Curtis et al., 1988), combinations involving fibrates and an inhibitor of HMG CoA reductase do not seem to be efficacious in this patient population (Illingworth and Bacon, 1989). Fibrates may have their greatest potential in combination therapy for patients with combined hyperlipidemia (East et al., 1988; Illingworth and O'Malley, 1990) but some combinations (e.g., lovasta-tin and gemfibrozil) are associated with an increased risk of side effects including myopathy. A more detailed discussion of combination drug therapy is presented elsewhere in this book (Hoeg).

IX. THE INFLUENCE OF FIBRATES ON PLATELET FUNCTION AND BLOOD COAGULATION

Abnormalities in platelet function, particularly increased platelet aggregation, and increased concentrations of fibrinogen and Factor VII may all contribute to an enhanced risk of atherosclerosis in humans. The influence of fibrate drugs on platelet aggregation in response to ADP, epinephrine, and colla-gen have been examined by several investigators (Monk and Todd, 1987; Todd and Ward, 1988; Balfour and Heel, 1990), and most, but not all, studies indicate that treatment with clofibrate, gemfibrozil, fenofibrate, and bezafibrate is associated with a reduction in platelet reactivity and aggre-gability.

   Treatment with clofibrate (O'Brien et al., 1978) and bezafibrate (Monk and Todd, 1988) have both been reported to reduce plasma concentrations of fibrinogen by up to 33%, in contrast, treatment with gemfibrozil resulted in either no change or a slight increase (Todd and Ward, 1988). Whether these differences are attributable to different effects of these drugs on fibrinogen concentrations or are attributable to variations in the patient population or the assay methods is unclear. Plasma concentrations of Factor VII are increased in patients with hypertriglyceridemia (Nordoy et al., 1990) and fall during effective hypotriglyceridemic therapy. To what extent changes in platelet function and blood coagulation in the Helsinki Heart Trial may have contributed to the decrease in cardiovascular morbidity and mortality observed in this study is not known, but, based on data from other studies, fibrates appear to induce potentially beneficial changes in platelet function and coagulation parameters.

X. THE INFLUENCE OF FIBRATE DRUGS ON BILIARY LITHOGENICITY

Clofibrate has been shown to increase biliary lithogenicity by increasing biliary cholesterol secretion and concurrently reducing bile acid excretion (Grundy et al., 1972); these changes have been associated with an increased incidence of gallstones during long-term therapy with clofibrate (Coronary Drug Project, 1977; Committee of Principal Investigators, 1978). Subsequent studies have indicated that the propensity to increase biliary lithogenicity occurs in hyperlipidemic patients treated with gemfibrozil, bezafibrate, fenofibrate, and ciprofibrate and appears to be a class effect which occurs with all fibrate drugs (Palmer, 1987). Despite the ability of fibrates to increase biliary lithogenicity, a statistically significant increase in cholecystectomies was not observed in the Helsinki Heart Study (Frick et al., 1987) in which patients received gemfibrozil or placebo for a treatment period of 5 years. Fibrate drugs should be used cautiously, if at all, in patients with preexistent gallstones in whom the increase in biliary lithogenicity may lead to more rapid stone formation, but in patients without preexistent biliary tract disease, the risk of developing gallstones is too low to contraindicate fibrate therapy in a patient in whom this class of drugs has an appropriate clinical indication.

XI. CLINICAL SIDE EFFECTS OF FIBRATE DRUGS

On the basis of placebo-controlled trials as well as long-term clinical use of fibrate drugs, clinically significant side effects appear to occur in 5–10% of treated patients but in the majority of cases are not of sufficient severity to warrant discontinuation of the drug (Monk and Todd, 1987; Todd and Ward, 1988; Balfour and Heel, 1990). Gastrointestinal side effects are the most common and occur in up to 5% of patients treated with fibrate drugs. Although direct comparisons of the frequency of side effects in the same

Table 9 Clinical Side Effects of Fibrates

Gastrointestinal: abdominal pain, nausea, eructation, flatulence, diarrhea, vomiting, gallstones.[a]
Integumentary: rash, urticaria, pruritus, hair loss, dermatitis, increased sweating.
Musculoskeletal: myalgias, fatigue.
Central nervous system: headache, impotence, insomnia, dizzyness, parasthesias, blurred vision.
Cardiovascular: chest pain, atrial and ventricular arrhythmias.[a]

[a]Documented only for clofibrate.

patients have not been conducted, the incidence of gastrointestinal side effects may be more common in patients treated with gemfibrozil as compared to clofibrate (Todd and Ward, 1988). Table 9 lists reported clinical side effects of fibric acid derivatives; with the exception of gastrointestinal side effects, the frequency of other reported adverse effects appears to be less than 1–2% and, in some studies, is similar to that seen in patients receiving placebo (Todd and Ward, 1988).

XII. THE EFFECTS OF FIBRATES ON CLINICAL LABORATORY VALUES

A number of biochemical changes have been reported in patients treated with fibrate drugs, but in patients with normal renal function who are receiving these drugs as monotherapy, the incidence of clinically significant biochemical side effects is low. Fibrates reduce serum concentrations of alkaline phosphatase and gamma glutamyl transferase (Monk and Todd, 1987; Blane, 1987; Todd and Ward, 1988). Minor increases in creatine kinase and in aminotransferases may also be observed, and some authors have reported slight decreases in the serum concentrations of uric acid and glucose. Table 10

Table 10 Reported Biochemical Changes During Therapy with Fibrates

↑ Aminotransferases, creatine kinase
↑ Urea, creatinine
Small ↓ in glucose, uric acid
↓ Alkaline phosphatase, gamma glutamyl transferase, bilirubin
↓ Hemoglobin, hematocrit, leukopenia
↓ Fibrinogen, ↓ platelet aggregation

summarizes reported biochemical changes observed during the treatment of adult patients with hyperlipidemia with fibrate drugs. Comparative studies to assess the frequency of these biochemical changes in patients treated with different fibrates have not been conducted, but based on published reports, these changes may be seen during treatment with any of the fibrate drugs in patients with normal renal function.

XIII. POTENTIAL DRUG INTERACTIONS WITH FIBRIC ACID DERIVATIVES

Fibrate drugs, particularly clofibrate and bezafibrate, may potentiate the action of warfarin anticoagulants, and close monitoring of the prothrombin time is advisable in patients treated with this anticoagulant during the initial months of treatment with fibrate drugs. Potential drug interactions between fibrates and bile acid sequestrants when administered concurrently have not been adequately examined, but in one study a 50% reduction in the absorption of bezafibrate was observed when this drug was taken at the same time as cholestyramine (Monk and Todd, 1987).

Several reports have indicated that the risk of myopathy is increased in patients with hyperlipidemia treated with the combination of lovastatin and gemfibrozil (Tobert, 1988; Illingworth and Bacon, 1989). This interaction may occur in up to 5% of the patients treated with this combination and has the potential to lead to rhabdomyolysis and acute renal failure. The risk appears to be greater in patients treated with higher doses of lovastatin and indicates that, despite the appeal of this combination for use in patients with combined hyperlipidemia (Garg and Grundy, 1989), gemfibrozil and lovastatin should only be used with extreme caution in highly selected patients; if used at all, careful clinical and biochemical monitoring of the patient is essential. At the present time, it is uncertain whether or not the risk of myopathy is increased during combination drug therapy with other fibrates and lovastatin or during combination therapy with fibrates and more hydrophilic HMG CoA reductase inhibitors such as pravastatin.

XIV. CONCLUSIONS

As a class, fibric acid derivatives represent an important group of drugs for the treatment of patients with hyperlipidemia. When used in the therapy of primary hypercholesterolemia the second-generation fibrate drugs (fenofibrate, bezafibrate, and ciprofibrate) are more effective than gemfibrozil or clofibrate, and, if available, the former three drugs could be used as potential first-choice agents in adult patients with singular elevations in the plasma concentrations of LDL cholesterol. The greatest potential usefulness of fibrate drugs, however, is in the treatment of patients with hypertriglyceridemia, and these agents, together with nicotinic acid, are the most effective drugs for reducing plasma concentrations of VLDL cholesterol. Fibrates are particularly effective in the therapy of patients with type III hyperlipidemia. The magnitude of change in LDL cholesterol in patients with combined hyperlipidemia is unpredictable, and in some patients decreases in VLDL concentrations are accompanied by a smaller reduction in LDL concentrations, whereas in other patients the concentrations of LDL may actually increase. Combined drug therapy with fibrates and bile acid sequestrants or potentially HMG CoA reductase inhibitors may be particularly effective in the treatment of this patient population, although the latter combination should be used very cautiously and with careful clinical and biochemical monitoring.

In the opinion of the author, fibrate drugs, particularly gemfibrozil, are the agents of choice for most adult patients with severe hypertriglyceridemia, many of whom have potential contraindications to the use of nicotinic acid. In addition to exerting favorable effects on the concentrations of triglyceride-rich lipoproteins, fibrates invariably increase the concentrations of HDL cholesterol in patients with preexistent hypertriglyceridemia, and in this patient population, use of gemfibrozil has been associated with a reduction in cardiovascular morbidity and mortality. Fibrates may also favorably influence platelet function and reduce the concentrations of fibrinogen and Factor VII; these changes may potentially also contribute to the antiatherogenic effects of these drugs.

Fibrates are not without side effects, and their use requires appropriate clinical and biochemical monitoring for efficacy and safety. The drugs should be used with caution in patients with impaired renal or hepatic function, in patients with hypoalbuminemia, or in patients with metabolic myopathies. As a class fibrates increase biliary lithogenicity and should be regarded as relatively contraindicated in patients with gallbladder disease or a strong family history of cholelithiasis.

The decision to begin treatment with a fibrate drug in a patient with hyperlipidemia should be made only after appropriate exclusion of secondary factors and should take into consideration the lipoprotein phenotype and genotype of the patient, relative contraindications to other hypolipidemic drugs, and the potential goals of therapy. Patients should be advised to return 6–8 weeks after beginning therapy, at which time an assessment of both clinical efficacy and safety should be performed. If an inadequate response is obtained after one or two follow-up visits on fibrate therapy, the drug should be discontinued, whereas if an appropriate response occurs, the patient should be followed at periodic intervals with appropriate monitoring for clinical and biochemical safety. If used in a responsible manner, fibrate drugs have an important role in the treatment of hyperlipidemia, particularly in the prevention of the sequellae of severe hypertriglyceridemia, and potentially in the prevention of atherosclerosis.

ACKNOWLEDGMENTS

This work was supported in part by National Institutes of Health Research Grants #HL28399, #HL37940, by the General Clinical Research Center's Program (RR334), and by the Clinical Nutrition Research Unit (P30 DK 40566).

REFERENCES

Albers, J. J., Cabana, V. G., Warnick, G. R., and Hazzard, W. R. (1975). Lp(a) lipoprotein: Relationship to sinking prebetalipoprotein, hyperlipoproteinemia and apolipoprotein B. *Metabolism* **24**:1047–1054.

Balfour, J. A., McTavish, D., and Heel, R. C. (1990). Fenofibrate: A review of its pharmacodynamic and pharmacokinetic properties and therapeutic use in dyslipidemia. *Drugs* **40**:260–290.

Berndt, J., Gaumert, R., and Still, J. (1978). Mode of action of lipid lowering agents clofibrate and BM15075 on cholesterol biosynthesis in rat liver. *Atherosclerosis* **30**:147–152.

Blane, G. F. (1987). Comparative toxicity and safety profile of fenofibrate and other fibric acid derivatives. *Am. J. Med.* **83**(Suppl. 5B):26–36.

Bridgeman, J. F., Rosen, S. M., and Thorp, J. M. (1972). Complications during clofibrate treatment on the nephrotic syndrome hyperlipoproteinemia. *Lancet* **2**:506–509.

Brown, W. V. (1989). Treatment of hypercholesterolemia with fenofibrate: A review. *Current Med. Res. and Opinion* **11**:321–330.

Committee of Principal Investigators. (1978). A cooperative trial in the primary prevention of the ischemic heart disease using clofibrate. *Br. Heart J.* **10**:1069–1118.

Committee of Principal Investigators. (1984). WHO cooperative trial on primary prevention of ischemic heart disease with clofibrate to lower serum cholesterol. *Lancet* **2**:600–604.

Coronary Drug Project Research Group. (1977). Gallbladder disease as a side effect of drugs influencing lipid metabolism. *N. Engl. J. Med.* **296**:1188–1190.

Curtis, L. D., Dickson, A. C., Ling, K. L. L. E., and Betteridge, J. (1988).

Combination treatment with cholestyramine and bezafibrate for heterozygous familial hypercholesterolemia. *Br. Med. J.* **297**:173–175.

Deckelbaum, R. J., Granot, E., Oschry, Y., Rose, L., and Eisenberg, S. (1984). Plasma triglyceride determines structure composition in low and high density lipoproteins. *Ateriosclerosis* **4**:225–232.

Desager, J. P., Costermans, J., Verberckmoes, R., and Harvengt, C. (1982). Effect of human dialysis on plasma kinetics of fenofibrate in chronic renal failure. *Nephron* **31**:51–54.

Digiulio, S., Boulu, R., Drueke, T., Nicolai, A., Zingraff, J., and Crosnier, J. (1977). Clofibrate treatment of hyperlipidemia in chronic renal failure. *Clin. Nephrol.* **8**:504–509.

East, C., Bilheimer, D. W., and Grundy, S. M. (1988). Combination drug therapy for familial combined hyperlipidemia. *Ann. Int. Med.* **109**:25–32.

Eisenberg, S., Gavish, D., and Kleinman, Y. (1986). Bezafibrate. In *Pharmacological Control of Hyperlipidemia*. Edited by R. Fears, R. I. Levy, J. Shepherd, C. J. Packard, N. E. Miller. Barcelona, J. R. Prouse Science Publishers, pp. 145–169.

Eisenberg, S., Gavish, D., Oschry, Y., Fainaru, M., and Deckelbaum, R. J. (1984). Abnormalities in very low, low, and high density lipoproteins in hypertriglyceridemia: Reversal toward normal with bezafibrate treatment. *J. Clin. Invest.* **74**:470–482.

Evans, J. R., Falland, S. C., and Cutler, R. E. (1987). The effect of renal function of the pharmacokinetics of gemfibrozil. *J. Clin. Pharmacol.* **27**:994–1000.

Franceschini, G., Sitori, M., Gianfrancheschini, G., Frosi, T., Montanari, G., and Sitori, C. O. (1985). Reversable increase of the apo CII/apo CIII ratio in the very low density lipoproteins after fenofibrate treatment in hypertriglyceridemic patients. *Artery* **12**:363–381.

Frick, M. H., Elo, O., Haapa, K., Heinenen, O. P., Heinsalmi, P., Helo, P., Huttunen, J. K., Kaitaniemi, P., Koskinen, P., and Manninen, V. (1987). Helsinki Heart Study: Primary prevention trial with gemfibrozil in middle-aged men with dyslipidemia. *N. Engl. J. Med.* **317**:1237–1245.

Fruchart, J. C., Davignon, J., Bard, J. M., Grothe, A. M., Richard, A., and Fievet, C. (1987). Effect of fenofibrate treatment on type III hyperlipoproteinemia. *Am. J. Med.* **83**(Suppl. 5B):71–74.

Garg, A., and Grundy, S. M. (1989). Gemfibrozil alone and in combination with lovastatin for treatment of hypertriglyceridemia in NIDDM. *Diabetes* **38**:364–372.

Garg, A., and Grundy, S. M. (1990). Management of dyslipidemia in NIDDM. *Diabetes Care* **13**:153–169.

Goldberg, A. C., Schonfeld, G., Anderson, C., and Gillingham, M. A. (1987). Fenofibrate effects the compositions of lipoproteins. *Am. J. Med.* **83**(Suppl. 5B):60–65.

Goldberg, A. C., Schonfeld, G., Feldman, E. B., Gingsberg, H. N., Hunninghake, D. B., Insell, W., Knopp, R. H., Kwiterovich, P. O., Mellies, M. J., Pickering,

J., and Samuel, P. (1989). Fenofibrate for the treatment of type IV and type V hyperlipoproteinemias: A double blind placebo-controlled multicenter U.S. study. *Clin. Therapeutics.* **11**:69–83.

Golper, T. A., Illingworth, D. R., Morris, C. D., and Bennet, W. M. (1989). Lovastatin in the treatment of multifactorial hyperlipidemia associated with proteinuria. *Am. J. Kidney Dis.* **13**:312–320.

Groggel, G. C., Cheung, A. K., Benigni, K. E., and Wilson, D. E. (1989). Treatment of nephrotic hyperlipoproteinemia with gemfibrozil. *Kidney Int.* **36**:266–271.

Grundy, S. M., Ahrens, E. H., Jr., and Salen, G. (1972). Mechanisms of action of clofibrate on cholesterol metabolism in patients with hyperlipidemia. *J. Lipid Res.* **13**:531–551.

Grundy, S. M., Goodman, D. S., Rifkind, B. M., and Kleeman, J. I. (1989). The place of HDL in cholesterol management. A perspective from the National Cholesteral Education Program. *Arch. Int. Med.* **149**:505–510.

Gugler, R., and Hartlapp, J. (1978). Clofibrate kinetics after single and multiple doses. *Clin. Pharmacol. Ther.* **24**:432–438.

Heller, F., and Harvengt, C. (1983). Effects of clofibrate, bezafibrate, fenofibrate and probucol on plasma lipolytic enzymes in normolipemic subjects. *Eur. J. Clin. Pharmacol.* **25**:57–63.

Houlston, R., Quiney, J., Watts, G. F., and Lewis, B. (1988). Gemfibrozil and the treatment of resistant familial hypercholesterolemia and type III hyperlipoproteinemia. *J. Roy. Soc. Med.* **81**:274–276.

Hunninghake, D. B., and Peters, J. R. (1987). Effect of fibric acid derivatives on blood lipid and lipoprotein levels. *Am. J. Med.* **83** (Suppl. 5B):44–49.

Illingworth, D. R., and Bacon, S. (1989). Influence of lovastatin plus gemfibrozil on plasma lipids and lipoproteins in patients with heterozygous familial hypercholesterolemia. *Circulation* **79**:590–596.

Illingworth, D. R., Olson, D. G., Cook, S. F., Wendell, H., and Connor, W. E. (1982). Ciprofibrate in the therapy of type II hypercholesterolemia: A double blind trial. *Atherosclerosis* **44**:211–221.

Illingworth, D. R., and O'Malley, J. P. (1990). The hypolipidemic effects of lovastatin and clofibrate alone and in combination in patients with type III hyperlipoproteinemia. *Metabolism* **39**:403–409.

Kesaniemi, Y. A., and Grundy, S. M. (1984). Influence of gemfibrozil and clofibrate on metabolism of cholesterol and plasma triglycerides in man. *JAMA* **251**:2241–2246.

Kissebah, A. H., Adams, B. W., Harrigan, P., and Wynn, V. (1974). The mechanism of clofibrate and tetranicotinile fructose on the kinetics of plasma free fatty acids and triglyceride transport in type IV and in type V hypertriglyceridemia. *Eur. J. Clin. Invest.* **4**:163–174.

Kissebah, A. H., Alfarsi, S., Adams, P. W., Seed, M., Falkard, J., and Wynn, V. (1976). Transport kinetics of plasma free fatty acids, very low density lipoprotein triglycerides and apoprotein B in patients with hypertriglyceridemia. Effects of gemfibrozil therapy. *Diabetalogia* **24**:199–218.

Kloer, H. U. (1987). Structure and biochemical effects of fenofibrate. *Am. J. Med.* **83**(Suppl. 5B):328.

Klosiewicz-Latoszek, L., Nowicka, G., Szostak, W. B., and Naruszewicz, M. (1987). Influence of bezafibrate and colestipol on LDL cholesterol, LDL apolipoprotein B and HDL cholesterol in hyperlipoproteinemia. *Atherosclerosis* **63**:203–209.

Kobayashi, M., Shigeta, Y., Hirata, Y., Omori, Y., Sakaoto, N., Namby, S., and Baba, S. (1988). Improvement of glucose tolerance in NIDDM by clofibrate: Randomized doubleblind study. *Diabetes Care* **11**:494–499.

Kostner, G. M. (1988). The affection of lipoprotein (a) by lipid lowering drugs. In *Recent Aspects of Diagnosis and Treatment of Lipoprotein Disorders*. Edited by K. Widhalm and H. K. Naito. New York, A. R. Liss, Inc., pp. 255–263.

Kritchevsky, D., Tepper, S. A., and Storey, J. A. (1979). Influence of procetofen on lipid metabolism in normocholesterolemic rats. *Pharmacol. Res. Commun.* **11**:635–641.

Leaf, D. A., Connor, W. E., Illingworth, D. R., Bacon, S. P., and Sexton, G. (1989). The hypolipidemic effects of gemfibrozil in type V hyperlipidemia. A double-blind crossover study. *JAMA* **262**:3154–3160.

Levy, R. I., Frederickson, D. S., and Shulman, R. (1972). Dietary and drug treatment of primary hyperlipoproteinemia. *Ann. Intern. Med.* **77**:267–294.

Lindner, M. A., and Illingworth, D. R. (1988). Expression of type III hyperlipoproteinemia in an adolescent patient with hypothyroidism. *J. Pediatrics* **71**:1–7.

Mahley, R. W., and Angelin, B. (1984). Type III hyperlipoproteinemia. Recent insights into the genetic defect of familial dysbetalipoproteinemia. *Adv. Int. Med.* **29**:385–411.

Malmendier, C. L., and Delecroix, C. (1985). Effects of fenofibrate on high and low density lipoprotein metabolism in heterozygous familial hypercholesterolemia. *Atherosclerosis* **55**:161–169.

Manninen, V., Elo, M. O., Frick, M. H., Haapa, K., Heinenen, O. P., Heinsalmi, P., Helo, P., Huttunen, J. K., Katianiemi, P., Koskinen, P., Manenpaa, H., Malkonen, M., Mantari, M., Norolo, S., Pasternack, A., Pikkarainen, J., Romo, M., Sjoblom, T., and Nikkila, E. A. (1988). Lipid alterations and decline in the incidence of coronary heart disease in the Helsinki Heart Study. *JAMA* **260**:641–651.

Manttari, M., Koskinen, P., Manninen, V., Huttunen, J. K., Frick, M. H., and Nikkila, E. A. (1990). The effect of gemfibrozil on the concentration and composition of serum lipoproteins. A controlled study with special reference to initial triglyceride levels. *Atherosclerosis* **81**:11–17.

Maxwell, R. E., Nawrocki, J. W., and Uhlendorf, P. D. (1983) Some comparative effects of gemfibrozil, clofibrate, bezafibrate, cholestyramine and compactin on sterol metabolism in rats. *Atherosclerosis* **48**:195–203.

Meinertz, H. (1986). Effects of gemfibrozil on plasma lipoproteins in patients with type II hypolipoproteinemia and familial hypercholesterolemia. In *Royal Soc. Med. Serv., Int. Congress and Symposium Series, 1987*. Further progress with gemfibrozil. London, Royal Soc. Med., pp. 15–21.

Monk, J. P., and Todd, P. A. (1987). Bezafibrate: A review of its pharmacodynamic and pharmacokinetic properties and therapeutic use in hyperlipidemia. *Drugs* **33**:539–576.

Nordoy, A., Illingworth, D. R., Connor, W. E., and Goodnight, S., Jr. (1990). Increased activity of Factor VII and Factor VII-phospholipid complex measured using a normotest system in subjects with hyperlipidemia. *Hemostasis* **20**:65–72.

Nye, E. R., and Sutherland, W. H. F. (1980). The treatment of hyperlipoproteinemia with gemfibrozil compared with placebo and clofibrate. *N. Z. Med. J.* **92**:345–349.

O'Brien, J. R., Ethrington, M. D., Jamieson, S., and Sussex, J. (1978). The effect of clofibrate on platelet function and other tests abnormal in atherosclerosis. *Thrombosis Hemostasis* **40**:75–82.

Packard, C. J., Clegg, R. J., Dominiczak, M. H., Lorimer, A. R., and Shepherd, J. (1986). Effects of bezafibrate on apolipoprotein B metabolism in type III hyperlipoproteinemic subjects. *J. Lipid Res.* **27**:930–938.

Pappu, A. S., Illingworth, D. R., and Bacon, S. (1989) Reduction in plasma low density lipoprotein cholesterol and urinary mevalonic acid by lovastatin in patients with heterozygous familial hypercholesterolemia. *Metabolism* **38**:542–549.

Palmer, R. H. (1987). Effects of fibric acid derivatives on biliary lipid composition. *Am. J. Med.* **83**(Suppl. 5B):37–43.

Posner, I., Wang, C. S., and McConathy, W. J. (1983). Kinetics of bovine, milk, lipoprotein lipase and the mechanism of enzyme activation by apolipoprotein CII. *Biochemistry* **22**:4041–4047.

Rabelink, A. J., Hene, R. J., Erkelens, D. W., Joles, J. A., and Koomans, H. A. (1988). Effects of simvastatin and cholestyramine on lipoprotein profile in hyperlipidemia of nephrotic syndrome. *Lancet* **2**:1335–1338.

Rabkin, S. W., Hayden, M., and Frohlich, J. (1988). Comparison of gemfibrozil and clofibrate on serum lipids in familial combined hyperlipidemia. A randomized placebo controlled double blind crossover clinical trial. *Atherosclerosis* **73**:233–240.

Rifkind, B. M. (1966). Effect of CPIB ester on plasma free fatty acid levels in man. *Metabolism* **15**:673–675.

Rouffy, J., Chanu, B., and Bakir, R. (1985). Comparative evaluation of the effects of ciprofibrate and fenofibrate on lipids, lipoproteins and apoproteins A and B. *Atherosclerosis* **54**:273–281.

Saku, K., Gartside, P. S., Hynd, B. A., and Kashyap, M. L. (1985). Mechanism of action of gemfibrozil on lipoprotein metabolism. *J. Clin. Invest.* **75**:1702–1712.

Saku, K., Sasaki, J., and Arakawa, K. (1989). Effects of slow release bezafibrate on serum lipids, lipoproteins, apolipoproteins and post-heparin lipolytic activities in patients with type IV and type V hypertriglyceridemia. *Clin. Therapeutics* **11**:331–340.

Schneider, A., Stange, E. F., Ditschuneit, H. H., and Ditschuneit, H. (1985). Fenofibrate treatment inhibits HMG CoA reductase activity in mononuclear cells from hyperlipoproteinemic patients. *Atherosclerosis* **56**:257–263.

Seed, M., Hoppichler, F., Reaveley, D., McCarthy, S., Thompson, G. R., Boerwinkle, E., and Utermann, G. (1990). Relation of serum lipoprotein (a) concentration and apolipoprotein (a) phenotype to Coronary Heart Disease in patients with familial hypercholesterolemia. *N. Engl. J. Med.* **322**:1494–1499.

Shepherd, J., Caslake, M. J., Lorimer, A. R., Vallance, B. D., and Packard, C. J. (1985). Fenofibrate reduces low density lipoprotein catabolism in hypertriglyceridemic subjects. *Arteriosclerosis* **5**:162–168.

Shepherd, J., and Packard, C. J. (1986). An overview of the effects of paracholorophenoxyisobuteric acids on lipoprotein metabolism. In *Pharmacological Control of Hyperlipidemia*. Edited by R. Fears, R. I. Levy, J. Shepherd, C. J. Packard, and N. E. Miller. Barcelona, J. R. Prouse Science Publishers, pp. 135–144.

Shepherd, J., Packard, C. J., and Stewart, J. M. (1984). Apolipoprotein A and B metabolism during bezafibrate therapy in hypertriglyceridemic subjects. *J. Clin. Invest.* **74**:2164–2177.

Steinmetz, J., Morin, C., Panek, E., Seist, G., and Drouin, P. (1981). Biological variations in hyperlipidemic children and adolescence treated with fenofibrate. *Clin. Chim. Acta.* **112**:43–53.

Stewart, J. M., Packard, C. J., Lorimer, A. R., Boag, D. E., and Shepherd, J. (1982). Effects of bezafibrate on receptor mediated and receptor independent low density lipoprotein catabolism in type II hyperlipoproteinemic subjects. *Atherosclerosis* **44**:355–364.

Thorp, J. M. (1962). Experimental evaluation of orally active combination of endosterone with ethylcholorophenoxyisobuterate. *Lancet* **1**:1323–1326.

Tobert, J. A. (1988). Efficacy and long term adverse effect pattern of lovastatin. *Am. J. Cardiol.* **62**:28J–34J.

Todd, P. A., and Ward, A. (1988). Gemfibrozil: a review of its pharmacodynamic and pharmacokinetic properties and therapeutic use in dyslipidemia. *Drugs* **36**:314–339.

Vega, G. L., and Grundy, S. M. (1985). Gemfibrozil therapy in primary hypertriglyceridemia associated with coronary heart disease. *JAMA* **253**:2398–2403.

Vega, G. L., and Grundy, S. M. (1988). Lovastatin therapy in nephrotic hyperlipidemia: effects on lipoprotein metabolism. *Kidney Int.* **33**:1160–1168.

Vega, J. L., and Grundy, S. M. (1989). Comparison of lovastatin and gemfibrozil in normolipidemic patients with hypoalphalipoproteinemia. *JAMA* **262**:3148–3153.

Wang, C. S., McConathy, W. J., Kloer, H. U., and Alaupovic, P. (1985). Modulation of lipoprotein lipase activity by apolipoproteins. Effect of apolipoprotein CIII. *J. Clin. Invest.* **75:**384–390.

Weisweiler, P., Merck, W., Janetschek, P., and Schwandt, P. (1984). Effect of fenofibrate on serum lipoproteins in subjects with familial hypercholesterolemia and combined hyperlipidemia. *Atherosclerosis* **53:**321–325.

Wheeler, K. A. H., West, R. J., Lloyd, J. K., and Barley, J. (1985). Doubleblind trial of bezafibrate in familial hypercholesterolemia. *Arch. Dis. Childhood* **60:**34–37.

Wysowski, D. K., Kennedy, D. L., and Gross, T. P. (1990). Prescribed use of cholesterol lowering drugs in the United States, 1978–1988. *JAMA* **263:**2185–2188.

7

HMG CoA Reductase Inhibitors: Clinical Applications and Therapeutic Potential

Scott M. Grundy

University of Texas
Southwestern Medical Center
Dallas, Texas

The management of hypercholesterolemia has been greatly facilitated by the discovery of inhibitors of 3-hydroxy-3-methyl glutaryl-coenzyme A (HMG CoA) reductase. The first drug of this type was called mevastatin and was isolated from extracts of *Penicillium citrinum* in 1976 by Endo et al. (Endo et al., 1976a). Mevastatin was subsequently shown to inhibit HMG CoA reductase (Endo et al., 1976b) and to lower serum cholesterol levels in dogs (Tsujita et al., 1979) and in humans (Shigematsu et al., 1979; Yamamoto et al., 1980; Mabuchi et al., 1981). A derivative of mevastatin, called lovastatin, was developed in the United States. This drug was shown to produce a marked lowering of serum cholesterol levels in normolipidemic subjects by Tobert et al. (1982) and in hypercholesterolemic patients in our laboratory (Bilheimer et al., 1983a,b; Grundy and Bilheimer, 1984; Grundy and Vega, 1985) and by Illingworth et al. (Illingworth and Sexton, 1984; Illingworth and Bacon, 1987; Illingworth, 1987). Subsequent larger clinical trials (Lovastatin Study Group, 1986; Havel et al., 1987), initiated by Merck and Company, confirmed the efficacy and general safety of lovastatin, and on the basis of these human studies and proven safety in laboratory animals, lovastatin was approved by the Food and Drug Administration (FDA) in 1987.

I. CHEMICAL STRUCTURES

The chemical structures of the HMG CoA reductase inhibitors are presented in Figure 1. One component of their structures is analogous to HMG CoA and is the active part of the molecule. Lovastatin is a methylated derivative of mevastatin, and simvastatin is its bimethylated derivative. Pravastatin has a hydroxy group in the place of the extra methyl group of lovastatin. These derivatives are all obtained from biological sources, whereas another compound, SRI-62320, is a synthetic molecule. Mevastatin, lovastatin, and simvastatin are administered in the lactone form, whereas pravastatin and SRI-62320 are given in the open acid form.

A question not entirely resolved is whether there are therapeutic advantages imparted by particular chemical structures among the HMG CoA reductase inhibitors. All of the inhibitors have an extremely high affinity for the enzyme; for instance, mevastatin has an affinity for HMG CoA reductase that

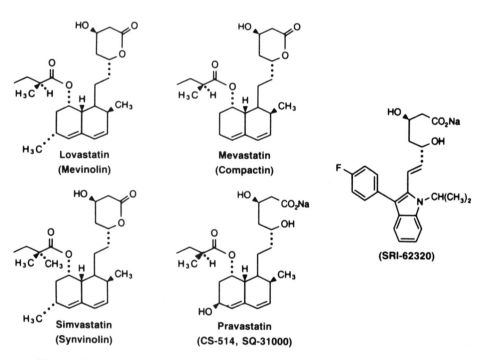

Figure 1 HMG CoA reductase inhibitors in clinic use or under development. Former names are shown in parentheses.

exceeds that of HMG CoA by 2900 times. Lovastatin binds to the enzyme with twice the affinity of mevastatin (Alberts et al., 1980), and simvastatin at four times (Hoffman et al., 1986). The greater binding affinity of simvastatin allows it to be given in lower doses than lovastatin, but this does not necessarily convey a therapeutic advantage, since potential side effects also may depend on the drug's action to inhibit HMG CoA reductase.

Perhaps a question of greater importance than potency is whether HMG CoA reductase inhibitors differ in tissue selectivity. Ideally, the inhibitors should act exclusively in the liver, because actions at other sites may produce side effects without therapeutic benefit. Some workers suggest that the lactone structure of lovastatin and simvastatin favors their accumulation in the liver by promoting first-pass clearance by the liver. Others claim instead that the open-acid group of pravastatin or its hydroxyl group help to exclude it from extrahepatic tissues and thereby minimize peripheral side effects. Neither of these claims has been validated, although the concept of tissue selectivity points to potential ways to maximize the therapeutic potential of drugs of this class.

A. Mechanisms of Action

The primary action of HMG CoA reductase inhibitors is to interfere with the synthesis of cholesterol by competitively inhibiting HMG CoA reductase. An intriguing question is how this action translates into a decrease in serum cholesterol levels. To examine this question, a brief review of cholesterol transport in plasma is required. Cholesterol is carried in three major lipoproteins: very low density lipoproteins (VLDL), low density lipoproteins (LDL), and high density lipoproteins (HDL). The major apolipoprotein of VLDL and LDL is apolipoprotein B-100 (apo B). The pathways of apo B–containing lipoproteins are shown in Figure 2. The liver secretes VLDL particles, which in turn are converted to VLDL remnants and on to LDL. VLDL and VLDL remnants contain apo Es and Cs in addition to apo B, but with hydrolysis of VLDL triglycerides, the former two species of apoproteins are removed, and LDL contains only apo B. Any of the lipoproteins in this catabolic cascade can be removed from the circulation by lipoprotein receptors. LDL receptors can remove all of these lipoproteins. These receptors recognize both apo B and apo E, and various types of VLDL particles that contain both types of apoproteins demonstrate a greater affinity for LDL receptors than LDL itself, which has only apo B. Liver cells, moreover, may possess other receptors that specifically recognize apo E. VLDL particles thus generally are removed directly by the liver more readily than LDL itself. In contrast, LDL, unlike

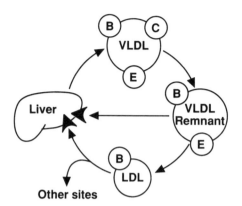

Figure 2 Pathways of lipoprotein metabolism. The liver produces triglyceride-rich lipoproteins, VLDL, which are degraded through the action of lipoprotein lipase to VLDL remnants. VLDL contain apolipoproteins B-100 (B), C-II and C-III (C), and E. As VLDL triglycerides undergo lipolysis, apo Cs are lost. VLDL remnants can either be removed directly by the liver, via LDL receptors, or they can be converted to LDL. In the process, VLDL remnants lose apo E. Most LDL is cleared by the liver; also a smaller fraction can be removed by extra hepatic tissues.

VLDL, can be removed by receptor-mediated clearance in other tissues, and in addition, a small portion of LDL is cleared by nonreceptor pathways.

The formation and catabolism of HDL are shown in Figure 3. Circulating HDL is thought to arise from nascent HDL particles, which are derived from several sources, i.e., the liver, gut, and possibly surface-coat lipids and apolipoproteins of other lipoproteins. Nascent HDL particles contain apo A-I and apo A-II as their major apoproteins. These lipoproteins can derive unesterified (free) cholesterol from extrahepatic tissues; this may be the first step in "reverse cholesterol transport," i.e., the transport of cholesterol from extrahepatic tissues to the liver for excretion. Acquisition of cholesterol ester converts nascent HDL into mature HDL particles; the latter include HDL_2 and HDL_3. HDL may be removed from the circulation either directly by the liver or by extrahepatic tissues, or HDL can transfer its cholesterol ester to triglyceride-rich lipoproteins in exchange for triglycerides. The functions of HDL are not fully understood, although many workers believe that these lipoproteins play a key role in reverse cholesterol transport.

How do HMG CoA reductase inhibitors affect these lipoprotein pathways? From a quantitative viewpoint, their major action is to reduce levels of LDL. Generally, they cause a 25–35% reduction in LDL cholesterol concentrations, and since LDL normally is the major cholesterol-carrying lipoprotein in

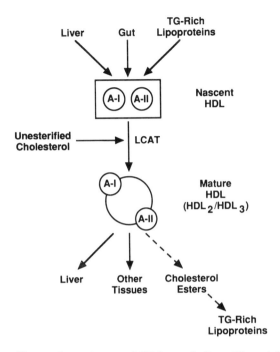

Figure 3 Pathways of HDL metabolism. The origins of HDL are complex. The liver, gut, triglyceride (TG)-rich lipoproteins appear to supply the essential components of HDL: apoproteins A-I and A-II, phospholipids, and unesterified cholesterol. The initial product is believed to be "nascent" HDL. More unesterified cholesterol may be derived from extrahepatic tissues, and through the action of an enzyme, LCAT, this extra cholesterol is esterified. The resulting spherical particle, which contains cholesterol ester, represents "mature" HDL; the latter can exist in two forms: HDL_2 and HDL_3. Whole HDL particles probably are removed directly by the liver and extrahepatic tissues, but some of the cholesterol esters of HDL can be transferred independently of whole particles to triglyceride (TG)-rich lipoproteins (dashed line).

plasma, the greatest reduction in serum total cholesterol occurs in this fraction. However, as a rule, levels of VLDL cholesterol fall during reductase-inhibitor therapy (Vega et al., 1988; Garg and Grundy, 1988; Vega and Grundy, 1988), and percentage reductions in VLDL are similar to those for LDL cholesterol. Any theory of the mechanism of action of HMG CoA reductase inhibitors therefore must explain the reduction in serum levels of *both* LDL and VLDL.

Studies carried out in tissue culture indicate that one consequence of inhibition of cholesterol synthesis is a stimulation of LDL receptor synthesis

(Goldstein and Brown, 1979). When intracellular levels of cholesterol decline, synthesis of LDL receptors is derepressed and LDL uptake enhanced. This response provides a means to restore intracellular content of cholesterol to an optimal level. Isotopic studies carried out in humans indicate that the fractional clearance rate (FCR) for LDL rises in some types of hypercholesterolemic patients during treatment with reductase inhibitors (Bilheimer et al., 1983a,b); this rise in FCR is consistent with an increase in LDL receptor activity. Such an increase could explain the fall in both VLDL cholesterol and LDL cholesterol levels because both VLDL and LDL are removed by LDL receptors (Fig. 2).

However, in a series of studies carried out in our laboratory, we observed that FCRs for LDL are not consistently raised by lovastatin therapy. For example, in patients with primary moderate hypercholesterolemia, the rate of conversion of VLDL to LDL is reduced (Grundy and Vega, 1985). Indeed, in a recent study, we observed that rates of formation of VLDL are reduced in patients with primary moderate hypercholesterolemia during pravastatin therapy (Vega et al., 1990). What is the meaning of this observation? Does it indicate that HMG CoA reductase inhibitors decrease secretion of lipoproteins by the liver? If so, is decreased secretion of lipoprotein a more important mechanism than stimulation of LDL receptor synthesis? This could be one explanation of the data. If cholesterol synthesis is reduced, the formation of apo B-containing lipoproteins also might be decreased. To date, however, there are no strong data to support the concept that the rates of cholesterol synthesis are linked closely to those of lipoprotein synthesis. We thus can ask whether apparent reductions in rates of synthesis of apo B—containing lipoproteins might have an alternative explanation.

Even so, we must ask whether an increase in formation of LDL receptors could be the primary action of HMG CoA reductase inhibitors and yet clearance rates for LDL not be enhanced. As indicated above, VLDL has a greater affinity for LDL receptors than LDL itself. An increase in LDL receptor activity theoretically should remove VLDL particles preferentially to removal of LDL particles. If this is true, the rate of conversion of VLDL (and VLDL remnants) to LDL should be reduced because of enhanced direct removal of remnant lipoproteins from the circulation. In other words, an increased activity of LDL receptors might reduce the conversion of VLDL to LDL because of greater direct removal of VLDL remnants. But how could an increase in LDL receptor activity explain a decrease in apparent formation of VLDL, as noted in our recent study (Vega et al., 1990)? This too could occur if a portion of newly secreted lipoproteins are rapidly hydrolyzed and removed by LDL receptors, too rapidly to be detected by isotope kinetic techniques. In other words, if some newly secreted VLDL are removed too rapidly to be detected, isotope kinetic data would suggest a decrease in production rate for VLDL. Thus, a reduction in levels of *both* VLDL and LDL and *apparent* decreases in production rates of both VLDL and LDL could be explained entirely by increased synthesis of LDL receptors.

In an attempt to determine whether HMG CoA reductase inhibitors *can* decrease formation of apo B–containing lipoproteins, we examined the actions of lovastatin in patients who have a complete absence of LDL receptors, namely, those with homozygous familial hypercholesterolemia (FH) (Uauy et al., 1988). If lovastatin were to inhibit the synthesis of apo B–containing lipoproteins, lovastatin therapy should reduce LDL levels in these patients, whereas if it acts exclusively by promoting LDL receptor activity, drug therapy should have no effect on LDL concentrations. In fact, our study (Uauy et al., 1988) revealed that lovastatin had no effect on LDL concentrations in homozygous FH patients, and we therefore concluded that the drug has little if any influence on synthesis and secretion of apo B–containing lipoproteins.

Still, one might ask whether the metabolism of lipoproteins could be so deranged in FH homozygotes that it obscures an action of HMG CoA reductase inhibitors to interfere with hepatic synthesis of lipoproteins. Some workers (Ginsberg et al., 1987) have questioned our interpretation of the isotope kinetic data (Uauy et al., 1988; Vega et al., 1990), and they contend that reductase inhibitors actually do inhibit the synthesis of apo B–containing lipoproteins. If their contention is correct, it would suggest a close link between the synthesis of cholesterol and hepatic formation of lipoproteins. To date, however, no such link has been identified, and corroborative data of other types must be obtained before this mechanism can be accepted. In our view, the best available data indicate that the major if not exclusive action of HMG CoA reductase inhibitors is to stimulate hepatic synthesis of LDL receptors.

In an early study from our laboratory (Grundy and Vega, 1985), lovastatin was observed to raise levels of HDL cholesterol. Although the magnitude of this response is not marked, it appears to be a true response. This finding was unexpected, and it raises the question of mechanism. For example, is the rise in HDL-cholesterol levels secondary to a reduction in VLDL and LDL levels, or is it due to a direct effect of lovastatin on HDL metabolism, independent of other lipoproteins? The former seems more likely. Inverse correlations between VLDL levels, and to some extent LDL levels, and concentrations of HDL cholesterol are known to exist. Thus, apo B–containing lipoproteins may act as sink for cholesterol esters carried by HDL, and when these lipoproteins are lowered, the level of HDL cholesterol will rise (see Fig. 3). The clinical significance of the rise in HDL cholesterol levels remains to be determined, but the same can be said for other lipid-lowering drugs that increase HDL levels.

II. PHARMACOKINETICS

The pharmacokinetics of HMG CoA reductase inhibitors represent a subject of considerable importance, but unfortunately, data on their absorption, metabolic conversions, and fates are limited and generally not published. Some information is available through the package insert for lovastatin (Mevacor, 1990). This information can be reviewed briefly, and unresolved questions can be examined.

A. Absorption

In laboratory animals, about 30% of a single dose of lovastatin is absorbed (Mevacor, 1990). The percentage absorption in humans is unknown, but if only 30% is absorbed, this represents a significant waste of expensive medication. Studies therefore are needed to determine percentage absorption in humans, and if they are low, on how to enhance absorption rates. Most of the newly absorbed drug apparently is removed rapidly in the first pass through the liver, and less than 5% of an oral dose enters the systemic circulation. The primary site of action of these drugs thus appears to be the liver. This does not mean of course that no secondary sites of action exist outside the liver.

B. Metabolic Conversion Products

Several of the HMG CoA reductase inhibitors are administered in the inactive lactone form (Fig. 1), but they are rapidly converted into the active form, the beta-hydroxyacid, in the liver. Lovastatin is hydroxylated at the 6-position, which is an active metabolite; two other active but unidentified metabolites have been recognized. Whether these various metabolites are more active than the parent compound is not known. Active metabolites of other HMG CoA reductase inhibitors must exist, but such have not been reported.

C. Excretion Pathways

The principal route of excretion of lovastatin, and presumably of other HMG CoA reductase inhibitors, is from liver into bile. Whether the major excretory product is the parent compound or various active metabolites needs to be determined. Less than 10% of lovastatin and its active products are excreted in the urine. A high fractional excretion into bile might be explained by the high affinity of the liver for these drugs, whereas the low excretion in urine may be the consequence of very low plasma concentrations of drug and metabolites.

D. Plasma Concentrations

HMG CoA reductase inhibitors are tightly bound to proteins in plasma, and free concentrations normally must be extremely low. This may be fortunate because any of the drug that enters extrahepatic tissues may produce side effects without the benefit of therapeutic efficacy. It thus appears advantageous to maintain as low a plasma concentration as possible. If so, we must ask what determines plasma concentrations of reductase inhibitors. First, the dose may be a factor; suggestive evidence indicates that the lower the dose, the lower the plasma level. Whether variability in fractional intestinal absorption affects blood levels is unknown. Second, the rate of biliary excretion of drug and metabolites appears to be a critical factor. Interference of biliary elimination seemingly results in very high blood levels. And third, do urinary excretion rates affect blood levels? Perhaps not in normal individuals, but in patients with reduced biliary excretion, urinary elimination may be a "safety valve" preventing development of toxic plasma levels.

E. Drug Interactions

Since HMG CoA reductase inhibitors are being used in individuals who are taking a variety of other drugs, the issue of drug interaction is assuming increasing importance. Two questions must be addressed: 1) Do HMG CoA reductase inhibitors enhance toxicity of other drugs? and 2) Do other drugs promote toxicity of reductase inhibitors? These questions have not been addressed in a systematic way, but some useful information has emerged (Mevacor, 1990). Preliminary testing suggests that lovastatin does not affect the pharmacokinetics of antipyrine in humans, which may be taken to mean that it does not influence the cytochrome P-450 system. Moreover, lovastatin apparently has no adverse effects on the pharmacology of propranolol and digoxin. Whether reductase inhibitors potentiate the toxicity of other drugs remains to be shown. On the other hand, any drug that raises plasma levels of HMG CoA reductase inhibitors can produce a toxic reaction from the latter. Drugs that interfere with biliary excretion could fall into this category. Alcohol, niacin, and cyclosporine are candidates for adverse interaction. The latter two drugs have precipitated severe muscle toxicity in patients treated with lovastatin. They presumably interfere with biliary excretion and raise blood levels of lovastatin. A toxic interaction also can occur between reductase inhibitors and gemfibrozil. Both drugs are potential muscle toxins, and when used together, the danger of severe myopathy is increased greatly.

III. SIDE EFFECTS

The HMG CoA reductase inhibitors have proven to be remarkably safe in most patients, but significant and even serious side effects have been recorded. A question that has not been resolved is whether all of the side effects of HMG CoA reductase inhibitors can be explained entirely by their action to competitively inhibit HMG CoA reductase. This is a question worthy of consideration. What then are the end products of the series of reactions initiated by the conversion of HMG CoA into mevalonic acid? They include cholesterol and its metabolic products—sex hormones, cortisol, and bile acids, dolichol, ubiquinone, and isopentyl adenine. The limited information available on effects of each of these products can be examined.

A. Cholesterol Synthesis

How much do HMG CoA reductase inhibitors reduce whole body cholesterol? Do they interfere with cholesterol synthesis to the extent that they produce a dangerous deficiency in body pools of cholesterol? When dogs are given very high doses of lovastatin, synthesis of cholesterol is severely inhibited, to the point that the central nervous system is deprived of cholesterol; consequently side effects of the central nervous system occur. A second adverse effect of high doses of lovastatin in dogs is cataract, and this too could be the result of a deficiency of cholesterol in lens-forming cells.

To determine whether lovastatin at therapeutic doses produces a marked reduction of synthesis of cholesterol in humans, we carried out cholesterol balance studies in patients with hypercholesterolemia (Grundy and Bilheimer, 1984). The data showed that in most patients lovastatin causes a moderate reduction, but not a severe decrease, in cholesterol synthesis. Other workers later reported similar results using different techniques for estimating cholesterol synthesis (Parker et al., 1984; Pappu et al., 1987). HMG CoA reductase inhibitor therapy thus does not markedly reduce cholesterol synthesis at therapeutic doses in humans. Even so, we might ask whether interference of cholesterol synthesis may have toxic effects in some patients.

For example, a few patients report insomnia when taking HMG CoA reductase inhibitors. Several investigators are convinced that it is a real side effect (Schaefer, 1988). Could insomnia be secondary to a mild inhibition of cholesterol synthesis in the CNS? This is a possibility. Reductase inhibitors also can give rise to myotoxicity and hepatotoxicity. Might these effects be due to a loss of cell membrane integrity because of a deficiency of cholesterol? This latter mechanism has not been documented, but since cholesterol is vital for all tissues, we might speculate whether inhibition of cholesterol synthesis might induce long-term side effects in some organs. This question needs further investigation; it is remarkable that HMG CoA reductase inhibitors to date have shown such a paucity of systemic side effects. This safety could be explained by their action being confined largely to the liver. Perhaps it is therefore not surprising that the most common side effect from HMG CoA reductase inhibitors is hepatotoxicity.

Fortunately, the fear that reductase inhibitors will cause cataract has not materialized. Careful follow-up of a large number of patients for several years failed to reveal an increased incidence of cataract (Tobert et al., 1990). For this reason, frequent slit-lamp examinations of most patients probably is not necessary. Still, it remains to be determined whether administration of HMG CoA reductase inhibitors for several years causes a gradual buildup of cataract. This question may require many years to answer, but from information to date, one need not restrict use of these drugs because of fear of cataracts.

B. Bile Acids

If the synthesis of cholesterol is curtailed by HMG CoA reductase inhibitors, should there not be a corresponding decrease in formation of bile acids? Our cholesterol-balance measurements indeed showed a moderate decrease in bile acid synthesis (Grundy and Bilheimer, 1984). This response theoretically could increase risk of cholesterol gallstone formation because insufficient bile acids might be available to solubilize the cholesterol in bile. In reality, the decrease in cholesterol synthesis causes a greater reduction in biliary cholesterol than in biliary bile acids, and saturation of bile with cholesterol actually decreases (Duane et al., 1988). Thus HMG CoA reductase inhibitors might actually be used to prevent development of gallstones in patients at high risk for cholesterol stones. Further research on this possibility is needed.

C. Adrenal and Gonadal Steroids

Although inhibition of cholesterol synthesis theoretically could reduce formation of adrenal and gonadal steroids, a series of studies (Illingworth and Corbin, 1985; Lovastatin Study Group, 1986; Thompson et al., 1986; Farnsworth et al., 1987; Havel et al., 1987) have failed to show a significant decrease in either type of steroid. This might be explained by an adequate availability of cholesterol in plasma lipoproteins to supply the sterol needed for their synthesis.

D. Dolichol Synthesis

Dolichol, a product of mevalonic acid, is required for glycoprotein synthesis. To date, no deficiencies of glycoproteins have been reported with reductase inhibitor therapy. A great many proteins in the body, however, contain carbohydrate moieties, and the potential for toxicity theoretically does exist. Since toxicity from decrease in glycoproteins has not emerged, perhaps synthesis of dolichol is not curtailed sufficiently to produce significant side effects. Nonetheless, the possibility of long-term side effects yet to be recognized should be kept in mind.

E. Ubiquinone Synthesis

Ubiquinone is employed by mitochondria for electron transport. If HMG CoA reductase inhibitors reduce formation of ubiquinone, the result could be interference with normal oxidative processes in muscle. No evidence has emerged that ubiquinone synthesis is directly curtailed by reductase inhibitors. In fact, one study (Mabuchi et al., 1981) failed to detect a reduction of plasma levels of ubiquinone in patients treated with mevastatin. It is intriguing to speculate, however, whether reduction in ubiquinone synthesis might account for development of myopathy occurring in some patients treated with HMG CoA reductase inhibitors.

F. Hepatotoxicity

Abnormalities in liver function tests have emerged as the most common side effects of reductase inhibitor therapy requiring discontinuation of the drug (Tobert et al., 1990). A small number of patients, perhaps one per 100, develop persistent increases in serum transaminases, exceeding three times normal, and these high levels disappear when the drug is discontinued. Increased transaminase levels often return to normal when drug therapy is reinstituted. The possibility of hepatotoxicity, although relatively rare, requires periodic testing for liver function abnormalities. What is the mechanism for this "hepatotoxicity"? One possibility is that reduced cholesterol synthesis in the liver provides insufficient cholesterol to maintain the structural integrity of cell membranes; if so, hepatocellular enzymes may "leak" into the circulation. Whether such a mechanism could cause hepatic inflammation or long-term, chronic liver disease is not known. For the present, therefore, reductase inhibitors should not be continued in the face of persistent elevation of liver enzymes. In addition, periodic testing for abnormal elevations of liver enzymes is indicated.

G. Myopathy

Evidence of abnormalities in skeletal muscle function manifests in several ways. Some patients taking HMG CoA reductase inhibitors complain of muscle aches and weakness without objective evidence of muscle toxicity, i.e., increased levels of creatine kinase. When this occurs, does it indicate true myopathy? Clinical practice suggests that subjective muscle dysfunction occurs too frequently to be unrelated to drug therapy, but a definite connection is difficult to prove. Some patients appear to improve by reduction of dose. Perhaps up to 10% of patients treated with reductase inhibitors develop transient high levels of creatine kinase. This is more "objective" evidence of true myopathy, but again, elevations of creatine kinase levels occur periodically from other causes, and an absolute link with the drug is difficult to prove. In some patients, however, creatine kinase levels are increased severalfold, and these elevations are accompanied by subjective muscle symptoms; in such patients, mild myopathy due to reductase inhibitor therapy is a reasonable presumption. Reduction in dose is indicated, and if signs and symptoms abate, the patient can be rechallanged with a higher dose later. If symptoms recur, the dose can be lowered or the drug discontinued.

Very rarely, in approximately one in 1000 patients, reductase inhibitor therapy produces severe myopathy (Tobert et al., 1990). This response can occur without obvious evidence of precipitating causes. Severe myopathy is manifest by marked weakness and discomfort of muscle, extreme elevations of creatine kinase, myoglobinuria, and even acute tubular necrosis. The mechanism for this reaction is not understood. It typically occurs with high plasma levels of reductase inhibitor and metabolites that presumably act directly upon muscle tissue. As suggested above, synthesis of ubiquinone may be inhibited, or a reduction in cholesterol synthesis may limit availability of cholesterol for muscle membranes. Whatever the mechanism, the disorder appears to be self-limiting. Discontinuation of the drug promptly reverses the myopathy.

Severe myopathy occurs most commonly when HMG CoA reductase inhibitors are given concomitantly with certain other agents or conditions. For example, fibric acids also can cause myopathy, and when they are combined with reductase inhibitors, severe myopathy can result (Mevacor, 1990).

Drugs that may interfere with excretion of reductase inhibitors by the liver, e.g., nicotinic acid, cyclosporine, and possibly tetracycline, also can raise drug levels and precipitate severe myopathy. Finally, risk of myopathy is raised in patients taking HMG CoA reductase inhibitors who are severely ill, especially in those having chronic renal failure.

IV. INDICATIONS FOR HMG CoA REDUCTASE INHIBITORS

With the development of a powerful new class of drugs for treatment of hypercholesterolemia, the issue arises as to which people are candidates for therapy with HMG CoA reductase inhibitors. For example, 20–25% of the total adult population has been designated as having high blood cholesterol by the National Cholesterol Education Program (Expert Panel, 1988). Most of these people presumably are at increased risk for CHD. Therefore, among this vast number of individuals with high cholesterol levels, who should receive HMG CoA reductase inhibitors for cholesterol lowering? Certainly the population of hypercholesterolemic individuals is not homogeneous, and thus when considering candidates for reductase inhibitor therapy, patients can be separated into several categories of dyslipidemia. For each category unique questions emerge pertaining to appropriate use of HMG CoA reductase inhibitors.

A. Familial Hypercholesterolemia

This disorder is characterized by an inherited deficiency of LDL receptors (Goldstein and Brown, 1983). Normally, one functional gene for the LDL receptor is inherited from each parent, and both genes must encode for the LDL receptor for serum cholesterol levels to remain in the normal range. In about one in 500 people, one inherited gene is abnormal and does not properly encode for LDL receptors. The number of LDL receptors consequently is half-normal, and LDL cholesterol levels are approximately doubled. The resulting severe hypercholesterolemia greatly increases risk for CHD. This condition is called heterozygous FH. Rarely a person inherits abnormal genes from both parents, and the affected patient can synthesize no functioning LDL receptors. In this disorder, called homozygous FH, levels of LDL are increased at least fourfold, and CHD and other atherosclerotic complications frequently develop in the teens.

Are patients with homozygous FH candidates for treatment with HMG CoA reductase inhibitors? Unfortunately, in most FH homozygotes, these drugs are largely ineffective. Since the primary action of reductase inhibitors is to enhance formation of LDL receptors, a lack of ability to synthesize receptors negates their effectiveness (Uauy et al., 1988). Some patients with homozygous FH can produce a few LDL receptors, and in these, HMG CoA reductase inhibitors are mildly effective (Yamamoto et al., 1980; Thompson et al., 1986; Laue et al., 1987). They are of little value, however, in most patients with homozygous FH.

In contrast, these drugs potently reduce LDL levels in FH heterozygotes (Mabuchi et al., 1981; Bilheimer et al., 1983a,b; Illingworth and Sexton, 1984; Havel et al., 1987). Seemingly, they can stimulate the one normal LDL receptor gene to supranormal activity. For example, lovastatin therapy at doses of 20 mg twice daily reduces LDL cholesterol levels by about 30%. At twice this dose, levels fall by 35–40%. The efficacy of reductase inhibitors in FH heterozygotes thus is not at question. The issue, rather, is which of these patients should be treated. Categories to consider are adult men, premenopausal women, postmenopausal women, and adolescents. Heterozygous FH children below age 10 rarely should be treated with these drugs.

Adult men with heterozygous FH are at high risk for CHD. They often are victims of coronary disease in their 30s or 40s, and sometimes even in their 20s. HMG CoA reductase inhibitors therefore clearly are indicated in adult men with heterozygous FH. LDL cholesterol levels typically fall 30% when these drugs are used alone. However, since LDL levels usually are 50–60% above those of normal people, LDL levels rarely are normalized by drug therapy in FH heterozygotes. On the other hand, several studies (Mabuchi et al., 1983; Illingworth, 1984; Grundy et al., 1985; Vega et al., 1989) have shown that when reductase inhibitors are combined with bile acid seques-trants, LDL cholesterol concentrations are reduced 50–60%, thus normalizing the levels. Interruption of the enterohepatic circulation (EHC) of bile acids therefore adds substantially to the LDL-lowering action of reductase in-hibitors. An alternate way to interrupt the EHC of bile acids is by the ileal exclusion operation. We have shown that this operation combined with reductase inhibitors markedly lowers LDL levels (Grundy et al., 1985). The operation has not been widely accepted as a means for lowering serum cholesterol, but in selected male patients with heterozygous FH, who must look forward to a lifetime of cholesterol-lowering treatment, the ileal exclu-sion operation combined with HMG CoA reductase inhibitors can be justified.

Premenopausal women with heterozygous FH are less prone to premature CHD than are men. Therefore, should premenopausal women be treated with HMG CoA reductase inhibitors? To assist in making a decision about such therapy in premenopausal women, they might be divided into high-risk and low-risk groups. High-risk women are defined as those with unusually high levels of cholesterol (e.g., persistently over 325 mg/dl) or those with other CHD risk factors; the latter include clinical manifestations of atherosclerotic disease (e.g., angina pectoris), cigarette smoking, hypertension that is not easily controlled, low HDL cholesterol (less than 35 mg/dl), and diabetes mellitus. For premenopausal women who are deemed to be at high risk, HMG CoA reductase inhibitors are justified. Again, combining a reductase inhibitor with bile acid sequestrants will facilitate LDL lowering. On the other hand, in the absence of these added risk factors, a more cautious approach should be taken. Bile acid sequestrants certainly are indicated in FH women as the first step of therapy. Over the next few years additional information will be gained about the safety of reductase inhibitors in women, and if they are shown to be largely safe, their use might be extended to premenopausal women with FH. Even now, for consideration of their use, "low-risk" premenopausal women might be divided into two age groups, less than 35 years and older. Older women clearly are better candidates than younger ones.

After menopause, FH women lose their special protection against CHD. They often develop clinical CHD in their late 40s or 50s. Therefore, can HMG CoA reductase inhibitors be justified in postmenopausal women with heterozygous FH? Since risk for CHD increases so markedly in these women, most can be treated with reductase inhibitors. Like their male counterparts, women will benefit by use of bile acid sequestrants together with reductase inhibitors. Limited evidence suggests that older women are at somewhat greater risk for severe myopathy during therapy with HMG CoA reductase inhibitors than are men. Consequently, women must be alerted to this possible side effect, and they should be monitored carefully and frequently.

At present, it is difficult to justify use of HMG CoA reductase inhibitors in most FH teenagers. Teenage girls with heterozygous FH rarely if ever are candidates for such therapy. Bile acid sequestrants, however, might be used in these girls if they have unusually high cholesterol levels, but reductase inhibitors should be reserved until adulthood. Unfortunately, teenage boys with heterozygous FH are *not* protected against accelerated coronary atherosclerosis. Consequently, a major effort should be made to lower their cholesterol levels. Bile acid sequestrants should be employed first, and in many cases, they will be sufficient therapy. HMG CoA reductase inhibitors should be avoided in most teenage boys until more data on their safety for this group become available. Still, if levels of LDL cholesterol are severely elevated, low doses of reductase inhibitors together with bile acid resins can be justified, although the patients must be monitored carefully for side effects.

B. Primary Severe Hypercholesterolemia (Non-FH)

Some adults have total cholesterol levels that are persistently over 300 mg/dl or LDL-cholesterol concentrations over 220 mg/dl, and yet they do not have classical features of heterozygous FH, i.e., tendon xanthomas and hypercholesterolemia in 50% of first-degree relatives. Male patients with primary severe hypercholesterolemia are without doubt at high risk for CHD, although clinical manifestations of coronary disease usually occur later than in FH heterozygotes. Many of these patients probably did not have marked hypercholesterolemia early in life, as do FH heterozygotes; consequently, they are not exposed to severely elevated levels of LDL for as long as FH patients and thus have a somewhat delayed onset of CHD. Again, it may be useful to distinguish between men and women when deciding whether to use HMG CoA reductase inhibitors for this category of elevated LDL.

Men with primary severe hypercholesterolemia without question are good candidates for reductase inhibitor therapy. The best approach is to start with bile acid sequestrants and to monitor the response. If the reduction in LDL levels is not adequate, reductase inhibitors can be added as a second drug. In this way, the dose of both types of drug can be kept relatively low, and side effects will be minimized. For women with severe hypercholesterolemia, the same approach can be taken as for FH women. Reductase inhibitors, however, may not be indicated in hypercholesterolemic women over age 65, particularly if they have no other risk factors. Before starting an HMG CoA reductase inhibitor in an older woman, she should be judged to be a good candidate to obtain long-term benefit from serum cholesterol lowering (Vega and Grundy, 1987). It is rarely justified to begin use of HMG CoA reductase inhibitors in women who are 40–80 years old and who have no signs of CHD.

C. Primary Moderate Hypercholesterolemia

This condition can be defined as a total cholesterol level in the range of 240–300 mg/dl (LDL cholesterol 160–220 mg/dl). Many cases of moderate hypercholesterolemia have a major dietary component, and they can be managed adequately by reduced intake of saturated fatty acids and cholesterol, weight reduction, and regular exercise. A genetic element nonetheless contributes to moderately elevated LDL cholesterol in many patients, and they will remain significantly hypercholesterolemic in spite of maximal dietary therapy. Consideration thus must be given to drug therapy in patients of this type. Three categories of patients—low-risk men, high-risk men, and women—can be considered for reductase inhibitor therapy.

Low-Risk Men

This group includes men without other CHD risk factors who have LDL cholesterol levels in the range of 160–220 mg/dl. This category includes nonsmokers and those without hypertension, low HDL cholesterol, obesity, or diabetes, and those without clinical evidence of CHD or strong family history of premature CHD. Since men of this type are commonly seen in clinical practice, we must ask whether they are appropriate candidates for treatment with HMG CoA reductase inhibitors. Although opinion differs, we believe that these drugs are not first-line therapy. A stronger argument can be made that low-risk men with moderate hypercholesterolemia *are* good candidates for bile acid sequestrants, particularly given in relatively low doses (e.g., 8–10 g/day). It must be emphasized that drug therapy of any type should not be started on the basis of a single cholesterol measurement. Apparently high levels of LDL cholesterol frequently are not confirmed by follow-up measurements. At least three elevated LDL cholesterol levels thus should be obtained while a patient is on maximal dietary therapy to document hypercholesterolemia before starting a patient on life-long cholesterol-lowering therapy.

High-Risk Men

This category includes men with established CHD, other atherosclerotic disease, or a family history of premature CHD, cigarette smokers, those with documented, persistent hypertension, reduced HDL cholesterol (<35 mg/dl), or diabetes mellitus. Patients with diabetes will be discussed in more detail later. Other high-risk men who maintain moderate hypercholesterolemia in spite of maximal dietary therapy are good candidates for HMG CoA reductase inhibitors. Several studies (Grundy and Vega, 1985; Hoeg et al., 1986; Vega et al., 1990) attest to the efficacy of reductase inhibitors in this condition. In such patients, a maximal reduction of LDL cholesterol level should be the goal of therapy. Addition of bile acid sequestrants as a second drug will help to achieve this goal (Vega and Grundy, 1987). This drug combination seems especially appropriate in men who have established CHD and in whom maximal lowering of LDL levels might promote regression of coronary lesions (Blankenhorn et al., 1987).

Women

When approaching therapy in women with moderately elevated LDL cholesterol, assessment of CHD risk likewise is in order. An enormous number of women in the United States have moderate hypercholesterolemia (Expert Panel, 1988), and certainly not all of these women are good candidates for reductase inhibitor therapy. Dietary therapy should be tried first

(Expert Panel, 1988). For postmenopausal women, standard estrogen replacement therapy may assist in LDL lowering and also may raise HDL. Benefit from doses of estrogens exceeding standard replacement is not documented and may increase breast cancer risk. If a cholesterol-lowering drug is deemed essential, bile acid sequestrants are the first line of therapy. If they fail to lower LDL cholesterol levels to the target goal, HMG CoA reductase inhibitors should be used in relatively low doses *in addition* to bile acid sequestrants, not in place of them.

D. Primary Mixed Hyperlipidemia

A portion of patients with primary hypercholesterolemia, perhaps 10–20%, have a concomitant increase in serum triglycerides. When total cholesterol levels exceed 240 mg/dl and triglyceride levels are between 250 and 500 mg/dl, the condition can be called primary mixed hyperlipidemia. The higher triglycerides are mainly in the VLDL fraction. When triglyceride levels substantially exceed 500 mg/dl, chylomicrons usually are present, and the lipoprotein pattern is called type 5 hyperlipoproteinemia. In this discussion, the term "mixed hyperlipidemia" will be restricted to triglyceride levels between 250 and 500 mg/dl in addition to elevated cholesterol. The mechanisms underlying mixed hyperlipidemia are variable. Some patients probably have familial combined hyperlipidemia, a disorder reported to be characterized by overproduction of apo B–containing lipoproteins (Grundy et al., 1987). Another cause of primary mixed hyperlipidemia is the simultaneous inheritance of two or more defects in lipoprotein metabolism, e.g., defective lipolysis of triglyceride-rich lipoproteins and reduced activity of LDL receptors. In the latter instance, primary mixed hyperlipidemia can be considered a polygenic disorder. Moreover, obesity often is a compounding factor raising both triglyceride and cholesterol levels.

Definitive therapy for primary mixed hyperlipidemia has not been developed. Perhaps the best drug is nicotinic acid. This drug interferes with secretion of lipoproteins by the liver, and thereby lowers both VLDL and LDL levels; at the same time, it raises HDL cholesterol concentrations. To date, however, nicotinic acid has not been tested systematically for treatment of mixed hyperlipidemia. This drug, furthermore, can cause a variety of side effects; these include gastrointestinal distress, flushing of the skin, itching, skin rash, hepatotoxicity, worsening of glucose tolerance, and hyperuricemia. Rarely, nicotinic acid causes acanthosis nigracans, arrhythmias, exacerbation of peptic ulcer or chronic bowel disease, or toxic amblyopia. Perhaps no more than 50% of patients can tolerate nicotinic acid in therapeutic doses on a long-term basis. Regular nicotinic acid is accompanied by less hepatotoxicity than sustained-release preparations. Nonetheless, for selected patients with mixed hyperlipidemia, nicotinic acid may be the drug of choice.

Another approach to mixed hyperlipidemia is to employ combined drug therapy. The combination of a fibric acid and bile acid sequestrant may be effective in some patients, but it will not normalize lipid levels in those with more severe hyperlipidemia (East et al., 1988). The combination of a fibric acid and HMG CoA reductase inhibitor is better for lipid lowering (East et al., 1988; Vega and Grundy, in press). Like nicotinic acid, this drug combination lowers both VLDL and LDL levels and raises HDL concentrations. Moreover, it generally is tolerated much better than nicotinic acid. Unfortunately, however, about one in 20 patients taking a fibric acid plus HMG CoA reductase inhibitor will develop severe myopathy and myoglobinuria. For this reason, the combination cannot be recommended for routine use and must be avoided except in highly selected cases.

Finally, consideration can be given to using an HMG CoA reductase inhibitor alone. We recently carried out a study on the effectiveness of lovastatin in patients with primary mixed hyperlipidemia (Vega and Grundy, in press). Lovastatin therapy produced a moderate reduction in VLDL triglyceride concentrations. It also markedly reduced both LDL cholesterol and total apo B levels. Although it failed to give a substantial increase in HDL-cholesterol levels, the favorable response in apo B–containing lipoproteins makes it a viable alternative to other lipid-lowering regimens for primary mixed hyperlipidemia. Indeed, use of an HMG CoA reductase inhibitor as a single agent may be the most practical mode of therapy for this condition.

E. Diabetic Dyslipidemia

One of the most common forms of secondary dyslipidemia is that induced by diabetes, especially non–insulin-dependent diabetes mellitus (NIDDM). Several lipoprotein abnormalities can occur in NIDDM (Howard, 1987). Hypertriglyceridemia is the most common, and elevated triglycerides often secondarily reduce HDL cholesterol levels. LDL cholesterol concentrations are not notably increased in many diabetic patients, but this appearance can be deceiving. In different diabetic populations, the frequency of CHD appears to be a function of LDL cholesterol levels (Garg and Grundy, 1990). Those populations having high rates of CHD typically have higher LDL concentrations than populations having low LDL levels. This relationship can be illustrated by comparing CHD rates in Pima Indians and Caucasian Americans (Ingelfinger et al., 1976). Pima Indian diabetics usually have total cholesterol levels in the range of 170–180 mg/dl (Howard et al., 1984), and they manifest little CHD (Ingelfinger et al., 1976). Caucasian diabetics in the United States in contrast have a mean total cholesterol of 210–220 mg/dl (Expert Panel, 1988), and their CHD rates are much higher than those of Pimas. Of interest, levels of triglycerides and HDL are similar for Pimas and Caucasians with NIDDM. This comparison suggests that differences in cholesterol levels determine relative risk for CHD to a greater extent in diabetic patients than do serum levels of triglycerides and HDL. The difference also suggests that lowering of cholesterol levels in Caucasians could yield a major decrease in CHD risk.

What then is the role of HMG CoA reductase inhibitors for treatment of diabetic dyslipidemia? They may be the drugs of choice since other drugs often are not satisfactory for diabetic patients. For example, although nicotinic acid has a favorable effect on diabetic dyslipidemia, it worsens glucose tolerance; therefore, it probably should not be used routinely in most diabetic patients. NIDDM patients also may be more prone to the other side effects of nicotinic acid (e.g., hyperuricemia). Bile acid sequestrants have two disadvantages: 1) they raise triglyceride levels, which already may be high in NIDDM patients, and 2) they promote constipation, which is common in diabetic patients. Like nicotinic acid, the fibric acids have the advantage of lowering triglyceride levels and raising HDL cholesterol, but in contrast to nicotinic acid, they do not reduce total apo B concentrations and can even increase LDL cholesterol levels when used in NIDDM patients with hypertriglyceridemia (Pyorala et al., 1987).

Because of the limitations of other lipid-lowering drugs in diabetic patients, HMG CoA reductase inhibitors probably are the best choice for treatment of dyslipidemia in most NIDDM patients. One study carried out in our laboratory (Garg and Grundy, 1988) supports this concept. In 16 diabetic patients, lovastatin therapy caused a marked lowering in plasma total cholesterol, LDL cholesterol, VLDL cholesterol, and LDL–apo B levels. These changes were accompanied by a moderate reduction in triglyceride levels and a modest rise in HDL cholesterol levels. Lovastatin therapy was well tolerated in this study, and no worsening of glucose tolerance was noted. None of our patients developed myopathy or significant abnormalities of liver function tests. Thus diabetic patients seemingly are not unusually prone to adverse responses from HMG CoA reductase inhibitors. Of interest, during lovastatin therapy total cholesterol and LDL cholesterol concentrations of our Caucasian patients fell into the range normally found in Pima Indians (Howard et al., 1984). If the low rates of CHD in Pimas truly can be explained by their relatively low concentrations of serum cholesterol, the reduction in cholesterol concentrations by lovastatin therapy in our Caucasian patients should be accompanied by a marked decrease in risk for CHD.

The potential usefulness of HMG CoA reductase inhibitors for reduction of CHD risk in diabetic patients is suggested by the observation that CHD is the number one killer of diabetic patients and approximately 50% of newly diagnosed cases of NIDDM already have evidence of CHD at time of diagnosis (Pyorala et al., 1987; Laakso et al., 1988). These observations indicate a need for early diagnosis of NIDDM and for early institution of cholesterol-lowering therapy. If HMG CoA reductase inhibitors prove to be safe in long-term therapy of NIDDM patients, they could constitute a major step forward in the prevention of CHD in these patients. Certainly, a clinical trial of reductase inhibitors for their effectiveness in reduction of CHD risk in NIDDM patients is needed.

F. Nephrotic Dyslipidemia

Another secondary dyslipidemia is that associated with the nephrotic syndrome. There is growing evidence that nephrotic dyslipidemia enhances the risk for CHD (Berlyne and Mallick, 1969; Mallick and Short, 1981). The major lipoprotein abnormality in the nephrotic syndrome is an elevation of serum LDL cholesterol (Baxter, 1962). This abnormality is considered by most investigators to be the result of overproduction of apo B–containing lipoproteins by the liver in response to loss of protein in the urine (Marsh, 1984). Another plasma lipid abnormality commonly observed in nephrotic patients is hypertriglyceridemia, and thus nephrotic dyslipidemia frequently is a mixed hyperlipidemia. Experience with lipid-lowering drugs in hyperlipidemic patients with the nephrotic syndrome is limited. Patients with nephrotic hypercholesterolemia have been shown to respond to bile acid sequestrants, but rarely do LDL cholesterol concentrations fall to the desirable range (Valeri et al., 1986; Rabelink et al., 1988). Fibric acid derivatives will lower triglyceride levels, but not LDL cholesterol or total apo B concentrations. Nicotinic acid might be the drug of choice for treatment of nephrotic dyslipidemia because it theoretically will reverse the underlying defect, namely, hepatic overproduction of lipoproteins. In spite of this potential, nicotinic acid has never been tested systematically in the nephrotic syndrome, and it could have too many side effects for most nephrotic patients. Probucol, another cholesterol-lowering drug, does produce some serum cholesterol lowering in nephrotic patients, but again, the reduction is modest. Thus, before the advent of HMG CoA reductase inhibitors, prospects for successful treatment of nephrotic dyslipidemia with drugs was bleak.

Several studies (Vega and Grundy, 1988; Rabelink et al., 1988; Golper et al., 1989) have revealed that HMG CoA reductase inhibitors will effectively lower cholesterol levels in nephrotic patients. A study from our laboratory

(Vega and Grundy, 1988) indicated that lovastatin will reduce serum levels of both LDL cholesterol and VLDL cholesterol in nephrotic dyslipidemia. Our results are consistent with the primary effect of lovastatin therapy being to increase the activity of LDL receptors. Other investigators have reported a similar favorable effect of both lovastatin (Golper et al., 1989) and simvastatin (Rabelink et al., 1988) in nephrotic hypercholesterolemia. To date, no serious side effects have been reported during treatment of nephrotic patients with HMG CoA reductase inhibitors. Still, the number of patients treated with reductase inhibitors has been relatively small, and further investigations are required before these drugs can be recommended without reservations in hyperlipidemic patients with nephrotic syndrome.

G. Hypoalphalipoproteinemia

A low level of HDL cholesterol (hypoalphalipoproteinemia) is a major risk factor for CHD. This relationship has been demonstrated most clearly in population studies (Miller and Miller, 1975; Castelli et al., 1977; Goldbourt et al., 1985). The mechanisms whereby a low HDL concentration raises the risk for CHD are not fully understood, but three theories have been set forth. First, a low HDL cholesterol often accompanies other CHD risk factors—smoking, obesity, lack of exercise, and diabetes mellitus; in these cases, a low HDL may not be directly atherogenic, but merely carry "guilt by association." Although at least part of the HDL–CHD link might be explained by this mechanism, other explanations likely pertain as well. Second, a low HDL cholesterol level can be secondary to high concentrations of apo B–containing lipoproteins, and these latter lipoproteins may be directly atherogenic; this too could account for the association between low HDL and CHD. And third, HDL directly protect against development of atherosclerosis, possibly by mobilizing cholesterol from the arterial wall. Regardless of mechanism, a low HDL level is at least a marker for increased CHD, and when it is present, attention must be given to the risk status of the patient.

If a low HDL is secondary to other CHD risk factors, the attempt should be made to modify these factors. Patients should be admonished to stop smoking, lose weight if they are obese, and exercise more. Moreover, if serum concentrations of apo B–containing lipoproteins are increased, they should be reduced—by diet if possible, and if not, by drug therapy. These two approaches generally will raise HDL cholesterol, at least to some extent. Finally, if drugs are to be employed, consideration can be given to which drugs may be appropriate.

The agent that has the greatest effect on HDL cholesterol levels probably is nicotinic acid (Shepherd et al., 1979; Atmeh et al., 1983), and it might be considered the drug of choice for treatment of dyslipidemic patients in whom a low HDL level is one abnormality. Although nicotinic acid probably should be tried first, many patients have significant side effects that preclude its long-term use. A second class of drugs that will raise HDL levels includes the fibric acids. Like nicotinic acid, the fibric acids exert this effect by reducing triglyceride-rich lipoproteins. In the Helsinki Heart Study (Frick et al., 1987; Manninen et al., 1988), the action of gemfibrozil to raise the HDL cholesterol was postulated to be one mechanism whereby gemfibrozil therapy reduces risk for CHD. Finally, HMG CoA reductase inhibitors can cause a modest rise in HDL cholesterol levels accompanying a decrease in concentration of apo B–containing lipoproteins. Although the degree of rise in HDL cholesterol level may be one indication of beneficial response to drug therapy, the extent of lowering of apo B–containing lipoproteins may be another. In general, nicotinic acid and gemfibrozil are good agents to lower triglyceride-rich lipoproteins and raise HDL cholesterol, although nicotinic acid generally produces the better response. HMG CoA reductase inhibitors usually give the best lowering of all apo B–containing lipoproteins, but the rise in HDL cholesterol levels often is modest.

An important but unresolved question is whether drug therapy is indicated for patients with low HDL cholesterol levels in whom concentrations of total cholesterol and triglycerides are in the "normal" range. There is growing evidence that such patients are at increased risk for CHD, and drug therapy may be particularly appropriate if a patient has existing atherosclerotic disease. Although nicotinic acid may be the drug of first choice for such patients, it is not always tolerated. For this reason, we recently carried out a study in which gemfibrozil and lovastatin therapies were compared in 22 normolipidemic patients who had hypoalphalipoproteinemia (Vega and Grundy, 1989). In this study, treatment with either gemfibrozil or lovastatin produced moderate increases in HDL cholesterol; for both, HDL levels increased about 11%. In addition, both drugs caused similar reductions of VLDL triglycerides and VLDL cholesterol concentrations. They differed in another important way, however. Gemfibrozil therapy did not cause a significant decrease in plasma levels of LDL cholesterol or total apo B. Lovastatin therapy, in contrast, caused marked decreases in both LDL cholesterol and total apo B concentrations. Further, lovastatin therapy caused greater improvement in the LDL/HDL ratio than did gemfibrozil. These results indicate that lovastatin therapy produces a better overall change in lipoprotein pattern in normolipidemic patients with low HDL cholesterol than gemfibrozil therapy. For this reason, if drug therapy is to be considered for normolipidemic patients with hypoalphalipoproteinemia, and if nicotinic acid cannot be tolerated, lovastatin would appear to be the drug of next choice.

V. CONCLUSIONS

In summary, HMG CoA reductase inhibitors represent a major advance in pharmacological control of dyslipidemia. Clearly, they are indicated in patients with severe hypercholesterolemia. But in addition, these drugs may have utility in other forms of dyslipidemia—mixed hyperlipidemia, diabetic dyslipidemia, nephrotic hypercholesterolemia, and hypoalphalipoprotein-emia. Further research, therefore, is indicated in these conditions to determine the role of HMG CoA reductase inhibitors.

REFERENCES

Alberts, A. W., Chen, J., Kuron, G., Hunt, V., et al. (1980). Mevinolin: A highly potent competitive inhibitor of hydroxy-methylglutaryl-coenzyme A reductase and a cholesterol lowering agent. *Proc. Natl. Acad. Sci. USA* **77**:3957–3961 (Abstract).

Atmeh, R. F., Shepherd, J., and Packard, C. J. (1983). Subpopulations of apolipoprotein A-I in human high-density lipoproteins: their metabolic properties and response to drug therapy. *Biochem. Biophys. Acta* **751**:175–188.

Baxter, J. H. (1962). Hyperlipoproteinemia in nephrosis. *Arch. Intern. Med.* **109**:742–757.

Berlyne, G. M., and Mallick, N. P. (1969). Ischaemic heart-disease as a complication of nephrotic syndrome. *Lancet* **2**:399–400.

Bilheimer, D. W., Grundy, S. M., Brown, M. S., and Goldstein, J. L. (1983a). Mevinolin and colestipol stimulate receptor-mediated clearance of low density lipoprotein from plasma in familial hypercholesterolemia heterozygotes. *Proc. Natl. Acad. Sci. USA* **80**:4124–4128.

Bilheimer, D. W., Grundy, S. M., Brown, M. S., and Goldstein, J. L. (1983b). Mevinolin stimulates receptor-mediated clearance of low density lipoprotein from plasma in familial hypercholesterolemia heterozygotes. *Trans. Assoc. Am. Physicians* **96**:1–9.

Blankenhorn, D. M., Nessim, S. A., Johnson, R. L., Sanmarco, M. E., Azen, S. P., and Cashin-Hemphill, L. (1987). Beneficial effects of combined colestipol-niacin therapy on coronary atherosclerosis and coronary venous bypass grafts. *JAMA* **257**:3233–3240.

Castelli, W. P., Doyle, J. T., Gordon, T., et al., (1977). HDL cholesterol and other lipids in coronary heart disease. The cooperative lipoprotein phenotyping study. *Circulation* **55**:767–772.

Denke, M. A., and Grundy, S. M. (1990). Hypercholesterolemia in the elderly: Resolving the treatment dilemma. *Ann. Intern. Med.* **112**:780–792.

Duane, W. C., Hunninghake, D. B., Freeman, M. L., Pooler, P. A., Schlasner, L. A., and Gebhard, R. L. (1988). Simvastatin, a competitive inhibitor of HMG-CoA reductase, lowers cholesterol saturation index of gallbladder bile. *Hepatology* **8**:1147–1150.

East, C., Bilheimer, D. W., and Grundy, S. M. (1988). Combination drug therapy for familial combined hyperlipidemia. *Ann. Intern. Med.* **109**:25–32

Endo, A., Kuroda, M., and Tsujita, Y. (1976a). ML-236A, ML-236B, and ML 236C, new inhibitors of cholesterogenesis produced by *Penicillum citrinum*. *J. Antibiot.* (Tokyo) **29**:1346–1348.

Endo, A., Kuroda, M., and Tanzawa, K. (1976b). Competitive inhibition of 3-hydroxy-3-methyl-glutaryl coenzyme: A reductase by ML-236A and ML-236B fungal metabolites, having hypocholesterolemic activity. *FEBS Lett.* **72**:323–326.

The Expert Panel. (1988). Report of the National Cholesterol Education Program Expert Panel on detection, evaluation, and treatment of high blood cholesterol in adults. *Arch. Intern. Med.* **148**:36–69.

Farnsworth, W. H., Hoeg, J. M., Maher, M., Brittain, E. H., Sherins, R. J., and Brewer, H. B., Jr. (1987). Testicular function in type II hyperlipoproteinemic patients treated with lovastatin (mevinolin) or neomycin. *J. Clin. Endocrinol. Metab.* **65**:546–550.

Frick, M. H., Elo, M. O., Haapa, K., et al. (1987). Helsinki Heart Study: Primary prevention trial with gemfibrozil in middle-aged men with dyslipidemia. *N. Engl. J. Med.* **317**:1237–1245.

Garg, A., and Grundy, S. M. (1988). Lovastatin for lowering cholesterol levels in non-insulin-dependent diabetes mellitus. *N. Engl. J. Med.* **318**:81–86.

Garg, A., and Grundy, S. M. (1989). Gemfibrozil alone and in combination with lovastatin for treatment of hypertriglyceridemia in NIDDM. *Diabetes* **38**:364–372.

Garg, A., and Grundy, S. M. (1990). Management of dyslipidemia in NIDDM. *Diabetes Care,* **13**:153–169.

Ginsberg, H. N., Le, N-A., Short, M. P., Ramakrishnan, R., and Desnick, R. J. (1987). Suppression of apolipoprotein B production during treatment of cholesteryl storage disease with lovastatin: Implications for regulation of apolipoprotein B synthesis. *J. Clin. Invest.* **80**:1692–1697.

Goldbourt, V., Holtzman, E., and Neufeld, H. N. (1985). Total and high density lipoprotein cholesterol in the serum and risk of mortality: Evidence of a threshold effect. *Br. Med. J.* **290**:1239–1243.

Goldstein, J. L., and Brown, M. S. (1979). The LDL receptor locus and the genetics of familial hypercholesterolemia. *Annu. Rev. Genet.* **13**:259–289.

Goldstein, J. L., and Brown, M. S. (1983). Familial hypercholesterolemia. In *The Metabolic Basis of Inherited Disease*. 5th Ed. Edited by J. B. Stanbury, J. B. Wyngaarden, D. S. Fredrickson, J. L. Goldstein, and M. S. Brown. New York, McGraw-Hill, pp. 672–713.

Golper, T. A.: Illingworth, D. R., Morris, C. D., and Bennett, W. M. (1989). Lovastatin in the treatment of multifactorial hyperlipidemia associated with proteinemia. *Am. J. Kidney Dis.* **13**:312–320.

Grundy, S. M., and Bilheimer, D. W. (1984). Influence of inhibition of 3-hydroxy-3-methylglutaryl-CoA by reductase by mevinolin in familial hypercholesterolemia heterozygotes: Effects on cholesterol balance. *Proc. Natl. Acad. Sci. USA* **81:**2538–2542.

Grundy, S. M., and Vega, G. L., (1985). Influence of mevinolin on metabolism of low density lipoproteins in primary moderate hypercholesterolemia. *J. Lipid Res.* **26:**1464–1475.

Grundy, S. M., Chait, A., and Brunzell, J. D. (1987). Familial combined hyperlipidemia workshop. *Arteriosclerosis* **7:**203–207.

Grundy, S. M., Vega, G. L., and Bilheimer, D. W. (1985). Influence of combined therapy with mevinolin and interruption of bile-acid reabsorption on low density lipoproteins in heterozygous familial hypercholesterolemia. *Ann. Intern. Med.* **103:**339–343.

Havel, R. J., Hunninghake, D. B., Illingworth, D. R., et al. (1987). Lovastatin (mevinolin) in the treatment of heterozygous familial hypercholesterolemia: A multicenter study. *Ann. Intern. Med.* **107:**609–615.

Hoeg, J. M., Maher, M. B., Zech, L. A., et al. (1986). Effectiveness of mevinolin on plasma lipoprotein concentrations in type II hyperlipoproteinemia. *Am. J. Cardiol.* **57:**933–939.

Hoffman, W. F., Alberts, A. W., Anderson, P. S., Chen, J. S., Smith, R. L., and Willard, A. K. (1986). 3-Hydroxy-3-methylglutaryl coenzyme A reductase inhibitors. 4. Side chain ester derivatives of mevinolin. *J. Med. Chem.* **29:**849–852.

Howard, B. V. (1987). Lipoprotein metabolism in diabetes mellitus. *J. Lipid Res.* **28:**613.

Howard, B. V., Knowler, W. C., Vasquez, B., Kennedy, A. L., Petitt, D. J., and Bennett, P. H. (1984). Plasma and lipoprotein cholesterol and triglyceride in the Pima Indian population; comparison of diabetics and nondiabetics. *Arteriosclerosis* **4:**462.

Illingworth, D. R. (1984). Mevinolin plus colestipol in therapy for severe heterozygous familial hypercholesterolemia. *Ann. Intern. Med.* **101:**598–604.

Illingworth, D. R. (1987). Long term administration of lovastatin in the treatment of hypercholesterolemia. *Eur. Heart J.* **8** (Suppl E):103–111.

Illingworth, D. R., and Bacon, S. (1987). Hypolipidemic effects of HMG-CoA reductase inhibitors in patients with hypercholesterolemia. *Am. J. Cardiol.* **60:**33G–42G.

Illingworth, D. R., and Corbin, D. (1985). The influence of mevinolin on the adrenal cortical response to corticotropin in heterozygous familial hypercholesterolemia. *Proc. Natl. Acad. Sci. USA* **82:**6291–6294.

Illingworth, D. R., and Sexton, G. J. (1984). Hypocholesterolemic effects of mevinolin in patients with heterozygous familial hypercholesterolemia. *J. Clin. Invest.* **74:**1972–1978.

Ingelfinger, J. A., Bennett, P. H., Liebow, I. M., and Miller, M. (1976). Coronary heart disease in Pima Indians: Electrocardiographic findings and postmortem evidence of myocardial infarction in a population with high prevalence of diabetes mellitus. *Diabetes* **25:**561–565.

Laakso, M., Ronnemaa, T., Pyorala, K., Kallio, V., Puukka, P., and Penttila, I.

(1988). Atherosclerotic vascular disease and its risk factors in non-insulin-dependent diabetic and nondiabetic subjects in Finland. *Diabetes Care* **11**:449–463.

Laue, L., Hoeg, J. M., Barnes, K., Loriaux, D. L., and Chrousos, G. P. (1987). The effect of mevinolin on steroidogenesis in patients with defects in the low density lipoprotein receptor pathway. *J. Clin. Endocrinol. Metab.* **64**:531–535.

The Lovastatin Study Group II. (1986). Therapeutic response to lovastatin (mevinolin) in nonfamilial hypercholesterolemia: A multicenter study. *JAMA* **256**:2829–2834.

Mabuchi, H., Haba, T., Tatami, R., et al. (1981). Effects of an inhibitor of 3-hydroxy-3-methylglutaryl coenzyme A reductase on serum lipoproteins and ubiquinone-10-levels in patients with familial hypercholesterolemia. *N. Engl. J. Med.* **305**:478–482.

Mabuchi, H., Sakai, T., Sakai, Y., et al. (1983), Reduction of serum cholesterol in heterozygous patients with familial hypercholesterolemia: Additive effects of compactin and cholestyramine. *N. Engl. J. Med.* **308**:609–613.

Mallick, N. P., and Short, C. D. (1981). The nephrotic syndrome and ischemic heart disease. *Nephron.* **27**:54–57.

Manninen, V., Elo, M. O., Frick, M. H., et al. (1988). Lipid alterations and decline in the incidence of coronary heart disease in the Helsinki Heart Study. *JAMA* **260**:641–651.

Marsh, J. B. (1984). Lipoprotein metabolism in experimental nephrosis. *J. Lipid Res.* **25**:1619–1623.

Mevacor (Lovastatin, MSD). (1990). United States Food and Drug Administration package insert. West Point, PA, Merck and Company.

Miller, G. J., and Miller, N. E. (1975). Plasma high density lipoprotein concentration and development of ischaemic heart disease. *Lancet* **1**:16–19.

Pappu, A. S., Bacon, S. P., and Illingworth, D. R. (1987). The influence of lovastatin (mevinolin) on 24 hour urinary mevalonate acid in familial hypercholesterolemia. *Clin Res.* **35**:62A.

Parker, T. S., McNamara, D. J., Brown, C. D., et al. (1984). Plasma mevalonate as a measure of cholesterol synthesis in man. *J. Clin. Invest.* **74**:795–804.

Pyorala, K., Laakso, M., and Uusitupa, M. (1987). Diabetes and atherosclerosis: An epidemiologic view. *Diabetes Metab. Rev.* **3**:463–524.

Rabelink, A. J., Erkelens, D. W., Hene, R. J., Joles, J. A., and Koomans, H. A. (1988). Effects of simvastatin and cholestyramine on lipoprotein profile in hyperlipidemia of nephrotic syndrome. *Lancet* **2**:1335–1338.

Schaefer, E. J. (1988). HMG CoA reductase inhibitors for hypercholesterolemia. *N. Engl. J. Med.* **319**:1222.

Shepherd, J., Packard, C. J., Patsch, J. R., Gotto, A. M., Jr., and Taunton, O. D. (1979). Effects of nicotinic acid on plasma high-density lipoprotein subfraction distribution and composition and on apolipoprotein A metabolism. *J. Clin. Invest.* **63**:858–867.

Shigematsu, H., Hata, Y., Yamamoto, M., et al. (1979). Treatment of hyper-cholesterolemia with a HMG CoA reductase inhibitor (CS-500). I. Phase I study in normal subjects. *Geriatr. Med.* (Japan) **17**:1564–1570.

Thompson, G. R., Ford, J., Jenkinson, M., and Trayner, I. (1986). Efficacy of mevinolin and adjunct therapy for refractory familial hypercholesterolemia. *Q. J. Med.* **60**:803–811.

Tobert, J. A., Bell, G. D., Birtwell, J., et al. (1982). Cholesterol-lowering effect of mevinolin, an inhibitor of 3-hydroxy-3-methylglutaryl coenzyme A reductase, in healthy volunteers. *J. Clin. Invest.* **69**:1913–919.

Tobert, J. A., Shear, C. L., Chremos, A. N., and Mantell, G. E. (1990). Clinical experience with lovastatin. *Amer. J. Cardiol.* **65**:23F–26F.

Tsujita, Y., Kuroda, M., Tanzawa, K., Kitano, N., and Endo, A. (1979). Hypolipidemic effects in dogs of ML-236B, a competitive inhibitor of 3-hydroxy-3-methylglutaryl coenzyme A reductase. *Atherosclerosis* **32**:307–313.

Uauy, R., Vega, G. L., Grundy, S. M., and Bilheimer, D. M. (1988). Lovastatin therapy in receptor-negative homozygous familial hypercholesterolemia: Lack of effect on low-density lipoprotein concentrations or turnover. *J. Pediatr.* **113**:387–392.

Valeri, A., Gelfand, J., Blum, C., and Appel, G. B. (1986). Treatment of the hyperlipidemia of the nephrotic syndrome: A controlled trial. *Am. J. Kid. Dis.* **8**:388–396.

Vega, G. L., and Grundy, S. M. (1987). Treatment of primary moderate hyper-cholesterolemia with lovastatin (mevinolin) and colestipol. *JAMA* **257**:33–38.

Vega, G. L., and Grundy, S. M. (1988). Lovastatin therapy in nephrotic hyperlipid-emia: Effects on lipoprotein metabolism. *Kidney Int.* **33**:1160–1168.

Vega, G. L., and Grundy, S. M. (1989). Comparison of lovastatin and gemfibrozil in normolipidemic patients with hypoalphalipoproteinemia. *JAMA* **262**:3148–3153.

Vega, G. L., and Grundy, S. M. (1990). Management of primary mixed hyperli-pidemia with lovastatin. *Arch. Int. Med.* **150**:1313–1319.

Vega, G. L., East, C., and Grundy, S. M. (1988). Lovastatin therapy in familial dysbetalipoproteinemia: effects on kinetics of apolipoprotein B. *Atherosclerosis* **70**:131–143.

Vega, G. L., East, C., and Grundy, S. M. (1989). Effects of combined therapy with lovastatin and colestipol in heterozygous FH: Effects on kinetics of apolipoprotein B. *Arteriosclerosis* **9**:I-135–I-144.

Vega, G. L., Krauss, R. M., and Grundy, S. M. (1990). Pravastatin therapy in primary moderate hypercholesterolemia: Changes in metabolism of apolipoprotein B-containing lipoproteins. *J. Intern. Med.* **227**:81–94.

Yamamoto, A., Sudo, H., and Endo, A. (1980). Therapeutic effects of ML-236B in primary hypercholesterolemia. *Atherosclerosis* **35**:259–266.

8

Probucol

Daniel Steinberg and Joseph L. Witztum
University of California, San Diego
La Jolla, California

I. INTRODUCTION

In this chapter we review the salient points regarding the pharmacology and clinical uses of probucol (Fig. 1). Even though this drug has been used clinically for lowering plasma cholesterol levels for almost 20 years, the exact mechanism of action remains uncertain. Probucol does not fit into any of the general categories of cholesterol-lowering agents (i.e., it is not a bile acid sequestrant, a reductase inhibitor, a fibric acid derivative, etc.). Recent studies have called attention to the antioxidant properties of the drug, but, as discussed below, there is still no evidence in man that this antioxidant property confers any additional benefit in management of hypercholesterolemia. A clear and comprehensive review has recently appeared (Buckley et al., 1989), which includes extensive documentation of the literature on probucol. We recommend that excellent review to those who want a complete survey. In this chapter, we confine ourselves primarily to some of the background relating directly or indirectly to the clinical uses of probucol.

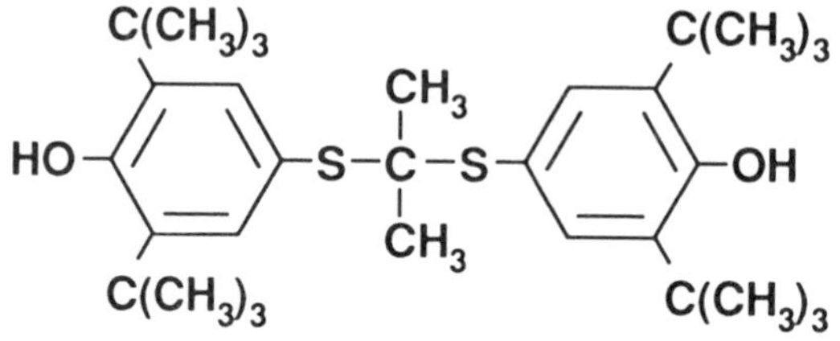

Figure 1 Structure of probucol:4,4'-isopropylidenedithio) bis (2,6-di-*t*-butylphe-nol). The two tertiarybutylphenol substituents, closely analogous in structure to *t*-butyl-hydroxytoluene, suggest a strong antioxidant potential.

II. MECHANISM OF ACTION

A. Effects on Plasma Lipoprotein Levels

Both in animals and in man the major effect of probucol is to decrease plasma cholesterol levels with little or no effect on triglyceride levels. Both LDL and HDL fall, the percentage decrease in HDL being generally equal to or greater than that in LDL (see Table 1). There still remains uncertainty about the underlying mechanism by which these changes are brought about.

The fall in LDL levels in patients is associated with an increase in its fractional catabolic rate (Nestel and Billington, 1981; Kesaniemi and Grundy, 1984). This is true also in patients with the homozygous form of familial hypercholesterolemia (Baker et al., 1982; Yamamoto et al., 1983), and since these patients lack the LDL receptor it appears that the increase in fractional catabolic rate can occur by way of receptor-independent pathways. However, the large increase in removal rate in patients with normal receptors, in which case only about one fourth of removal is receptor-independent, suggests that receptor-dependent uptake is also enhanced. An increase in fractional catabolic rate has also been reported in LDL receptor–deficient rabbits (Naruszewicz et al., 1984). In the studies of Naruszewicz et al. it was shown that LDL taken from a probucol-treated donor animal and injected into an untreated recipient animal showed a higher fractional catabolic rate than the normal LDL. Thus, there is evidence that the treatment with probucol leads to a modification of the LDL molecule such that its intrinsic removal rate is increased. There are a number of changes in the composition of LDL associated with probucol treatment (Lock et al., 1983; Naruszewicz et al., 1984) as is the case with a number of other drugs used in the treatment of hypercholesterolemia (Witz-tum et al., 1985; Young et al., 1989). Whether it is these changes in composition or the presence of the probucol molecule itself in the LDL particle that increases its catabolic rate remains to be established.

Table 1 Effects of Probucol on Lipoprotein Levels

No. of patients	Total cholesterol	LDL cholesterol	HDL cholesterol	Ref.
Used as a single agent:				
30	−14	−17	−25	LeLorier et al., 1977
27	−13	−16	−14	Riesen et al., 1980
19	−11	−8	−26	Mellies et al., 1980
20	−13	−13	−21	Hunninghake et al., 1980
31	−10	−9	−30	Davignon et al., 1988
47	−14	−12	−32	Dujovne et al., 1984
32	−11	−10	−23	Hulve and Tikkanen, 1988
17	−15	−14	−29	Witztum et al., 1989b
80	−11	−9	−27	Pietro et al., 1989
Used with bile sequestrant resin:				
17	−17	−9	−25	Current report
47	−10	−6	−29	Dujovne et al., 1984
44	−26	−21	−29	Kuo et al., 1986
Used with lovastatin:				
8	−11	−8	−33	Lees et al., 1986
17	−6	0	−24	Witztum et al., 1989b

Shown are selected studies from the literature of the effects of probucol on plasma lipoprotein levels. Results shown are the changes (% change from baseline) observed in response to probucol administration compared to preprobucol values. In these studies all patients had hypercholesterolemia with Type II or IIB phenotypes.

It should be noted that the responses of the receptor-deficient (WHHL) rabbit are variable for reasons not yet clarified. Carew et al. (1987), using a protocol essentially the same as that used by Naruszewicz et al. (1984), found a much smaller effect of probucol treatment (using the same dosage, i.e., 1% by weight in the diet) on LDL levels in WHHL rabbits and therefore, not unexpectedly, very little effect on the fractional catabolic rate of LDL.

A small effect on the rate of cholesterol biosynthesis has been observed in vitro (Anastasi et al., 1980; Barnhart et al., 1988) but there are no in vivo studies or clinical studies to further assess this effect. The absence of any effects on triglyceride levels speaks somewhat against inhibition of cholesterol synthesis as a major mechanism of action, since in that case one might expect a decrease in VLDL production and VLDL levels as well, at least in some patients.

As mentioned above, the drop in HDL levels frequently exceeds the drop in LDL levels. Total HDL cholesterol can fall as much as 20–30%, and this response is quite consistent in clinical practice (see Table 1). In addition to decreased HDL cholesterol levels, a reduction in average HDL particle size has also been reported (Yamamoto et al., 1986; Johansson and Walldius, 1988). It has been suggested that this is related to changes in reverse cholesterol transport (see below). Plasma levels of apoprotein AI also drop (Atmeh et al., 1983; Helve and Tikkanen, 1988), but there is disagreement with regard to effects on apoprotein AII levels (Mellies et al., 1980; Schonfeld et al., 1982; Atmeh et al., 1983).

The fractional catabolic rate of apo AI is decreased by probucol treatment, implying a decrease in the rate of production (Atmeh et al., 1983; Giada et al., 1986), but it is not clear how this decrease is brought about. Recent studies, discussed below, show that treatment with probucol enhances cholesteryl ester transfer protein (CETP) activity (Sirtori et al., 1988; Franceschini et al., 1989) and indeed causes an increase in the net plasma concentration of CETP protein (McPherson et al., 1990). It is not clear as yet which response is primary and which secondary. For example, an increase in CETP activity could account for a decrease in the concentration of cholesterol esters in the HDL fraction by increasing the rate of its transfer to VLDL and LDL. This could occur even without any change in the apoprotein content of HDL. On the other hand, there might be a secondary response in lipoprotein production and/or removal rates. Conversely, a primary effect on HDL concentration, secondary to a change in HDL production, could possibly result in a compensatory change in CETP activity. The increase in CETP activity might represent an attempt to keep the net rate of cholesteryl ester transfer constant despite a drop in HDL concentration. Further studies are needed.

B. Is Reverse Cholesterol Transport Reduced by Treatment with Probucol?

This is the crucial question that must be asked in face of the marked decrease in total HDL concentration during probucol treatment. In view of the strong negative correlation between levels of HDL and risk of coronary heart disease, there is an understandable tendency, irrespective of mechanisms, to be concerned about interventions that lower HDL levels. A variety of experimental studies have made a strong case for HDL (or some subfraction thereof) as either the primary or intermediary carrier for cholesterol transport from the periphery back to the liver for reutilization or excretion in the bile (reverse cholesterol transport) (Small, 1988; Gwynne, 1989). Unfortunately, there is surprisingly limited evidence in vivo that would let us evaluate the importance of HDL concentration as a potential rate-limiting factor in reverse cholesterol transport. In fact we do not even have reliable quantitative information on *rates* of reverse cholesterol transport in animals in vivo and certainly none in man. The technical problems faced are very difficult, and the lag in obtaining the needed in vivo information is understandable. Probucol, by providing an agent that perturbs the system, may be useful in ultimately developing a quantitative approach to assessing reverse cholesterol transport.

Meanwhile, what can we say about the question of whether the net effects of probucol are harmful or beneficial? In three independent studies of the treatment of patients with familial hypercholesterolemia, it has been noted that both cutaneous and tendinous xanthomata regressed to a greater extent than would have been expected on the basis of the decrease in total cholesterol and LDL cholesterol. In the study by Baker et al. (1982), eight of nine patients showed moderate or marked regression after 13–16 months of treatment and four showed complete disappearance of their xanthomata. Buxtorf et al. (1985) also observed regression, particularly in xanthelasma, over a year of treatment. Yamamoto et al. (1986) again observed striking regression of cutaneous xanthomata and also quantified regression of tendon xanthomata using xerography. Now, it is true that regression of xanthomata has been noted in patients treated in a number of ways for their hypercholesterolemia, and it is not really possible with the semi-quantitative observations in hand to be certain whether the regression in probucol-treated patients is or is not greater than expected on the basis of the degree of lowering of their LDL levels. The distinct impression, however, is that there is a discordance and that something additional is happening under treatment with probucol to amplify the effects of cholesterol lowering. At least there is nothing to suggest that the drop in HDL level has prevented regression of xanthomata. Indeed, Yamamoto et al. (1986) found that the regression of tendinous xanthomata correlated positively with the extent to which HDL levels fell!

To these clinical data we must add the experimental findings of Carew et al. (1987) and Kita et al. (1987) in LDL receptor-deficient rabbits. Both groups observed a striking decrease in the rate of progression of atherosclerotic lesions in WHHL rabbits treated with probucol. In the study of Carew et al. this occurred even though HDL levels fell along with a fall in cholesterol. Carew et al. (1987) controlled for the decrease in total cholesterol levels by treating a control group with small doses of lovastatin just sufficient to keep the cholesterol levels in the two groups comparable. In the Kita studies there was no such control, but there was a relatively small decrease in cholesterol level probably insufficient to account for the striking inhibition of progression of lesions.

There is currently a great deal of interest in the heterogeneity of the HDL fraction and the possibility that certain components may be much more critical in reverse cholesterol transport than others. Epidemiological studies suggest that a high concentration of the HDL_2 subfraction correlates best with protection against coronary heart disease, more so than changes in the concentration of HDL_3 (Gofman et al., 1966). Recent experimental findings suggest, however, that the situation is much more complicated because there are *many* types of particles that make up "HDL" (Cheung et al., 1987; Castro et al., 1988). With further refinement of methodology it may be possible to make more sense of the clinical and epidemiological findings. In any case, the effects of probucol on subclasses of HDL have been inconsistent. Some investigators report a greater lowering of the HDL_2 subfraction (Matsuzawa et al., 1988; Sirtori et al., 1988), others report a greater decrease in the HDL_3 subfraction (Atmeh et al., 1983), and others report variable results (Helve et al., 1988).

As discussed above, there is now evidence for an increase in the transfer of cholesteryl ester from HDL to lighter lipoprotein fractions under treatment with probucol (Sirtori et al., 1988; Franceschini et al., 1989), and this is evidently attributable to a net increase in plasma concentrations of the cholesteryl ester transfer protein (McPherson et al., 1990). What we badly need to know is whether the rate-limiting step in reverse cholesterol transport is the transfer of cholesterol from the cells to the lipoprotein molecule or the rate of esterification and transfer of the cholesterol ester to lower density lipoprotein fractions. In the absence of quantitative measurements, we must defer judgment on just what is happening with respect to reverse cholesterol transport when we treat with probucol.

C. Probucol as an Antioxidant

Over the past decade considerable evidence has accumulated to suggest that LDL must undergo modifications in its structure in order to become a truly atherogenic lipoprotein (Brown and Goldstein, 1983; Steinberg et al., 1989). The best documented modification that may play a role in atherogenesis is oxidation of the LDL particle. The nature of this hypothesis and the evidence—still limited—supporting it have been reviewed recently and need not be covered here in any detail (Steinberg et al., 1989). We can summarize briefly by pointing out several properties of oxidatively modified LDL that are not shared by native LDL and that could contribute to accelerated atherogenesis:

1. It is taken up much more rapidly by macrophages and can therefore generate foam cells.
2. It acts as a chemoattractant specific to monocytes and could recruit

arterial monocytes into the subendothelial space. These are believed to be the major precursors of the foam cells that characterize the early fatty streak lesions.

3. It inhibits the motility of tissue macrophages and might prevent their getting back out of the subendothelial space into the blood again.

4. It is cytotoxic, at least in the absence of other serum proteins, and might damage endothelial cells or other cells in the developing arterial lesion (Chisolm and Morel, 1988).

5. It appears to activate endothelial cells and possibly macrophages as well (Berliner et al., 1990).

Parthasarathy and co-workers (1986) called attention to the potency of probucol as an antioxidant. Its potential as an antioxidant was evident from its structure (Fig. 1), and, interestingly, it develops that this compound was originally synthesized at Dow Chemical because of their interest in rubber manufacturing and the need for antioxidants during that manufacturing process. When the William S. Merrell Company was acquired by Dow Chemical, a series of compounds was tested for possible cholesterol-lowering potential and probucol was one of them!

Possibly the most direct evidence suggesting that probucol might slow the atherosclerotic process by virtue of its antioxidant properties has come from studies of LDL receptor-deficient rabbits (Carew et al., 1987; Kita et al., 1987). At a very high dosage (1% w/w in the diet) it did in fact slow the progression of the disease. Wissler and Vesselinovitch (1983) reported that probucol inhibited atherosclerosis in nonhuman primates, but significant lowering of cholesterol occurred. Furthermore, it remains a possibility that the slowing of progression of lesions under treatment with probucol in the receptor-deficient rabbits may have been due in part to other mechanisms of action. For example, Ku et al. (1990a) have shown that probucol inhibits the release of interleukin-1 from mouse peritoneal macrophages. Also, the effects on CETP discussed above could possibly have contributed, although this was not measured in the rabbit studies. Yamamoto and co-workers (1988) reported that probucol could inhibit the uptake of acetylated LDL by macrophages, which could of course contribute to an antiatherosclerotic effect, but other investigators have not been able to confirm that finding (Carew et al., 1987; Nagano et al., 1989; Ku et al., 1990b). It should be noted that a negative report has appeared with regard to the ability of probucol to inhibit atherosclerosis in cholesterol-fed rabbits (Stein et al., 1989), while another group has reported an inhibition (Daugherty et al., 1989). And no studies have yet been carried out in man to determine whether antioxidant compounds do in fact influence the atherogenic process. A study to test the effects of probucol on vascular disease, utilizing femoral angiography, is in process in Sweden

(Walldius et al., 1988). However, this study involves substantial alterations in lipoprotein levels, and it is unlikely that the outcome can be interpreted as a test of the antioxidant hypothesis. Until that kind of evidence becomes available, the decision to use probucol must be based entirely on its effects on plasma lipoproteins, the benefit to be gained therefrom, and the balance between such benefits and any potential adverse side effects.

Before leaving the subject of the antioxidant properties of probucol, it should be pointed out that these may have potential benefits in direction other than that of atherogenesis. For example, Chisolm and Morel (1988) have shown that probucol acts as an antioxidant in streptozotocin-treated rats to protect lipoproteins against oxidation and thus prevent cytotoxicity that might result. A protective effect of probucol against alloxan-induced diabetes in rats has also been reported (Matsushita et al., 1989). Drash and co-workers have reported preliminary studies suggesting that probucol might actually slow the progression of diabetes mellitus in rats that have a genetic predisposition to develop diabetes (Drash et al., 1988). Bird et al. (1988) showed that pretreatment with probucol significantly reduced the extent of reperfusion ischemic injury to the rat kidney.

III. SIDE EFFECTS AND TOXICITY

The current recommended dose of probucol is 500 mg twice daily. This dosage is associated with few serious side effects or toxicity. The most frequent side effects are gastrointestinal in nature, with loose stools or occasional diarrhea reported most commonly, but abdominal bloating, heartburn, and flatulence are also reported (Glueck et al., 1982; Tedeschi et al., 1982). In fact, the tendency to produce loose stools can act to counteract the constipating effect of the bile resins, when these agents are given concomitantly.

In addition, headaches, dizziness, musculoskeletal, and other minor effects have been reported. In various published reports, the overall rate of reported side effects has been 3–20%. Based on data from early large-scale clinical trials, 3–8% of patients have had probucol discontinued because of side effects (Heel et al., 1978; Miettinen et al., 1986). However, it has been our experience in clinical practice that it is quite unusual to have to discontinue probucol because of side effects.

Probucol has the distinct ability to increase the QTc interval of the electrocardiogram in some patients. Early toxicology studies in dogs receiving probucol for up to 2 years evidenced an increased incidence of sudden death. At first this was thought to be species specific, due to sensitization of canine myocardium to epinephrine-induced ventricular fibrillation (Marshall and Lewis, 1973). Subsequent studies in rhesus monkeys also revealed an increased frequency of arrhythmias and even sudden death (Eder, 1982). However, in monkeys probucol was fed together with a high fat, atherogenic diet. Because of the extreme lipophilic nature of probucol, it is likely that this protocol led to enhanced absorption and relatively elevated plasma levels, at least postprandially. QTc prolongation was documented in monkeys given probucol concomitantly with a high fat diet (Eder, 1982), but when given separately in time from the diet, no QTc prolongation or cardiotoxicity was observed (Marshall, 1982; Wissler and Vesselinovitch, 1983). Although the relevance of these findings to humans is unclear, as noted below, the official prescribing information recommends that probucol be administered only to individuals on a low fat diet.

There seems little doubt that in some patients prolongation of the QTc interval has occurred in response to probucol (Dujovne et al., 1984). In some studies this appears to be related to plasma probucol concentrations (Troendle et al., 1982), but as probucol is probably absorbed in chylomicrons, fasting probucol levels may not adequately reflect peak plasma levels. Although prolonged QTc intervals have been reported in as many as 50% of patients treated, no evidence for clinical consequences have been reported in man. In most patients affected, the prolongation of the QTc interval is in the order of 10–25 msec and rarely exceeds an absolute QTc interval of 440 msec (Naukkarinen et al., 1989). Although there are no data to suggest that the probucol-related prolongation of the QTc interval is clinically important in the average patient, in any individual with cardiac disease at risk of developing a prolonged QTc interval, or in those taking other agents known to prolong this interval, probucol should be given with great caution and the EKG should be monitored. Probucol should not be given to individuals with greater than 15% prolongation of the QTc interval.

IV. CLINICAL APPLICATIONS

A. Used as Single Drug

The primary effect of probucol is to lower total plasma cholesterol, which it does by lowering both LDL and HDL levels. (Results of representative studies reported in the literature are given in Table 1.) On average it lowers LDL cholesterol levels 10–20%. However, such mean changes can be misleading, as characteristically there is great variability in response, with occasional subjects having marked degrees of LDL lowering, while many have little or no LDL response at all. The reasons for this are unknown but

Nestruck et al. (1987) have suggested that patients with the apo E phenotype E_4/E_4 are more responsive than those with other apo E phenotypes.

In contrast to the variable effect on LDL levels, probucol profoundly lowers HDL levels in almost all patients, even in those in whom it fails to affect LDL levels (see Table 1). It is primarily because of the uncertainty of the consequences of the profound HDL-lowering effect that most investigators do not currently regard probucol as a first-line drug for the treatment of hypercholesterolemia due to elevated LDL levels. Despite this, interest remains high in probucol because, among all known hypolipidemic agents, it alone has been reported to be effective in treating subjects homozygous for familial hypercholesterolemia. In such subjects, probucol lowers LDL levels only modestly, but despite this, appears to cause a dramatic reduction in size of their xanthomata, as discussed above. As noted above, probucol lowers LDL levels 10–20% in most studies, whether patients have familial or nonfamilial hypercholesterolemia. In contrast, HDL levels fall 20–30% or more in nearly everyone. Further research is needed to clarify the meaning of this fall in HDL. As discussed above, it need not indicate an adverse effect on reverse cholesterol transport.

B. Used in Combination with Other Drugs

The efficacy of probucol as a primary LDL-lowering agent has been compared directly with that of most of the other commonly used hypolipidemic agents (reviewed in detail in Buckley et al., 1989). In most of these studies probucol as monotherapy was far less effective than monotherapy with bile acid–binding resins or lovastatin. Thus, while probucol produces average decreases of LDL of only 10–20%, bile sequestrants lower LDL 25–35% and HMG-CoA reductase inhibitors lower LDL 35–45% (reviewed in Witztum, 1989a). However, addition of probucol to the regimen of patients already on a maximally tolerated dose of a bile acid-binding resin can sometimes lower LDL levels still further (see Table 1). An example of this is shown in Figure 2. In this study 14 Type II patients, who already were on maximally tolerated doses of colestipol (20–30 g/day) were given placebo or probucol in a blinded crossover design. Figure 2 compares the additional changes in LDL cholesterol and HDL cholesterol produced by placebo or probucol. For the group as a whole, LDL levels were lowered an additional 9% by probucol. However, seven subjects had a greater than 10% reduction in LDL cholesterol levels, and in these "responders," there was an average reduction of 21% (range 11–47%). In contrast, half the patients showed no further drop in LDL. Note that despite the variable effects on LDL levels, HDL levels fell in nearly

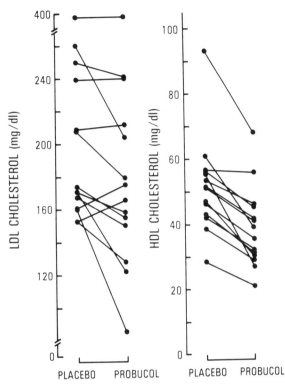

Figure 2 Mean levels of LDL cholesterol and HDL cholesterol for each individual during placebo and probucol periods. Each person was already on a maximally tolerated dose of colestipol and subsequently took probucol (1 g/day) or placebo for a 3-month period in a double-blind crossover trial with 1 month washout interval. For each person the value graphed represents the average of three values obtained at monthly intervals during each period. (Data from Witztum and Schonfeld, unpublished observations.)

everyone, averaging 25%. Plasma apo AI levels fell in every subject, while apo AII did not, resulting in a fall of the AI/AII ratio in 13 of the 14 subjects. This suggests a drop primarily in HDL_2 levels. Others have reported similar results (Dujovne et al., 1984; Kuo et al., 1986).

While the addition of probucol to a bile resin may lower LDL further in 50% of patients, addition of probucol to a patient already on lovastatin appears to add little to therapy in terms of lowering LDL (see Table 1). This is

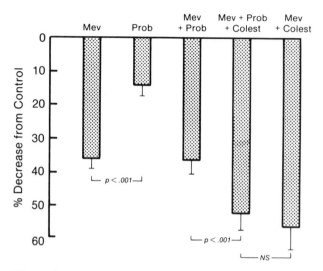

Figure 3 Effect of each drug period on LDL cholesterol levels in 17 heterozygous FH subjects. Each person participated in each drug period, which lasted 3–6 months. For each drug period, the mean percent change ($\pm$ SEM) versus the control period is shown. Mev = lovastatin 40 mg/day; Prob = probucol, 1 g/day; Colest = colestipol HCl, 20 g/day. (Reproduced with permission from Witztum et al., 1989b.)

illustrated in Figure 3, taken from our recent report directly comparing the efficacy of probucol versus lovastatin used alone or in combination with a bile acid–sequestering agent (Witztum et al., 1989b). Probucol was less effective than lovastatin in lowering LDL levels and added little when added in combination with lovastatin, or when added in combination with lovastatin and colestipol. In contrast, it dramatically lowered HDL levels, even preventing the increased HDL levels frequently seen with lovastatin and colestipol therapy. In fact, only after 6 months off the drug did HDL levels return to control valves.

There are few reports, with only a few patients, comparing the combination of probucol and gemfibrozil (or clofibrate), but surprisingly, the combination has been reported to lower HDL levels even more than when probucol was used alone (Davignon et al., 1986). Similarly, there are virtually no prospective data on the efficacy of probucol plus nicotinic acid. This would be of interest as nicotinic acid is normally quite potent in raising HDL levels.

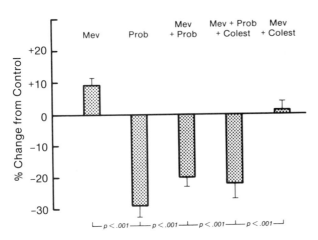

Figure 4 Effect of each drug period on HDL cholesterol levels in the same study described in legend to Figure 3. (Reproduced with permission from Witztum et al., 1989b.)

C. Indications for Use of Probucol

For all these reasons, we and other investigators most often limit use of probucol to a second-line agent to be used in combination with a bile sequestrant, but only when lovastatin or nicotinic acid cannot be used. Finally, as discussed earlier, probucol has been documented to be a potent lipophilic antioxidant. Its rather dramatic ability to cause reduction of xanthomata in homozygous FH patients has been attributed in part to this property. The studies of Carew et al. (1987) and Kita et al. (1987), as well as the earlier studies of Kritchevsky et al. (1971) and Wissler and Vesselinovitch (1983), all support an antiatherosclerotic effect of probucol therapy in experimental animal models of atherosclerosis. The use of probucol as an antioxidant to prevent atherosclerosis *in humans* lacks any data at present and must await further clinical trials. However, for the rare patient with homozygous FH, use of probucol is indicated. For the severe heterozygous FH patient, particularly those with xanthomata, it might be rational to include probucol therapy as adjunctive therapy, in addition to other effective hypolipidemic agents. Similarly, for the occasional non-FH, high-risk patient, its use could be considered on an individual basis. This latter recommendation must be considered as experimental and should be applied only to severely affected and/or very high risk patients. Clearly the use of probucol or other antioxidants as adjunctive

therapy to prevent LDL oxidation in the prevention or amelioration of atherosclerosis remains a highly speculative area of current research.

V. SUMMARY

Probucol is a highly lipophilic drug transported primarily in the lipoprotein
fractions of plasma. Its ability to decrease plasma cholesterol levels was
discovered by empirical screening, and the mechanism of action is still not
entirely certain. The drug is moderately effective at lowering LDL levels in
some patients, but it also lowers HDL levels to a similar or even greater
degree in all patients. This latter effect of the drug is of some concern because
of the well-documented inverse correlation between HDL levels and coronary
heart disease risk. However, patients under treatment with probucol actually
show an increase in the rate of cholesteryl ester transfer from HDL to other
lipoprotein fractions, due to an increase in the plasma concentrations of
cholesteryl ester transfer protein, and actual regression of cutaneous and
tendinous xanthomata has been observed in treated patients. These findings
together with some in vitro findings suggest that the drop in HDL concentration need not reflect a decrease in reverse cholesterol transport. No long-term
clinical intervention studies using probucol have been reported thus far, but a
study is currently in progress in Scandinavia. Although the drug has been
associated with cardiac deaths in dogs and in monkeys under certain circum-
stances, this effect appears to be species specific and no serious cardiotoxicity
has been reported in man. Nevertheless, because it does cause a lengthening
of the QTc interval in many patients, it should not be given to individuals with
baseline prolongation of QTc.

The mechanism of action by which probucol lowers LDL levels remains
uncertain. The fractional rate of disappearance of LDL has been observed to
increase both in patients and in experimental animals, and there is some
evidence that probucol alters the physical and biological properties of LDL so
that its disappearance is enhanced, possibly by both receptor-independent and
receptor-dependent pathways.

Currently there is a great deal of interest in a new hypothesis for atherogenesis—the so-called oxidative modification hypothesis. Low density lipoprotein after oxidation is potentially more atherogenic than native LDL in a
number of ways. Probucol, in addition to lowering LDL levels, has been
shown to be a potent antioxidant and to protect LDL against oxidation.
Experimental studies show that the drug significantly slows the progression of
atherosclerosis in LDL receptor-deficient rabbits, but there are no studies in

man to confirm this. Additional animal studies and, ultimately, clinical studies will be needed before this new hypothesis can be fully evaluated.

The advantages of probucol are that it is easy to administer and there are relatively few side effects. Response varies considerably from patient to patient, and the response in each individual patient must be assessed before deciding to continue the drug or not. The LDL responses to bile acid sequestrants, to nicotinic acid, and to HMG-CoA reductase inhibitors are all greater than those to probucol. Probucol should be considered only for patients who cannot take one of the first-line drugs or as a second drug in combination therapy.

REFERENCES

Anastasi, A., Betteridge, D. J., and Galton, D. J. (1980). Effect of probucol and other drugs on sterol synthesis in human lymphocytes. In *Diet and Drugs in Atherosclerosis*. Edited by G., Noseda, B., Lewis, and R., Paoletti. New York, Raven Press, pp. 161–163.

Atmeh, R. F., Stewart, J. M., Boag, D., Packard, C. J., Lorimer, A. R., and Shepherd, J. (1983). The hypolipidemic action of probucol: A study of its effects on high and low density lipoproteins. *J. Lipid Res.* **24**:588–595.

Baker, S. G., Joffe, B. I. Mendelsohn, D., and Seftel, H. C. (1982). Treatment of homozygous familial hypercholesterolemia with probucol. *South African Medical Journal* **62**:7–11.

Barnhart, J. W., Li, D. L., and Cheng, W. D. (1988). Probucol enhances cholesterol transport in cultured rat hepatocytes. *Am. J. Cardiol.* **62**:52B–56B.

Berliner, J. A., Territo, M. C., Sevanian, A., Ramin, S., Kim, J. A., Barnshad, B., Esterson, M., and Fogelman, A. M. (1990). Minimally modified low density lipoprotein stimulates monocyte endothelial interactions. *J. Clin. Invest.* **85**:1260–1266.

Bird, J. E., Milhoan, K., Wilson, C. B., Young, S. G., Mundy, C. A., Parthasarathy, S., and Blantz, R. C. (1988). Ischemic acute renal failure and antioxidant therapy in the rat. The relation between glomerular and tubular dysfunction. *J. Clin. Invest.* **81**:1630–1638.

Brown, M. S., and Goldstein, J. L. (1983). Lipoprotein metabolism in the macrophage: Implications for cholesterol deposition in atherosclerosis. *Ann. Review Biochem.* **52**:223–261.

Buckley, M. M.-T., Goa, K. L., Price, A. H., and Brogden, R. N. (1989). Probucol. A reappraisal of its pharmacological properties and therapeutic use in hypercholesterolemia. *Drugs* **37**:761–800.

Buxtorf, J. C., Jacotot, B., Beaumont, V., and Beaumont, J. L. (1985). Action du probucol dans les hypercholestérolémies familiales de Type II. *Semaine des Hôpitaux Paris* **61**:837–840.

Carew, T. E., Schwenke, D. C., and Steinberg, D. (1987). Antiatherogenic effect of probucol unrelated to its hypocholesterolemic effect: Evidence that antioxidants in vivo can selectively inhibit low density lipoprotein degradation in macrophage-rich fatty streaks and slow the progression of atherosclerosis in the Watanabe heritable hyperlipidemic rabbit. *Proc. Natl. Acad. Sci. USA* **84**:7725–7729.

Castro, G. R., and Fielding, C. J. (1988) Early incorporation of cell-derived cholesterol into pre-beta-migrating high-density lipoprotein. *Biochemistry* **27**:25–29.

Cheung, M. C., Segrest, J. P., Albers, J. J., Cone, J. T., Brouillette, C. G., Chung, B. H., Kashyap, M., Glasscock, M. A., and Anantharamaiah, G. M. (1987). Characterization of high density lipoprotein subspecies: structural studies by single vertical spin ultracentrifugation and immunoaffinity chromatography. *J. Lipid Res.* **28**:913–929.

Chisolm, G. M., and Morel, D. W. (1988). Lipoprotein oxidation and cytotoxicity. Effect of probucol on streptozotocin-treated rats. *Am. J. Cardiol.* **62**:20B–26B.

Daugherty, A., Zweifel, B. S., and Schonfeld, G. (1989). Probucol attenuates the development of aortic atherosclerosis in cholesterol-fed rabbits. *Br. J. Pharmacol.* **98**:612–618.

Davignon, J., Nestruck, A. C., Alaupovic, P., and Bouthillier, D. (1986). Severe hypoalphalipoproteinemia induced by a combination of probucol and clofibrate. *Adv. Exp. Med. Biol.* **201**:111–125.

Davignon, J., Xhignesse, M., Mailloux, H., Nestruck, A. C., Lussier-Cacan, S., Roederer, G., and Pfister, P. (1988). Comparative study of lovastatin versus probucol in the treatment of hypercholesterolemia. In *Atherosclerosis Reviews*. Vol. 18. Edited by J. Stokes III and M. Mancini. New York, Raven Press, pp. 139–151.

Drash, A. L., Rudert, W. A., Borquaye, S., Wang, R., and Lieberman, I. (1988). Effect of probucol on development of diabetes mellitus in BB rats. *Am. J. Cardiol.* **62**:27B–30B.

Dujovne, C. A., Krehbiel, P., Decoursey, S., Jackson, B., Chernoff, S. B., Pitterman, A., and Garty, M. (1984). Probucol with colestipol in the treatment of hypercholesterolemia. *Ann. Int. Med.* **100**:477–482.

Eder, H. A. (1982). The effect of diet on the transport of probucol in monkeys. *Artery* **10**:105–107.

Franceschini, G., Sirtori, M., Vaccarino, V., Gianfranceschi, G., Rezzonico, L., Chiesa, G., and Sirtori, C. R. (1989). Mechanisms of HDL reduction after probucol: Changes in HDL subfractions and increased reverse cholesteryl ester transfer. *Arteriosclerosis* **9**:462–469.

Giada, F., Valerio, G., Bicego, L., Padrini, R., Moretto, R., Baiocchi, M. R., and Fellin, R. (1986). Probucol with cholestyramine in the treatment of familial hypercholesterolemia: Effects on lipoprotein and serum probucol levels. *Current Therapeutic Research* **40**:975–986.

Glueck, C. J. (1982). Colestipol and probucol: Treatment of primary and familial hypercholesterolemia and amelioration of atherosclerosis. *Ann. Int. Med.* **96**:475–482.

Gofman, J. W., Young, W., and Tandy, R. (1966). Ischemic heart disease, atherosclerosis and longevity. *Circulation* **34**:679–697.

Gwynne, J. T. (1989). High-density lipoprotein cholesterol levels as a marker of reverse cholesterol transport. *Am. J. Cardiol.* **64**:10G–17G.

Heel, R. C., Brogden, R. N., Speight, T. M., and Avery, G. S. (1978). Probucol: A review of its pharmacological properties and therapeutic use in patients with hypercholesterolemia. *Drugs* **15**:409–428.

Helve, E., and Tikkanen, M. J. (1988) Comparison of lovastatin and probucol in treatment of familial and non-familial hypercholesterolemia: Different effects on lipoprotein profiles. *Atherosclerosis* **72**:189–197.

Hunninghake, E., Bell, C., and Olson, L. (1980). Effects of probucol on plasma lipids and lipoproteins in type IIb hyperlipoproteinemia. *Atherosclerosis* **37**:469–474.

Johansson, J., and Walldius, G. (1988). Probucol-induced change in HDL particle size in man. Presented at the 8th International Symposium on Atherosclerosis, Venice, October 7–8, 1988.

Kesaniemi, Y. A., and Grundy, S. M. (1984). Influence of probucol on cholesterol and lipoprotein metabolism in man. *J. Lipid Res.* **25**:780–790.

Kita, T., Nagano, Y., Yokode, M., Ishii, K., Kume, N., Ooshima, A., Yoshida, H., and Kawai, C. (1987). Probucol prevents the progression of atherosclerosis in Watanabe heritable hyperlipidemic rabbit, an animal model for familial hypercholesterolemia. *Proc. Natl. Acad. Sci. USA* **84**:5928–5931.

Kritchevsky, D., Kim, H. K., and Tepper, S. A. (1971). Influence of 4,4'(isopropylidenedithio)bis(2,6-di-t-butylphenol)(DH-581) on experimental atherosclerosis in rabbits. *Proc. Soc. Exp. Biol. Med.* **136**:1216.

Ku, G., Doherty, N. S., Schmidt, L. F., Jackson, R. L., and Dinerstein, R. J. (1990a). Ex vivo lipopolysaccharide-induced interleukin-1 secretion from murine peritoneal macrophages inhibited by probucol, a hypocholesterolemic agent with antioxidant properties. *FASEB J.* **4**:1645–1653.

Ku, G., Schroeder, K., Schmidt, L. F., Jackson, R. L., and Doherty, N. S. (1990b). Probucol does not alter acetylated low density lipoprotein uptake by murine peritoneal macrophages. *Atherosclerosis* **80**:191–197.

Kuo, P. T., Wilson, A. C., Kostis, J. B., and Moreyra, A. E. (1986). Effects of combined probucol-colestipol treatment for familial hypercholesterolemia and coronary artery disease. *Am. J. Cardiol.* **57**:43H–48H.

Lees, A. M., Stein, S. W., and Lees, R. S. (1986). Therapy of hypercholesterolemia with mevinolin and other lipid lowering drugs. *Circulation* **74-II**:200.

LeLorier, J., Dubreuil-Quidoz, S., Lussier, Cacan, S., Huang, Y. S., and Davignon, J. (1977). Diet and probucol in lowering cholesterol concentrations. Additive effects on plasma cholesterol concentrations in familial type II hyperlipoproteinemia. *Arch. Int. Med.* **137**:1429–1434.

Lock, D. R., Kuisk, I., Gonen, B., Patsch, W., and Schonfeld, G. (1983). Effect of probucol on the composition of lipoproteins and on VLDL apoprotein B turnover. *Atherosclerosis* **47**:271–278.

Marshall, F. N. (1982). Pharmacology and toxicology of probucol. *Artery* **10:**7–21.

Marshall, F. N., and Lewis, J. E. (1973). Sensitization to epinephrine-induced ventricular fibrillation produced by probucol in dogs. *Toxicol. Appl. Pharmacol.* **24:**594–602.

Matsushita, M., Yoshino, G., Iwai, M., Matsuba, K., Morita, M., Iwatani, I., Yoshida, M., Kazumi, T., and Baba, S. (1989). Protective effect of probucol on alloxan diabetes in rats. *Diabetes Res. Clin. Pract.* **7:**313–316.

Matsuzawa, Y., Yamashita, S., Funahashi, T., Yamamoto, A., and Tarui, S. (1988). Selective reduction of cholesterol in HDL_2 fraction by probucol in familial hyper-cholesterolemia and hyper HDL_2 cholesterolemia with abnormal cholesteryl ester transfer. *Am. J. Cardiol.* **62:** 66B–72B.

McPherson, R., Hogue, M., Milne, R. W., Tall, A. R., and Marcel, Y. (1990). *Arteriosclerosis,* in press.

Mellies, M. J., Gartside, P. S., Glatfelter, L., Vink, P., Guy, G., Schonfeld, G., and Glueck, C. J. (1980). Effects of probucol on plasma cholesterol, high and low density lipoprotein cholesterol, and apolipoproteins A1 and A2 in adults with primary familial hypercholesterolemia. *Metabolism* **29:**956–963.

Miettinen, T. A., Huttunen, J. K., Naukkarinen, V., Strandberg, T., and Vannanen, H. (1986) Long-term use of probucol in the multifactorial primary prevention of vascular disease. *Am. J. Cardiol.* **57:**49H–54H.

Nagano, Y., Kita, T., Yokode, M., Ishii, K., Kume, N., Otani, H., Arai, H., and Kawai, C. (1989). Probucol does not affect lipoprotein metabolism in macrophages of Watanabe heritable hyperlipidemic rabbits. *Arteriosclerosis* **9:**453–461.

Naruszewicz, M., Carew, T. E., Pittman, R. C., Witztum, J. L., and Steinberg, D. (1984). A novel mechanism by which probucol lowers low density lipoprotein levels demonstrated in the LDL receptor-deficient rabbit. *J. Lipid Res.* **25:**1206–1213.

Naukkarinen, V., Strandberg, T., Vanhanen, H., and Miettinen, T. A. (1989). Probucol-induced electrocardiographic changes in a five-year primary prevention of vascular diseases. *Current Therapeutic Research* **45:**232–237.

Nestel, P. J., and Billington, T. (1981). Effects of probucol on low density lipoprotein removal and high density lipoprotein synthesis. *Atherosclerosis* **38:**203–209.

Nestruck, A. C., Bouthillier, D., Sing, C. F., and Davignon, J. (1987). Apolipoprotein E polymorphism and plasma cholesterol response to probucol. *Metabolism* **36:**743–747.

Parthasarathy, W., Young, S. G., Witztum, J. L., Pittman, R. C., and Steinberg, D. (1986). Probucol inhibits oxidative modification of low density lipoprotein. *J. Clin. Invest.* **77:**641–644.

Pietro, D. A., Alexander, S., Mantell, G., Staggers, J. E., and Cook, T. J. (1989). Effects of simvastatin and probucol in hypercholesterolemia (Simvastatin Multicenter Study Group II). *Am. J. Cardiol.* **63:**682–686.

Riesen, W. F., Keller, M., and Mordasini, R. (1980). Probucol in hypercholesterolemia. A double blind study. *Atherosclerosis* **36:**201–207.

Schonfeld, G., Witztum, J., and Basich, P. (1982). Probucol further lowers the serum cholesterol of colestipol-treated patients with hypercholesterolemia. *Artery* **10**:99–104.

Sirtori, C. R., Sirtori, M., Calabresi, L., and Franceschini, G. (1988). Changes in high-density lipoprotein subfraction distribution and increased cholesteryl ester transfer after probucol. *Am. J. Cardiol.* **62**:73B–76B.

Small, D. M. (1988). Mechanisms of reversed cholesterol transport. *Agents and Actions* (Suppl.) **26**:135–146.

Stein, Y., Stein, O., Delplanque, B., Fesmire, J. D., Lee, D. M., and Alaupovic, P. (1989). Lack of effect of probucol on atheroma formation in cholesterol-fed rabbits kept at comparable plasma cholesterol levels. *Atherosclerosis* **75**:145–155.

Steinberg, D., Parthasarathy, S., Carew, T. E., Khoo, J. C., and Witztum, J. L. (1989). Beyond cholesterol: Modifications of low-density lipoprotein that increase its atherogenicity. *New Engl. J. Med.* **320**:915–924.

Tedeschi, R. E., Martz, B. L., Taylor, H. A., and Cerimele, B. J. (1982). Safety and effectiveness of probucol as a cholesterol lowering agent. *Artery* **10**:22–34.

Troendle, G., Gueriguian, J., Sobel, S., and Johnson, M. (1982). Correspondence. Probucol and the QT interval. *Lancet* **1**:1179.

Walldius, G., Carlson, L. A., Erickson, U., Olsson, A. G., Johansson, J., Molgaard, J., Nilsson, S., Stenport, G., Kaijser, L., and Lassvik, C. (1988). Development of femoral atherosclerosis in hypercholesterolemic patients during treatment with cholestyramine and probucol/placebo: Probucol Quantitative Regression Swedish Trial (PQRST): A status report. *Am. J. Cardiol.* **62**:37B–43B.

Wissler, R. W., and Vesselinovitch, D. (1983). Combined effects of cholestyramine and probucol on regression of atherosclerosis in rhesus monkey aortas. *Appl. Pathol.* **1**:89–96.

Wiztum, J. L. (1989a). Current approaches to drug therapy for the hypercholesterolemic patient. *Circulation* **80**:1101–1114.

Witztum, J. L., Simmons, D., Steinberg, D., Beltz, W. F., Weinreb, R., Young, S. G., Lester, P., Kelly, N., and Juliano, J. (1989b). Intensive combination drug therapy of familial hypercholesterolemia with lovastatin, probucol and colestipol hydrochloride. *Circulation* **79**:16–28.

Witztum, J. L., Young, S. G., Elam, R. L., Carew, T. E., and Fisher, M. (1985). Cholestyramine-induced changes in low density lipoprotein composition and metabolism: I. Studies in the guinea pigs. *J. Lipid Res.* **26**:92–103.

Yamamoto, A., Matsuzawa, Y., Kishino, B., Hayashi, R., Hirobe, K., and Kikkawa, T. (1983). Effects of probucol on homozygous cases of familial hypercholesterolemia. *Atherosclerosis* **48**:157–166.

Yamamoto, A., Matsuzawa, Y., Yokoyama, S., Funahashi, T., Yamamura, T., and Kishino, B. (1986). Effects of probucol on xanthoma regression in familial hypercholesterolemia. *Am. J. Cardiol.* **57**:29H–35H.

Yamamoto, A., Hara, H., Takaichi, S., Wakasugi, J., and Tomikawa, M. (1988).

Effect of probucol on macrophages, leading to regression of xanthomas and atheromatous vascular lesions. *Am. J. Cardiol.* **62:**31B–36B.

Young, S. G., Witztum, J. L., Krauss, R., Lindgren, F. (1985). Colestipol induced changes in LDL composition and metabolism. II: Studies in man. *J. Lipid Res.* **30:**225–239.

9

Nicotinic Acid and Its Derivatives

W. Virgil Brown, William James Howard, and Laraine Field
Medlantic Research Foundation
Washington, D.C.

I. HISTORY

At the beginning of the 20th century, nicotinic acid (niacin) or its amide derivative, nicotinamide (vitamin B_3) were discovered to be essential dietary components (Darby et al., 1975). Their deficiency underlay pellagra, a disease with signs and symptoms affecting the skin, gastrointestinal tract, and central nervous system. In the mammalian liver, nicotinic acid is rapidly converted to nicotinamide, which in turn is the substrate for NAD (nicotinamide adenine dinucleotide) as well as NADP (nicotinamide adenine dinucleotide phosphate). These physiologically important derivatives act as hydrogen transferring coenzymes for a series of dehydrogenases (Fig. 1). The Recommended Dietary Allowance is less than 20 mg per day and therefore, doses of nicotinic acid which greatly exceed this have pharmacologic effects which go beyond its role in normal physiologic processes.

High doses of nicotinic acid were first demonstrated to lower serum cholesterol by Altschul in 1955 (Altschul et al., 1955). Hypothesizing that oxidation of cholesterol might be driven by excessive nicotinic acid, doses of 1–4 g were given over periods of 3–24 h in both animals and humans. Serum

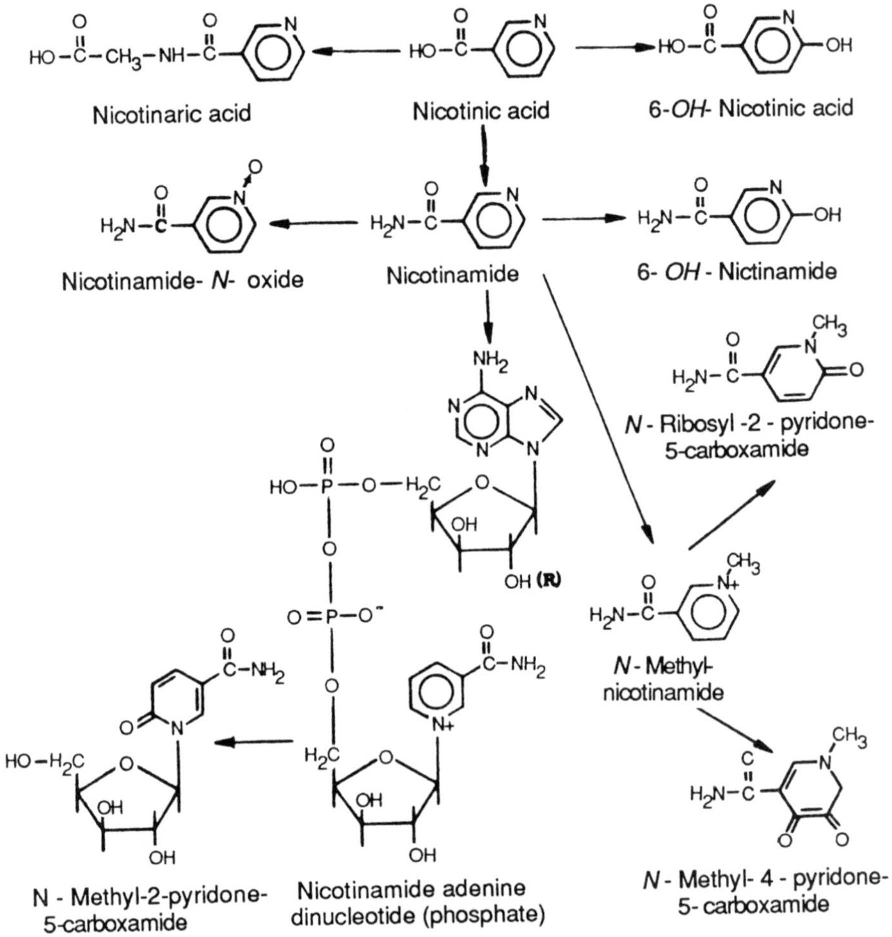

Figure 1 Nicotinic acid metabolism.

cholesterol levels fell between 8 and 22%, with the greatest effect observed in hypercholesterolemic humans. It was quickly discovered that the chronic daily use of nicotinic acid in this range produced reduction in serum cholesterol up to 50% and in total lipids (reflecting triglycerides) in the same range (Gurian and Adlersberg, 1959). Parsons reported experience with 50 hypercholesterolemic patients treated with nicotinic acid for over one year (Parsons, 1961a). He described a reduction of total cholesterol of 23–29% with a decrease in esterified lipids (primarily triglycerides) as well as beta lipoprotein (low-density lipoproteins, LDL) and an increase in Alpha I lipoprotein (high-density lipoproteins, HDL). In patients with xanthomata tuberosum (currently known as dysbetalipoproteinemia), a dramatic decrease in cholesterol from over 700 mg/dl to less than 200 mg/dl was found. Most of the adverse effects currently known were also described in this classic work including flushing of the skin, heartburn, nausea, activation of peptic ulcer, diarrhea, dryness of skin acanthosis nigricans, increased uric acid and hepatic dysfunction (Parsons, 1961b). A marked acute suppression of plasma free fatty acids was noted by Carlson and Oro (1962) and the reduction of this important substrate for cholesterol and triglyceride synthesis in the liver was suggested as the mechanism of action.

During the past 30 years, nicotinic acid has been used in multiple clinical trials and has been demonstrated to have high efficacy in reducing lipids, and specifically the lipoproteins containing the apolipoprotein B which elevation is associated with vascular disease. Additionally, it reproducibly raises high-density lipoprotein cholesterol and the apoproteins contained therein. Unfortunately, the multiple annoying and serious side effects have markedly suppressed its acceptability by patient and physician alike. However, our very large knowledge base and the demonstrated efficacy in altering lipoproteins toward more favorable patterns as well as the growing body of evidence that vascular disease prevention may be associated with niacin therapy caused the National Cholesterol Education Program's Adult Treatment Panel to recommend niacin as a drug of first choice (NCEP Expert Panel, 1988).

II. PHARMACOLOGY

Crystalline nicotinic acid is rapidly absorbed and rapidly excreted in the urine. After an oral dose of 1 g, peak plasma levels of approximately 10–40 μg/ml are reached after 30–60 minutes (Carlson et al., 1968). The plasma half life is approximately 1 h with 80–90% of an oral dose recovered in the urine during the first 24 h (Hotz, 1983). Metabolites such as NAD are concentrated in the erythrocytes, thus the total blood level of nicotinic acid and its metabolic products may be 100 times higher than serum levels.

The distribution of the metabolic products of nicotinic acid depend greatly on the dose level (Fig. 1). At usual dietary intakes, the major excretory products found in the urine include n-methylnicotinamide and n-methyl-2-pyridone carboxamide (Cayen, 1985). When gram quantities are given for pharmacologic effect, the major metabolic product becomes the glycine derivative nicotinuric acid (Mrochek et al., 1976). Only after the capacity of the liver to conjugate nicotinic acid is exceeded does the unchanged compound begin to appear in the urine. At dose levels of 3–6 g/day, this may approach 20% of the total excreted load. At low-dose levels, almost all nicotinic acid is rapidly amidated but very little nicotinamide appears in the urine due to the *n*-methylation and oxidation to the pyridone derivatives (Fig. 1).

Although rapid metabolism makes correlations difficult, it appears that plasma concentrations of only 0.5 to 2 μg/ml of free nicotinic acid are required to produce maximal pharmacological effects (Weiner, 1979). Due to the rapid absorption and excretion, large oral doses are required to maintain concentrations in this range for prolonged periods. Consequently, a variety of techniques have been used to slow the bioavailability of nicotinic acid. These include delayed absorption from the intestine and slow release from its esters with polyhydric alcohols (Hotz, 1983). Examples of the latter include tetra-nicotinoyl fructose (Bradilan), pentaerythritol tetranicotinate (Niceritrol), nicotinic acid hexaester of sorbitol (Sorbinicate), and mesoinositol tetranico-tinate (Hexanicit). These derivatives are absorbed primarily intact from the gastrointestinal tract and are hydrolyzed to free nicotinic acid by esterases in plasma and in various tissues. These are relatively slow reactions and the maximum plasma concentration is achieved only after 2–4 h following oral dosage. Accordingly, the plasma concentration is only 20–50% of that achieved with the crystalline nicotinic acid but the duration of a concentration adequate to have pharmacological effects may be markedly prolonged. A similar effect has been achieved by linking nicotinic acid to the lipid-lowering drug clofibric acid through an ethylene glycol bridge forming a double ester. This drug is known as etofibrate (Ortega et al., 1980). The plasma half life of nicotinic acid is increased since the hydrolysis of this compound is relatively slow in tissues. Another approach to delaying the release and metabolism of nicotinic has been through the use of beta-pyridylcarbinol which is oxidized to nicotinic acid in the liver providing the pharmacological effects (Hotz, 1983). Although this appears to work in experimental animals, it has not been carried forward to full development for prescription use.

III. MECHANISM OF ACTION

The fall in plasma cholesterol with nicotinic acid therapy is due to a decline in VLDL, IDL, and LDL (Grundy et al., 1981; Knopp et al., 1985). Reduction in VLDL synthesis has been found in clinical studies (Grundy et al., 1981). The fall in IDL and LDL are secondary effects since these lipoproteins are sequential products of the delipidation of plasma VLDL. Some increase in removal of entire VLDL particles during processing to LDL has also been found (Grundy et al., 1981). On the other hand, most evidence suggests that LDL clearance rates do not change (Froberg et al., 1971). Concomitant with the VLDL fall, plasma triglyceride concentrations also are reduced in normal individuals and those with elevated triglycerides. This fall is compatible with a reduction in hepatic synthesis of triglycerides and a concomitant fall in VLDL secretion. Kinetic studies using radiolabeled lipoproteins have demonstrated reduced VLDL triglyceride production rates and smaller increases in VLDL triglyceride clearance (Grundy et al., 1981).

Although reduced cholesterol synthesis may result, the major alteration in lipid metabolism is reduced triglyceride synthesis. The early report by Carlson and Oro (1962) of suppression of free fatty acid mobilization from adipose tissue stores, seemed to provide a logical explanation since the plasma free fatty acid is normally the major substrate for hepatic triglyceride production. Subsequently, the transient nature of this suppression was revealed (Carlson and Olsson, 1984). Although triglycerides may remain depressed 12 to 24 hours after a 1 g dose of niacin, the fall in free fatty acids is usually maximum during the first hour, and by 2 to 3 hours, the levels are usually back to baseline and continue to rise with a significant overshoot (Carlson and Oro, 1962). Studies of rat adipose tissue after longer term treatment show no evidence of suppressed free fatty acid release. It has also been noted that other drugs, such as aspirin or 5-fluoro nicotinic acid, which produce a more prolonged reduction in free-fatty acids fail to result in a significant plasma triglyceride reduction (Carlson and Olsson, 1984). At present, the biochemical mechanisms underlying the reduced synthesis and secretion of triglycerides by the niacin exposed liver cell are not understood.

The protein components of VLDL and LDL also are reduced during niacin treatment. Apo B, Apo CI, Apo CII, Apo CIII, and Apo E have all been found to fall (Wahlberg et al., 1988). In a group of 24 hyperlipoproteinemic subjects, niacin (in a dose of 1 g four times daily) reduced the mean serum level of these apolipoproteins by 30–40% concomitant with a mean reduction in VLDL triglyceride by 57% and LDL cholesterol by 29%. The change in Apo B correlated well with the fall in LDL cholesterol and the change in the ApoCs with VLDL triglyceride reduction. This indicates that the composition of these lipoproteins must undergo little change with regard to the major lipid or protein components.

In contrast to VLDL and LDL, HDL cholesterol shows a significant rise (10–40%) in normal and hyperlipoproteinemic persons (Alderman, 1989; Knopp et al., 1985; Luria, 1988). The major apolipoprotein of HDL, Apo AI also increases due to reduced catabolism of HDL particles (Blum et al., 1977; Shepherd et al., 1979). Patients with elevated triglycerides often have the greatest rise in HDL. Since HDL clearance usually is accelerated in hypertriglyceridemia, reducing the elevated VLDL levels with niacin may cause a dramatic rise in HDL by correcting the abnormal rapid clearance.

Another lipoprotein Lp(a) has been of interest recently. Case-controlled studies have shown that elevated levels of this lipoprotein are associated with the prevalence of coronary heart disease (Hoeffler et al., 1988). The efficacy of drug regimens reducing Lp(a) has been tested by several groups. In one study, elevated Lp(a) levels were not significantly reduced by niacin (Kostner et al., 1984). However, Carson et al. (1989) found that in patients with elevated LDL and/or elevated VLDL, Lp(a) was reduced with niacin at doses of 4 g daily. Lp(a) fell most dramatically (38%) in patients with very high triglyceride levels. Lp(a) was also reduced by a combination of niacin and neomycin in studies by Guvakav et al. (1985). The mechanism or the clinical benefit of this effect is not known.

IV. CLINICAL EFFICACY

At the usual therapeutic doses of 2–8 g/day, nicotinic acid produces a reduction in total serum cholesterol of 15–30% and a reduction in triglycerides in the range 20–60% (Figge et al., 1988). The success in reducing these lipoproteins is determined by the nature of the underlying lipoprotein disorder but individual variability in response is considerable. At doses of approximately 1 g/day, minimal changes in total plasma cholesterol and triglyceride have been noted but the increase in HDL may be quite significant (Alderman, 1989). The potential benefit of this increase in HDL at low-dose nicotinic acid therapy has not been tested in adequate clinical trials with cardiovascular endpoints. The full response in VLDL and LDL reduction is usually seen after 3–6 weeks of treatment. HDL, however, seems to respond more slowly and increases may continue for several months. It is useful to consider the efficacy of nicotinic acid in each of the common lipoprotein disorders. The following discussion of the expected alteration in lipoprotein levels is derived from a synopsis of the literature and personal experience. It is assumed that the full effect of good adherence to a diet reduced in saturated fat and cholesterol has been achieved before treatment with niacin is begun.

A. Elevated LDL (Type II Hyperlipoproteinemia)

In patients with significantly elevated LDL cholesterol (above 190 mg/dl) a fall of 20–25% is usually observed in those who comply with regimens of 3–9 g of niacin daily (Figge et al., 1988). This is usually true for LDL elevations produced by major gene defects such as heterozygous familial hypercholesterolemia or by polygenic disorders. Such individuals usually have normal triglyceride levels and only a 20% reduction in triglycerides is expected with niacin treatment. In patients with combined disorders, where both VLDL and LDL are elevated, the percentage change in triglyceride is usually larger with 30–50% reductions commonly seen in patients whose total plasma triglycerides exceed 300 mg/dl. In these patients, the LDL reduction may be less dramatic with only a 5 to 20% fall.

Niacin is not the drug of first choice in patients with elevated LDL and normal triglycerides. The bile acid binding resins or HMG CoA reductase inhibitors are generally more effective. However, it is a good second-line drug when therapy with these other agents is not possible.

B. Familial Combined Hyperlipoproteinemia

In this disorder, VLDL or LDL or both lipoproteins may be elevated in a given patient at any specific time. Total plasma cholesterol reductions of 30% can be expected with niacin therapy and reductions in VLDL triglycerides by 30–50% are common (Carlson and Olsson, 1990; Olsson, et al., 1986). HDL cholesterol tends to rise 10–30%. Niacin is the drug of first choice in such patients when there are no contraindications.

C. Disbetalipoproteinemia (Type III Hyperlipoproteinemia)

This disorder involves abnormal processing of VLDL with an accumulation remnant lipoproteins which are both cholesterol and triglyceride-rich LDL cholesterol may actually be quite normal. Niacin reduces these VLDL and IDL particles by 50–60% and often raises HDL cholesterol by 30% (Carlson and Olsson, 1990). Niacin may be the drug of first choice in this disorder.

D. VLDL Elevations (Type IV Hyperlipoproteinemia)

This common abnormality involving triglyceride levels of 300–800 mg/dl is usually explained by increased VLDL of normal composition. LDL is often normal or low and HDL is usually reduced. Niacin may be expected to reduce the plasma triglycerides by 40–60% with the concomitant rise in HDL cholesterol by 25–50%. For reasons that are unclear, LDL cholesterol may not change or may show a modest rise. It is quite unusual for the LDL to rise outside desirable limits in such patients with niacin therapy. Niacin should be considered in the initial treatment of these individuals. Elevations of chylomicrons and VLDL (Type V hyperlipoproteinemia) are found in patients with severe hypertriglyceridemia (>1000 mg/dl). Although niacin does not appear to affect fat absorption, chylomicron formation or the lipase enzymes involved in their clearance, chylomicrons fall when such patients are treated with niacin. This is apparently due to the reduced VLDL entering plasma to compete with the lipolytic sites which are involved in the degradation of both lipoproteins. In fact, in these patients the most dramatic triglyceride reductions are observed, often in excess of 65% (Carlson et al., 1977). Low levels of LDL and HDL are common and both tend to rise toward the normal range with treatment.

V. CLINICAL USE

Niacin, a white crystalline powder, is normally provided in tablets of 50 to 500 mg. It is supplied by many manufacturers in over-the-counter preparations and is also available as a prescription drug from several pharmaceutical houses. The rapid absorption and metabolism has led to the development of a variety of delayed release preparations. This is achieved in some preparations by including various binding agents and thereby reducing the rate of solution within and absorption from the intestinal tract. Another technique used to delay the metabolic release of niacin is the esterification to a variety of polyhydric alcohols such as pentaerythritol, inositol, fructose, or sorbitol. These derivatives are apparently absorbed in the unhydrolyzed form from the intestinal tract and are further metabolized slowly by various tissue esterases. Preparations of the latter type are not currently available in the United States. Although reducing the initial side effect of cutaneous flushing, the long-term side effects and tolerance of the slow-release forms of niacin do not appear to offer significant advantage over the regular niacin (Knopp et al., 1985).

Therapy with niacin must be started at a low dose given 3 or 4 times daily. A common schedule is to begin with 100 mg tablets following meals and to repeatedly double the dose at intervals of 3–7 days if flushing episodes have abated. After reaching a total daily dose of 1.5 g/day, it is advisable to allow the patient to stabilize for approximately 4 weeks when the lipoprotein levels should be re-evaluated and the patient examined for adverse reactions including clinical chemistry tests (ASAT, ALAT, glucose and uric acid). If an adequate reduction of cholesterol or triglyceride has not been achieved and no side effects are evident, the dose can be doubled to approximately 3 g/day. The patient should be monitored 4 to 6 weeks after each dose increase. Significant reduction in triglycerides and LDL cholesterol should be seen with dose levels of 3 g/day and only in the minority of patients should it be necessary to increase the dose to 4.5 or 6 g per day. The incidence of systemic side effects (see below) increases markedly at doses above 3 g/day. In some studies, niacin has been used at doses of 8–12 g/day (Illingworth et al., 1981; Kane et al., 1981; Nessim et al., 1983) and many patients will tolerate such high intake. However, it is not clear that such doses were needed to achieve the desired lipoprotein reductions. Instead of using very high doses, combining additional cholesterol reducing medications with different mechanisms of action may produce a more effective and a safer long-term regimen for the patient.

Many of the annoying side effects (see below) may be avoided by artful clinical use. For example, administering aspirin or other cyclooxygenase inhibitors in small doses twice daily during the phase of graduated niacin dosing often prevents the cutaneous side effects (Jay et al., 1990). Administration after a meal and the avoidance of hot liquids in conjunction with niacin intake may reduce the abdominal discomfort experienced by some patients. It is also very important to remind the patient that strict adherence to the regimen will maintain the tachyphylaxis to the flushing reaction. Omitting one or two doses may lead to a marked cutaneous flush with the next dose. Discontinuing the medication even for a few days requires repeating the graduated administration schedule used initially.

Continued monitoring of the lipoproteins at one- or two-month intervals may show continued improvement in the HDL level for at least six months (Alderman, 1989). In choosing the niacin preparation, it is important to consider the source. Since the quality of the preparations and the cost can vary markedly. For example, high-quality niacin at a dose of 3 g/day may be purchased for less than $10.00 per month, whereas other preparations may exceed this price by 10–20-fold. It is our clinical experience that abdominal discomfort is produced by certain brands and not by others. This may have to do with the content of excipients or the quality of the tablet preparation. Improper manufacturing can result in tablets that do not dissolve, with patients reporting the medication actually appearing in the stool. Some of the sustained release forms have also been found to dissolve so slowly that only a portion of the niacin contained therein is available for absorption.

VI. ADVERSE REACTIONS

There are many adverse reactions to niacin therapy and its successful use requires systematic and careful monitoring of the patient's progress. Fortunately, the most common of these are only annoying (cutaneous flushing, abdominal discomfort) and usually they can be avoided or ameliorated. However, certain side effects are serious and potentially fatal (Table 1).

Table 1 Adverse Reactions Observed with Niacin Therapy

Adverse reaction	Estimated frequency	
Skin:		
Cutaneous flushing	Very common	≥90%
Pruritus	Common	(10–50%)
Rash	Common	(5–30%)
Dry skin	Less common	(5–10%)
Acanthosis nigricans	Less common	(<5%)
Gastrointestinal:		
Abdominal pain	Common	(10–20%)
Nausea	Common	(5–10%)
Vomiting	Less common	(1–5%)
Anorexia	Less common	(1–5%)
Diarrhea	Less common	(1–5%)
Liver:		
Elevated ASAT and ALAT	Common	(5–10%)
Elevated alkaline phosphatase	Less common	(1–3%)
Elevated bilirubin	Rare	(<1%)
Heart:		
Cardiac arrhythmias	Less common	(1–5%)
Muscle:		
Myopathic changes	Rare	(<1%)
Eye:		
Cystic maculopathy	Rare	(<1%)
Metabolic:		
Elevated uric acid	Common	(5–10%)
Abnormal GTT	Common	(5–10%)
Elevated fasting glucose	Common	(5–10%)
Weight loss	Less common	(1–5%)

The frequency estimates refer to patients taking crystalline niacin in the dose range of 3–6 g/day for several months or longer. Gastrointestinal side effects may be two or three times more common with delayed release forms.

A. Skin

Cutaneous flushing has been reported in more than 90% of patients beginning niacin therapy in some studies. The onset is usually within one hour after the dose and begins with a sensation of sudden unexplained warmth. The skin may appear reddened over the upper trunk and face, sometimes involving the total body. This results from marked vasodilatation which may be sufficient to cause a drop in blood pressure with lightheadedness. Recently, this vasodilatation has been attributed to the endogenous release of the prostaglandin PGD_2 (Morrow et al., 1989). This vasodilatory compound is rapidly converted to a metabolic product $9A,11B-PGF_2$ which has been shown to rise several hundredfold in the serum of patients concomitant with niacin absorption. This is consistent with the ameliorating effect of predosing with cyclooxygenase inhibitors (Morrow et al., 1989). Other cutaneous side effects include pruritus, which may occur only acutely with the flushing episode or may be a more chronic problem. Finally, hyperpigmentation in the folds about the neck and axillae (acanthosis nigricans) is occasionally seen after long-term therapy at high doses.

B. Gastrointestinal

Abdominal discomfort shortly after taking niacin is a frequent complaint, particularly on an empty stomach or concomitant with hot liquids. To some individuals, this may lead to nausea and vomiting. Rarely, a patient may note diarrhea. It is very important to explore any history of gastrointestinal disorders before beginning niacin since inflammatory diseases of the intestinal tract may be exacerbated by this therapy. Although there is not clear evidence that niacin causes peptic ulcer disease, it can certainly aggravate a pre-existing condition. Unfortunately, slow-release preparations of niacin may not reduce the gastrointestinal side effects and in one study have been found to increase the frequency of intestinal complaints (Knopp et al., 1985).

C. Liver

Liver dysfunction is noted in 3–5% of patients taking 3 g or more of niacin daily. There may be no symptoms or the patient may feel lethargic and mildly nauseated. AST and ALT are usually the first chemical abnormalities detected but in some patients, the disorder may be so severe that jaundice appears, and in a few cases, hepatic failure has occurred (Christiansen et al., 1961; Clementz and Holmes, 1987; Patterson et al., 1983). Some reports of hepatic failure have been associated with the use of delayed release forms of niacin (Christiansen et al., 1961; Mullin et al., 1989). A marked and unexplained further reduction in lipoprotein levels may be the first sign of hepatic dysfunction, consistent with the hepatic origin of VLDL and LDL. With the appearance of mild liver dysfunction, reducing the dose by 50% may result in a return to normal liver tests and continued treatment with this agent. Careful monitoring of such patients is necessary.

D. Muscle

Myopathic changes with myalgias and increased serum creatine phosphokinase (CPK) and AST are a rare problem. Several case reports have appeared in which the signs and symptoms disappeared on discontinuing nicotinic acid (Goldstein, 1989; Litin and Anderson, 1989; Reaven and Witztum, 1988). However, it is quite infrequent as indicated by no cases being observed during the coronary drug project in which 3 g/day of nicotinic acid was administered to over 750 patients for 5 years. In the majority of these cases, other drugs with known myopathic effects have been present including ethanol, gemfibrozil, and lovastatin. Animal studies indicate effects on muscle metabolism by nicotinic acid (Lowell and Goodman, 1987) and thus some synergism with other agents must be considered as probable.

E. Eye

Rarely patients report loss of visual acuity in the pericentral visual field (Gass, 1973; Millay et al., 1988). This is usually due to a condition called cystic maculopathy which is thought to be secondary to the accumulation of fluid within the retinal tissue. Patients complain of a doughnut-shaped blurring of vision with a stellate pattern of blurring radiating out from this central region. The disorder is usually bilateral and on ophthalmological examination, macular swelling and cystic lesions located in a sunburst shape may be observed. Millay et al., on systematic examination of patients taking 3–6 g of niacin daily, found an incidence of cystoid maculopathy in approximately 0.7% of patients (Millay et al., 1988). No subclinical findings were reported, indicating that ophthalmological exams are not useful in the asymptomatic patient. Fortunately, this disorder usually disappears completely on discontinuation of niacin.

F. Heart

Some patients note palpitations and rapid pulse during the flushing episodes due to the vasodilatation. However, more severe cardiac arrhythmias have been noted with niacin therapy. In the coronary drug project, there was an excess incidence of atrial fibrillation and other arrhythmias in the niacin group (The Coronary Drug Project Group, 1975). Possible explanations include changes in free fatty acid metabolism and direct myopathic changes as noted above for skeletal muscle. Although the great majority of patients will have no cardiac signs or symptoms with niacin therapy, individuals with rhythm disturbances should be treated with great caution.

G. Metabolic Changes

Elevated uric acid levels may appear in patients who have normal levels prior to therapy and patients with hyperuricemia usually show significant further increases. This is probably a renal effect due to the need to excrete a large load of nicotinuric acid. The actual precipitation of a gouty attack following the institution of nicotinic acid therapy is relatively uncommon but has been reported (The Coronary Drug Project Group, 1975). Clearly, uric acid levels need to be monitored during the first few months on nicotinic acid treatment. Patients with significant hyperuricemia or gouty arthritis should not be treated with this agent.

Decreased glucose tolerance has been reported and rarely the appearance of frank diabetes follows niacin treatment. In the Coronary Drug Project, there was a significant increase in the fasting plasma glucose and in the 1 hour postchallenge glucose compared with placebo-treated controls (The Coronary Drug Project Group, 1975). Since most patients have no abnormality even on large doses of niacin, this side effect may be selective for individuals with subclinical diabetes. At present, it is not clear whether niacin may interfere with insulin secretion or increase insulin resistance, however, patients with known glucose intolerance or strong family histories of diabetes should be treated with caution. On the other hand, patients with frank diabetes mellitus and severe hypertriglyceridemia have been treated with niacin therapy quite successfully and in many (perhaps most) of these individuals, the control of blood glucose is not significantly altered (Parsons, 1961b). If niacin treatment is chosen for such patients, careful monitoring of the diabetic status must be undertaken.

VII. COMBINATION THERAPY

Nicotinic acid alone may produce satisfactory reduction in serum triglycerides and cholesterol. However, many patients with severe elevations of LDL cholesterol often remain in the high-risk range after the full effect of high-dose niacin therapy. In such patients, the addition of a second lipid-lowering medication may produce desirable levels of LDL cholesterol. Alternatively, when other drug regimens prove only partially effective, niacin may be added.

A. Niacin Plus Bile-Acid Binding Resins

Several studies have now reported the combined use of niacin and either colestipol or cholestyramine (Illingworth et al., 1981; Kane et al., 1981; Nessim et al., 1983). The LDL reduction of 20–25% seen with each agent alone is at least additive with total declines in excess of 50% reported in patients with familial hypercholesterolemia (Kane et al., 1981) and in those with idiopathic or polygenic disorders causing the high LDL concentrations. In some patients, the initial treatment with bile-acid binding resins induces an increase in triglycerides. This is ameliorated with niacin therapy which usually produces reductions below those initially observed. Thus, in patients with both elevated LDL and VLDL, niacin, followed by cholestyramine treatment, may produce optimal lipid reductions. The side effects observed in such patients have been those usually seen with the drugs used individually.

B. Niacin Plus Fibric Acid Derivatives

No systematic controlled trials have been published in which niacin or fibric acid derivatives (clofibrate, gemfibrozil, fenofibrate, etc.) have been compared with a combination of the two. Case reports indicate some additive effect but also reports of myopathic changes with this combination have appeared. The combination of clofibrate and niacin was used successfully in the Stockholm Heart Study (Carlson and Rosenhamer, 1988) over a five-year period with few reported adverse reactions (see below). Niacin and fenofibrate treatment in 42 patients resulted in dropouts due to improvements in the angiographic findings of femoral artery arteriosclerosis was reported by these investigators after one year of treatment with this combination in the remaining patients (Olsson et al., 1990).

C. Niacin and Reductase Inhibitors

The addition of niacin to the regimen of lovastatin-treated patients appears to produce an additional reduction in LDL cholesterol. However, myopathy has been reported in a few cases and a possible interaction of the two drugs producing this side effect has been postulated (Reaven and Witztum, 1988). This has proved to be a very potent combination, producing a 50% mean reduction in LDL cholesterol in patients with heterozygous familial hypercholesterolemia (Malloy et al., 1987). The effect was comparable to colestipol plus lovastatin in the same patients. A further reduction of 35% was achieved with a combination of all three agents. In this study, the LDL cholesterol was reduced from a mean value of 323 mg/dl on diet alone to 161 mg/dl with lovastatin and niacin and to 103 mg/dl when colestipol was added—an overall reduction of 70% (Malloy et al., 1987).

D. Niacin Plus Neomycin

Neomycin has been used for many years to reduce cholesterol. This agent apparently inhibits absorption of both dietary cholesterol and bile acids. Although poorly absorbed by most, certain patients with increased absorption of decreased clearance of this antibiotic are subject to kidney and eighth nerve damage. For this reason, it should not be used in routine practice, however, it has been useful in specialized lipid clinics. Hoeg et al. combined this agent with niacin in patients with elevated LDL cholesterol using a double-blind randomized placebo-controlled cross-over design (Hoeg et al., 1984). In 25 subjects, neomycin was found to reduce LDL cholesterol by 29%. On introduction of niacin, only 14 of the 25 were able to tolerate the agent due to adverse reactions but in these 14, a further 25% reduction of LDL cholesterol was achieved. These patients also experienced a 32% rise in HDL cholesterol on institution of niacin therapy. Overall, the combination produced a 45% reduction in LDL cholesterol as compared with the baseline diet. Lp(a) was also reduced by 24% by neomycin 2 g/day and 45% by the combination of neomycin 2 g/day and niacin 3 g/day (Guvakav et al., 1985) in this study. However, the possible benefit of changing the concentrations of Lp(a) has not yet been demonstrated in clinical trials.

E. Niacin Plus Probucol

Probucol lowers LDL cholesterol by 10–25% in many patients but also lowers HDL cholesterol by a comparable or greater amount. Recently, clinical experience with 19 patients treated sequentially with diet, niacin, and the combination of niacin and probucol was reported (Cohen and Morgan, 1988). At baseline, the mean cholesterol was 352 mg/dl in these patients. Dietary therapy produced a 15% reduction; niacin a further 14% reduction and the addition of probucol a further 21% reduction, leading to a final mean total cholesterol of 202 mg/dl. Lipoprotein levels were not reported. This combination may prove to be clinically useful but additional studies with adequate control regimens and evaluation of lipoprotein changes are needed.

VIII. NIACIN AND VASCULAR DISEASE

Niacin has been used in a variety of clinical trials attempting to demonstrate a reduction in cardiovascular endpoints. A few of these have used niacin as the primary intervention, but most recent studies have explored the potential benefits of combinations of niacin with one or two other agents. These are of interest because they give insights into the ultimate benefit of long-term treatment with niacin and also provide information on the adverse events which may occur with its prolonged clinical use. Some of these studies have explored the relationship between the appearance of vascular disease end-points and a variety of lipoprotein parameters. These findings are helping to build useful hypotheses about mechanisms by which the various lipoproteins may be damaging the vascular wall.

In attempting to interpret large trials for relevance to the clinical use of niacin, one must remember that the analyses usually are based on "intention to treat." That is, the data obtained on the participants are analyzed as though the full dose of drug was taken as prescribed and no other differences existed between the controls and the treated group. Patients are treated according to the study regimen whether they respond with cholesterol reduction or not. The degree of lipoprotein change and any consequences are, in truth, blunted by lack of adherence to the regimen or the introduction of lipid-lowering therapy in the control group. Secondly, the benefits are judged over a relatively short period of time (2 to 7 years), not the lifetime of treatment that one anticipates in the individual patient. Since the patients are blinded to both the regimen and results, there is no sharing of the lipid response information to provide the positive reinforcement often needed to sustain compliance. In clinical practice, those not responding could be changed to other medication. The results from a clinical trial provide evidence for efficacy which is the minimum one should expect in a truly compliant patient who is thoughtfully treated and systematically followed for many years.

A. The Coronary Drug Project

This large project attempted to test the efficacy and safety of several lipid-influencing drugs in the long-term therapy of coronary heart disease in men with proven previous myocardial infarction (Coronary Drug Project Group, 1975). Five drug regimens were compared with a placebo-controlled group in a double-blind, randomized design. A total of 1,119 men were assigned to niacin (3 g/day) and were compared over a five-year period with a placebo group comprised of 2,789 men. All were 30–64 years at the beginning of the trial.

Of patients taking niacin, 10% dropped out versus only 7.5% of the placebo-treated group. Of the remaining niacin-treated patients, 78% took at least 80% of their prescribed medicine for the full five years of the study versus 90% of those taking placebo and remaining in the trial. The niacin-treated group sustained a mean reduction in total plasma cholesterol of 10% and in triglycerides of 26% compared with the placebo-treated group. No difference was found in total death or in cardiovascular death rates at the end of the five years. However, a significant reduction in definite nonfatal myocardial infarction was observed: 8.9% versus 12.2% in the placebo-treated group. The combined endpoint used in the Lipid Research Clinic Coronary Primary Prevention Trial (Lipid Research Clinic Program) of coronary death and definite nonfatal myocardial infarction was also reduced significantly (22.8 vs. 26.2%). Definite or suspected fatal or nonfatal strokes or intermittent cerebral ischemic attacks, as a group, were reduced as well. Other cardiovascular endpoints were also found to be reduced significantly including the appearance of new angina pectoris (38.1 vs. 48.7%) and the need for coronary heart disease surgery (1.3 vs. 3.2%).

Certain adverse effects also reached statistically significant numbers. Atrial fibrillation occurred in 4.7% of the niacin group as opposed to 2.9% in the placebo-treated group and other cardiac arrhythmias were significantly increased as well (32.7 vs. 28.2%). Over the course of the trial, there was a slight but statistically significant increase in uric acid levels and acute gouty arthritis was slightly more frequent, 6.4% versus 4.3%. There was also evidence for some change in glucose tolerance. The percentage of individuals with fasting plasma glucose greater than 120 was 23.8% in the niacin-treated group as opposed to 15.9% in the placebo-treated group and those with plasma glucose in excess of 240 one hour after a glucose load was 18.9% versus 12.9%. There was no significant difference in those developing glucosuria (4.2 vs. 3.9%). Other expected side effects appearing frequently included abdominal pain, nausea, flushing of the skin, pruritus, and skin rash.

Although the Coronary Drug Project did not demonstrate a significant effect of niacin treatment on total mortality at the end of five years, the results were different when the vital status of all participants was determined after approximately 15 years from the beginning of the study or nine years after termination of the study (Canner et al., 1986). Mortality in the niacin-treated group was found to be 11% lower than in the placebo-treated group due to a highly significant decline in coronary heart disease death. This was observed although niacin had been discontinued in the great majority of patients after five years. This result cannot be viewed with the same weight as a positive result addressing the specific major hypothesis tested by a clinical trial. However, it is an interesting observation that five years of niacin treatment appeared to carry over for such a long period of time. One can only speculate as to the potential result of having treated this population for the entire 15 years.

B. The Stockholm Ischemic Heart Disease Study

This study examined the effect of niacin and clofibrate in a randomized open trial in a group of 555 consecutive survivors of myocardial infarction in a single hospital in Stockholm (Carlson and Rosenhamer, 1988). These subjects (80% men and 20% women) were randomly assigned to a control group (n = 276) or a treatment group (n = 279). Of these patients, 83% had experienced a single myocardial infarction and 17% had had two or more occurrences. Patients with "extreme hyperlipidemia" and "familial hypercholesterolemia" or with other serious illnesses were excluded. After four months of diet therapy, the patients were assigned to the treated group (Clofibrate 1 g twice daily) and two months later were placed on a long-acting ester of nicotinic acid (pentaerytrityltetranicotinate) at a dose of 1 g three times daily. Matching placebos were administered in a similar fashion to the control group. A total of 59% of the patients took at least 1.5 g of each medication daily throughout the study. In the treatment group, 6% withdrew during the five years of the trial. Total serum cholesterol was reduced by 13% and serum triglycerides by 19% as compared with the placebo-treated group.

At the end of five years, a 26% reduction in total mortality and a 36% reduction in ischemic heart disease mortality was observed. Both factors were statistically significant. The inclusion of older patients was unique to this study of lipid-lowering therapy in coronary heart disease. Those individuals who entered the study between ages 60 and 70 had a 28% decline in total mortality, a finding significant by the statistical criteria used. Nonfatal myocardial infarction was reduced by 30% overall but this did not reach statistical significance with the small number of observations. The very large and rapid impact of this treatment on cardiovascular death was surprising, particularly in light of the relatively small reduction of total plasma cholesterol and triglycerides. It is possible that some additional effects on other physiological systems such as clotting parameters may have been altered by this drug combination. Unfortunately, LDL cholesterol and HDL cholesterol values were not available. Changes in these parameters may have been more predictive of the positive outcome.

During the five years of the study, 26% of the patients taking clofibrate and niacin withdrew for a variety of reasons including subjective side effects. This compared with only 12% withdrawing in the placebo group. Five cases of biliary disease appeared in the treated group, whereas, no cases were observed in the control group, although this was not statistically significant.

C. Cholesterol Lowering Atherosclerosis Study (CLAS)

In this study, niacin was used in combination with colestipol to produce dramatic changes in both low-density and high-density lipoproteins (Blankenhorn et al., 1987). CLAS was a randomized, placebo-controlled, selectively blinded trial of 162 men who had previously had venous bypass grafts of the coronary tree. All were between 40 and 59 years of age and had undergone the surgery at least three months prior to admission to the study. At baseline, plasma cholesterol levels were in the range 185–350 mg/dl. This trial used carefully systematized angiography to evaluate the status of both native vessels and the bypass grafts at entry and again two years later. The major endpoint was a change in the status of each lesion detected at the baseline angiogram.

The 80 patients were placed on a very low saturated fat, low cholesterol diet, colestipol (30 g/day) and niacin (3–12 g/day). The latter was titrated individually on the basis of blood cholesterol response and tolerance. The medications were distributed as three doses with meals. The 82 men in the control group were instructed in a less demanding diet change and placebos. A mean reduction in LDL cholesterol of 43% and a mean rise in HDL cholesterol of 37% was achieved in the colestipol/niacin-treated group.

The baseline and repeat angiograms were read by a team of experts who were blinded to the sequence of the angiography. The change at each lesion sight was given a score and then combined into a "global score" to determine progress of lesion development, stability or possible regression. After two years, the treated group showed a highly significant shift toward stability and reduced rate of progression as compared with the placebo group. The subjects had a significant reduction in new lesions, new closures, and number of lesions with increased stenosis. When the grafts were evaluated, the number of subjects with new lesions, closures and any adverse change were also significantly fewer in the drug-treated group. This study presented the first strongly positive result demonstrating that changes in lipoprotein levels with drug therapy can alter the progression of the angiographically demonstrated coronary artery atherosclerosis.

In a subsequent report, a detailed analysis of the relationship between changes in lipoprotein lipids and apolipoproteins AI, B, and CIII were related to the angiographic findings (Blankenhorn et al., 1990). Although virtually all of the lipids lipoproteins and apolipoproteins changed dramatically with drug treatment, the only change which distinguished those who showed progression of coronary arteriosclerosis as opposed to those who did not progress was the content of a minor apolipoprotein, ApoC III, in the high-density lipoprotein fraction. This small molecular-weight apolipoprotein is known to inhibit lipoprotein lipase (Brown and Baginsky, 1972) and to be related to the rate at which both VLDL and HDL cholesterol is removed from the bloodstream (Ginsberg et al., 1986; Le et al., 1988). The ApoC III content was less in those drug-treated patients who showed progression of lesions and an increase in this apoprotein was predictive of less progression. It is not clear why this specific index was the strongest predictor of arteriosclerotic change in the coronary arteries of the drug-treated patients. Much further research is necessary to confirm and to explain this relationship.

D. The Familial Atherosclerosis Treatment Study (FATS)

A second angiographic demonstration of modifying coronary artery disease progression was recently reported. The Familial Atherosclerosis Treatment Study (FATS) involved the assignment of 146 men with proven coronary artery disease to three groups (Brown et al., 1990). All were less than 62 years of age and had apolipoprotein B levels in excess of 125 mg/dl. All participants had at least one coronary artery lesion occluding 50% or more of the diameter of the artery or three lesions each causing at least 30% stenosis. All patients had a family history of cardiovascular disease in at least one male relative before age 56 or one female relative before age 70. Previous revascularization procedures were an exclusion, therefore, in contrast to the CLAS study all coronary arteries evaluated involved native vessels with original lesions. The men were randomly assigned to two treatment groups and a placebo-controlled group by double-blind strategy. The two treatment groups included one receiving niacin and colestipol and a second was prescribed lovastatin and colestipol. In the niacin-treated group, the dose was increased to 1 g three times daily. In those patients with LDL cholesterol remaining greater than 120 mg/dl, the dose was increased to 1.5 g four times daily. In the lovastatin-treated group, a dose of 20 mg twice daily was increased to 40 mg twice daily if LDL cholesterol did not fall below 120 mg/dl. In both treatment groups, colestipol at a dose of 10 g, three times daily was administered. In the control group, only placebo was administered unless the LDL cholesterol exceeded the 90th percentile for age. For those with higher LDL concentrations, colestipol was administered at increasing doses to reduce the LDL below this value. Arteriographic projections were recorded on film by a standardized protocol at baseline and again 2.5 years later. Tracings of the lesions were digitized by computer and quantitative parameters involving the minimum diameter and nearby "normal diameters" were quantitated using a standard catheter measure as a scaling factor. This quantitative technique added greatly to the power of the study.

In the niacin/colestipol-treated group, the LDL cholesterol fell 32% and the HDL cholesterol rose 43%. When compared with conventional therapy, the niacin/colestipol-treated group showed a mean widening of the vessel diameter at the stenotic lesions whereas the control group showed progression of stenosis. This change was most dramatic when those lesions with greater than 50% stenosis were compared. Comparable improvement in the coronary angiogram was found in the lovastatin/colestipol-treated group where the LDL cholesterol was even more dramatically reduced (46%) although the HDL cholesterol rise was less (15%). It is interesting that clinical signs and symptoms worsened significantly in 13 of the 52 control patients whereas only 2 of the 48 patients treated with niacin and colestipol had new clinical signs of coronary artery disease.

The use of niacin and colestipol was associated with the expected adverse reactions including a mean rise in uric acid from 6.9 to 7.5 mmol/L, the development of gout in two patients, and a moderate rise in the serum aspartate aminotransferase level (mean increase 20%). Three patients developed acanthosis nigricans and four complained of a pruritic skin rash. Two patients had worsening of their blood sugar level requiring antidiabetic drugs during the trial. As with the CLAS study, this study provides objective evidence that niacin in conjunction with a bile-acid binding resin can produce significant protection from progression of coronary artery disease. The lipoprotein parameters, whose changes best correlated with reduced rates of stenosis, included reduction in LDL and HDL cholesterol.

IX. SUMMARY

Niacin is one of the oldest drugs used to reduce plasma cholesterol. As more knowledge has been gained about lipoprotein metabolism, the effects of niacin treatment have been appreciated to reduce those lipoproteins which may be causative in the development of arteriosclerosis, namely LDL, IDL, VLDL, and Lp(a). This drug also raises HDL which may prove beneficial as well. Only low doses (1 g/day) are required to produce this effect. The combination of niacin with other lipid-lowering medications provides marked reductions of LDL often in excess of 50%. This type of therapy can bring the high concentrations of LDL found in familial hypercholesterolemia to within a desirable range.

The Coronary Drug Project gave strong evidence that the incidence of recurrent myocardial infarction could be reduced by niacin as the only intervention and long-term follow-up of that cohort indicated that exposure to this therapy for five years was associated with improved survival over 15 years. Recent trials have found niacin in combination with other agents to reduce the rate of progression of coronary artery lesions.

The successful clinical use of niacin requires the careful selection of the appropriate patient and education of that patient regarding the potential of adverse effects and methods of avoiding these. Flushing of the skin will occur in the great majority of those treated. Gastrointestinal side effects include abdominal pain, nausea, vomiting, and rarely, diarrhea. Liver dysfunction is usually mild and reversible. Rare cases of hepatocellular failure have been reported. Cardiac arrhythmias are an uncommon side effect and myopathic changes in skeletal muscle are quite rare. The latter appear to be more common when fibric acid therapy or heavy alcohol use are also present. Hyperuricemia and abnormal glucose tolerance accompany niacin therapy in patients with a predisposition to these disorders.

REFERENCES

Alderman, J. D. (1989). Effect of a modified, well tolerated niacin regimen on serum total cholesterol, high density lipoprotein cholesterol and the cholesterol to high density lipoprotein ratio. *Am. J. Cardiol.* **64:**725–729.

Altschul, R., Hoffer, A., and Stephen, J. D. (1955). Influence of nicotinic acid on cholesterol in man. *Arch. Biochem.* **54:**558–559.

Blankenhorn, D. H., Nessim, S. A., Johnson, R. L., San Marco, M. E., Azen, S. P., and Cashin-Hemphill, L. (1987). Beneficial effects of combined colestipol-niacin therapy on coronary artherosclerosis and coronary venous bypass grafts. *JAMA* **257:**3233–3240.

Blankenhorn, D. H., Alaupovic, P., Wickhom, E., Chin, H. P., and Azen, S. P. (1990). Prediction of angiographic change in native human coronary arteries and aorto coronary bypass grafts. Lipid and non lipid factors. *Circulation* **81:**470–476.

Blum, C. E., Levy, R. I., Eisenberg, S., Hall, M., Geobel, R. N., and Berman, M. (1977). HDL metabolism in man. *J. Clin. Invest.* **60:**795–807.

Brown, G., Albers, J., Fisher, L., Schaefer, S., Lin, J.-T, Kaplan, C., Zhao, X-Q, Bisson, B., Fitzpatrick, V., and Dodge, H. (1990). Regression of Coronary Artery Disease as a result of intensive lipid-lowering therapy in men with high levels of apolipoprotein B. *New Engl. J. Med.* **323:**1289–1298.

Brown, W. V., and Baginsky, M. L. (1972). Inhibition of lipoprotein lipase activity by an apolipoprotein of human very low density lipoprotein. *Biochem. Biophys. Res. Commun.* **46:**375–382.

Canner, P. L. and the Coronary Drug Project Research Group. (1986). Mortality in Coronary Drug Project patients during a nine-year past-treatment period. *J. Am. Coll. Cardiol.* **8:**1245–1255.

Carlson, L. A., and Oro, L. (1962). The effect of nicotinic acid on the plasma free fatty acids. *Acta Med. Scand.* **172:**641–645.

Carlson, L. A., Oro, L., and Ostman, J. (1968). Effect of a single dose of nicotinic acid on plasma lipids in patients with hyperlipoproteinemia. *Acta Med. Scand.* **183:**457–465.

Carlson, L. A., Olsson, A. G., and Ballantyne, D. (1977). On the rise in low density and high density lipoproteins in response to the treatment of hypertriglyceridemia in type IV and type V hyperlipoproteinemia. *Atherosclerosis* **26:**603–609.

Carlson, L. A., and Olsson, A. G. (1984). Effect of nicotinic acid on serum lipids and lipoproteins. In *Treatment of Hyperlipoproteinemia*. Edited by A. G. Olsson. New York, Raven Press, pp. 115–119.

Carlson, L. A., and Rosenhamer, G. (1988). Reduction in mortality in the Stockholm Ischaemic Heart Disease Secondary Prevention Study by combined treatment with clofibrate and nicotinic acid. *Acta Med. Scand.* **223:**405–414.

Carlson, L. A., Hamsten, A., and Asplund, A. (1989). Pronounced lowering of serum levels of lipoprotein Lp(a) in hyperlipidemic subjects treated with nicotinic acid. *J. Int. Med.* **226:**271–276.

Carlson, L. A., and Olsson, A. G. (1990). Effects of hyperlipidemic drugs on serum; lipoproteins. In *Progress in Biochemical Pharmacology*. Edited by S. Eisenberg. New York, S. Karger, AG 15; 238–257.

Cayen, M. N. (1985). Disposition, metabolism and pharmakinetics of anti-hyperlipidemic agents in laboratory animals and man. *Pharm. Ther.* **29:**157–204.

Christiansen, N. A., Achor, R. W. P., Berge, K. G., and Mason, H. L. (1961). Nicotinic acid treatment of hypercholesterolemia—Comparison of plain and sustained action preparations and report of two cases of jaundice. *J. Am. Med. Assoc.* **177:**546–550.

Clementz, G. L., and Holmes, A. W. (1987). Nicotinic acid-induced fulminant hepatic failure. *J. Clin. Gastroenterol.* **9:**582–584.

Cohen, L., and Morgan, J. (1988). Effectiveness of individualized long-term therapy with niacin and probucol in reduction of serum cholesterol. *J. Fam. Practice* **26:**145–150.

The Coronary Drug Project Group. (1975). Clofibrate and niacin in coronary heart disease. *J. Am. Med. Assoc.* **231:**360–381.

Darby, W. J., McNutt, K. W., and Tod Hunter, E. N. (1975). Niacin. *Nutr. Rev.* **33:**289–297.

Expert Panel. (1988). Report of the National Cholesterol Education Program Expert Panel on Detection, Evaluation and Treatment of High Blood Cholesterol in Adults. *Arch. Intern. Med.* **148:**36–39.

Figge, H. L., Figge, J., Souney, P. F., Mutnick, A. H., and Sacks, F. (1988). Nicotinic acid: A review of its clinical use in the treatment of lipid disorders. *Pharmacotherapy* **8:**287–294.

Froberg, S. O., Boberg, J., Carlson, L. A., and Erickkson, M. (1971). *Metabolic Effects of Nicotinic Acid and its Derivatives*. Hans Huber Publishers, pp. 167–181.

Gass, J. D. M. (1973). Nicotinic acid maculopathy. *Am. J. Ophthalmol.* **76:**500–510.

Ginsberg, H. N., Le, N. A., Goldberg, I. J., Gibson, J. C., Rubinstein, A., Wang-Iverson, P., Norum, R., and Brown, W. V. (1986). Apolipoprotein B metabolism in subjects with deficiency of apolipoprotein CIII and AI: Evidence that apolipoprotein CIII inhibits lipoprotein lipase in vivo. *J. Clin. Invest.* **78:**1287–1295.

Goldstern, M. (1989). Nicotinic acid-associated myopathy. *Am. J. Med.* **87:**248.

Grundy, S. M., Mok, H. Y. I, Zech, L., and Berman, M. (1981). Influence of nicotinic acid on metabolism of cholesterol and triglyceride in man. *J. Lipid Res.* **22:**24–36.

Gurian, A., and Adlersberg, D. (1959). The effect of large doses of nicotinic acid on circulating lipids and carbohydrate tolerance. *Am. J. Med. Sci.* **237:**12.

Guvakav, A., Hoeg, J. M., Kostner, G., Papadopoulos, N. M., and Brewer, H. B., Jr. (1985). Levels of lipoprotein Lp(a) decline with neomycin and niacin treatment. *Atherosclerosis* **57:**293–301.

Hoeg, J. M., Maher, M. B., Bou, E., Zech, L. A., Bailey, K. R., Gregg, R. E., Sprecher, D. L., Susser, J. K., Pikus, A. M., and Brewer, H. B. (1984). Normalization of plasma lipoprotein concentrations in patients with Type I hyperlipoproteinemia by combined use of neomycin and niacin. *Circulation* **70:**1004–1011.

Hotz, W. (1983). Nicotinic acid and its derivatives: A short survey. *Adv. Lipid Res.* **20:**195–217.

Illingworth, D. R., Phillipson, B. E., Rapp, J. H., and Connor, W. E. (1981). Colestipol plus nicotinic acid in the treatment of heterozygous familial hypercholesterolemia. *Lancet* **1:**296–298.

Jay, R. H., Dickson, A. C., and Betteridge, D. J. (1990). Effects of aspirin upon the flushing reaction induced by niceritrol. *Br. J. Clin. Pharm.* **29:**120–122.

Kane, J. P., Mallay, J. J., and Tun, P. (1981). Normalization of low-density lipoprotein levels in heterozygous familial hypercholesterolemia with combined drug regimen. *N. Engl. J. Med.* **304:**2541–258.

Knopp, R. H., Ginsberg, J., Albers, J. J., Hoff, C., Ogilvie, J. T., Warnick, G. R., Burrows, E., Retzlaff, B., and Poole, M. (1985). Contrasting effects of unmodified and time-release forms of niacin or lipoproteins in hyperlipidemic subjects: Clues to mechanism of action of niacin. *Metabolism* **34:**642–650.

Kostner, G., Klein, G., and Krempler, F. (1984). Can Serum Lp(a) concentration be lowered by drugs and or diet? In *Treatment of Hyperlipoproteinemia.* Edited by L. A. Carlson and A. G. Olsson. New York, Raven Press, pp. 154–156.

Le, N. A., Gibson, J. C., and Ginsberg, H. N. (1988). Independent regulation of plasma apolipoproteins CII and CIII concentrations in very low density and high density lipoproteins. Implication for the regulation of catabolism of these lipoproteins. *J. Lipid Res.* **29:**669–677.

Lipid Research Clinics Program. (1984). The Lipid Research Clinic Coronary Primary Prevention Trial Results I. Reduction in incidence of coronary heart disease. *J. Am. Med. Assoc.* **251:**351–364.

Litin, S. C., and Anderson, C. F. (1989). Nicotinic acid—associated myopathy: A reported three cases. *Am. J. Med.* **86:**481–483.

Lowell, B. B., and Goodman, M. N. (1987). Protein sparing in skeletal muscle during prolonged starvation—dependence on lipid fuel availability. *Diabetes* **36:**14–19.

Luria, M. H. (1988). Effect of low dose niacin on high-density lipoprotein cholesterol and total cholesterol high-density lipoprotein cholesterol ratio. *Arch. Intern. Med.* **148:**2493–2495.

Malloy, M. J., Kane, J. P., Kunitake, S. T., and Tun, P. (1987). Complementarity of colestipol, niacin and lovastatin in the treatment of severe familial hypercholesterolemia. *Ann. Intern. Med.* **107:**616–623.

Millay, R. H., Klein, M. L., and Illingworth, D. R. (1988). Niacin maculopathy. *Ophthalmology* **95**:930–936.

Morrow, J. D., Parsons, W. G., III, and Roberts, L. J., II. (1989). Release of markedly increased quantities of prostaglandin D2 in Vivo in humans following the administration of nicotinic acid. *Prostaglandins* **38**:263–274.

Mrochek, J. E., Jolley, R. I., and Young, D. S. (1976). Metabolic response on humans to ingestion of nicotinic acid and nicotinamide. *Clin. Chem.* **22**:1821–1827.

Mullin, G. E., Greenson, J. K., and Mitchell, M. C. (1989). Fulminant hepatic failure after ingestion of sustained-release nicotinic acid. *Ann. Intern. Med.* **111**:253–255.

Nessim, S. A., Chin, H. P., Alaupovic, P., and Blankenhorn, D. H. (1983). Combined therapy of niacin, colestipol and fat controlled diet on men with coronary bypass: Effect on blood lipids and apolipoproteins. *Arteriosclerosis* **3**:568–573.

Olsson, A. G., Walldus, G., and Wahlberg, G. (1986). Nicotinic acid and its analogues—mechanisms of action, effects and clinical usage. In *Pharmacological Control of Hyperlipidemia*. Edited by R. Fears. Barcelona, Spain, J. R. Prous Science Publishers, pp. 217–230.

Olsson, A. G., Ruhn, G., and Erikson, U. (1990). The effect of serum lipid regulation on the development of femoral atherosclerosis in hyperlipidemia: a non-randomized controlled study. *J. Intern. Med.* **227**:381–390.

Ortega, M. P., Sunkel, C., Armijo, M., and Priego, J. G. (1980). Effects of Etofibrate on platelet function: in vitro studies in human plasma. *Thrombo. Res.* **19**:409–416.

Parsons, W. B., Jr. (1961a). Progress report with review of studies regarding mechanism of action. *Arch. Intern. Med.* **107**:639–652.

Parsons, W. B., Jr. (1961b). Studies of nicotinic acid use in hypercholesterolemia: Changes in hepatic function, carbohydrate tolerance and uric acid metabolism. *Arch. Intern. Med.* **107**:653–667.

Patterson, D. J., Dew, E. W., Gyorkey, F., and Graham, D. Y. (1983). Niacin hepatitis. *South Med. J.* **76**:239–241.

Reaven, P., and Witztum, J. L. (1988). Lovastatin, nicotinic acid and rhabdomyolysis. *Annal Intern. Med.* **109**:597–595.

Shepherd, J., Packard, C. J., Patsch, J. R., Gotto, A. M., and Tounton, O. D. (1979). Effects of nicotinic acid therapy on plasma high density subfraction and composition and on apolipoprotein A metabolism. *J. Clin. Invest.* **63**:858–867.

Wahlberg, G., Holmquist, L., Walldins, G., and Annuzzi, G. (1988). Effects of nicotinic acid on concentrations of serum apolipoproteins. B, CI, CII, CIII and E in the hyperlipidemic patients. *Acta Med. Scand.* **224**:319–327.

Weiner, M. (1979). Clinical pharmacology and pharmakinetics of nicotinic acid. *Drug Metab. Rev.* **9**:99–106.

10

Combination Drug Therapy

Jeffrey M. Hoeg
National Heart, Lung, and Blood Institute
National Institutes of Health
Bethesda, Maryland

I. INTRODUCTION

Most patients who require treatment to reduce their cardiovascular disease risk by modifying their plasma lipoprotein concentrations respond to either diet-only therapy or to dietary modification in concert with a single hypolipidemic drug. However, certain patients in virtually every clinical practice will not achieve the desired levels of plasma lipoprotein concentrations with the use of a single pharmacological agent. The inability of single agents to sufficiently affect the plasma lipoprotein concentrations in selected hypercholesterolemic patients has led, over the past decade, to a series of studies evaluating combinations of drug therapies. These investigations indicate that some drug therapy combinations are superior to others with respect to both efficacy and tolerability.

Recent clinical trials indicate other advantages to using combinations of drugs to treat hyperlipidemia. In addition to providing improved efficacy, drug combinations can often permit the use of lower doses of each of the agents. Lower doses, in turn, limit both the appearance and the severity of adverse side effects. Futhermore, the use of combination therapy may lead to lowered cost to the patient since the doses of the more expensive medications can be reduced. These additional benefits of combination therapy invite serious consideration for the use of this approach in selected patients.

However, not all combinations of hypolipidemic drugs can be recommended. Some combinations are not particularly effective in reducing the total and low density lipoprotein cholesterol concentrations in certain subsets of hyperlipidemic patients. Other combinations provide little, if any, additional benefit compared to monotherapy. In addition, some drug combinations have been implicated in producing potentially serious adverse side effects not frequently observed when the drugs are given as monotherapy. The goal of this chapter is to summarize the experience of using combinations of lipid-lowering drugs to manage the hypercholesterolemic patient. At least 17 different combinations of hypolipidemic agents have been systematically studied over the past 10 years and provide a framework from which to select the best hypolipidemic drug combination for a given patient. Considering the fast pace of development, the best currently available combinations will undergo further refinement for both patient selection and dosage regimens. Additionally, even better combinations of agents will become available. Therefore the use of combination therapy to treat hypercholesterolemia will play an increasingly important role in routine clinical practice.

II. EFFICACY OF COMBINATION DRUG THERAPY

The majority of patients requiring intervention to reduce cardiovascular disease risk will respond to dietary treatment either alone or in conjunction with drug monotherapy. Standard therapy will generally lead to the recommended goals for therapy outlined by the Adult Treatment Guidelines Panel of the National Cholesterol Education Program (Expert Panel, 1988). Only a small fraction of hypercholesterolemic patients will require consideration for combination drug therapy. Patients with the heterozygous form of familial hypercholesterolemia figure prominently among the individuals who do not reach the designated goal LDL cholesterol concentrations. Goldstein and coworkers first demonstrated that 5% of patients under age 60 admitted to Seattle hospitals with myocardial infarctions manifested this autosomal codominant inborn error of metabolism (Goldstein et al., 1973a,b). Although this represents one of the most commonly recognized genetic diseases, fewer than 1 in 20 hypercholesterolemic patients will manifest this condition. However, many, if not most, patients experiencing difficulty in reducing their total and LDL cholesterol concentrations will have inherited one allele with one of the several mutations in the LDL receptor gene that can lead to this condition (Goldstein and Brown, 1989). In addition, both men and women heterozygous for this disease have a markedly increased risk for premature cardiovascular disease (Stone et al., 1974). The widepread recognition of the seriousness of this disease as well as the difficulty in modulating the plasma lipoproteins in this condition by dietary therapy has led to a series of investigations that have evaluated the efficacy of therapy in these patients. Therefore, most of the clinical trials that have been conducted utilizing combinations of hypolipidemic drugs have focused upon this patient population.

Table 1 summarizes the results of 28 different clinical trials using 17 different drug combinations. The effects of these different combinations of drug therapy in affecting the concentrations of total, LDL, and HDL cholesterol concentrations are shown. Most of these studies have been conducted in patients with heterozygous familial hypercholesterolemia who had markedly elevated LDL cholesterol concentrations. An elevation in the LDL concentration defines the type II hyperlipoproteinemia phenotype (Fredrickson et al., 1967). For comparison among the different studies, it is useful to express the effects of treatment based upon the percent change from baseline therapy. However, it must be stated that the principal goal of therapy in these patients is to reduce the LDL cholesterol concentration to specific goal levels based upon the presence of cardiovascular disease or other risk factors (Expert Panel, 1988). Unfortunately, many clinical trials do not report the individual responses to treatment that would permit evaluation of the data with respect to the guideline recommendations.

The responses to combined drug therapy in patients with an elevated LDL cholesterol concentration vary considerably among the different clinical trials (see Table 1). The percent total cholesterol and LDL cholesterol reductions ranged from 11 to 55% and 12 to 61%, respectively. The wide ranges in response to these different combinations of treatment were also observed with the HDL cholesterol concentrations. Combination of colestipol with probucol *reduced* the HDL cholesterol concentration by 29%, whereas the cholestyramine and compactin combination *increased* the HDL levels by 44%. These results indicate that these 17 different treatment regimens were quite heterogeneous as to their effects on the plasma lipoprotein concentrations.

However, several important trends in efficacy are apparent. First, the bile acid sequestrants cholestyramine and colestipol are quite effective when used in combination with drugs that have complementary mechanisms of action. In fact, 23 of the 28 clinical trials summarized have used one of these two compounds. Second, the combinations of a bile acid sequestrant with either

Table 1 Efficacy of Combined Drug Treatment in Modifying Plasma Concentrations of Total, LDL, and HDL Cholesterol

Drug combination	% Change			Ref.
	Total	LDL	HDL	
Cholestyramine +				
Compactin	−36	−51	+44	Mabuchi et al., 1983
Neomycin	−28	−33	−11	Hoeg et al., 1984
Niacin	−26	−32	+23	Angelin et al., 1986
Lovastatin	−51	−61	+21	Leren et al., 1988
Bezafibrate	−35	−39	+2	Curtis et al., 1988
	−26	−37	+15	Series et al., 1989
Colestipol +				
Niacin	−41	−48	+25	Packard et al., 1980
	−45	−54	+15	Kane et al., 1981
	−40	−47	+32	Illingworth et al., 1981
	−45	−55	+17	Kuo et al., 1981
	−29	−40	+33	Nessim et al., 1983
	−31	−37	+25	Malloy et al., 1987
Lovastatin	−45	−54	−2	Illingworth et al., 1984
	−46	−59	0	Witztum et al., 1989
+ Niacin	−55	−66	+32	Malloy et al., 1987
Simvastatin	−47	−57	+6	Weisweiler, 1988
Clofibrate	−20	−28	+9	Hunninghake et al., 1981
	−11	−12	+25	Hunninghake et al., 1981
	−21	NR	NR	Das, 1986
Fenofibrate	−39	−54	+15	Heller et al., 1981
	−29	−32	+29	Weisweiler et al., 1986
	−30	−37	+23	Weisweiler, 1989
Probucol	−28	−29	−29	Dujovne et al., 1984, 1986
Niacin +				
Neomycin	−36	−45	+13	Hoeg et al., 1984
Lovastatin +				
Neomycin	−28	−32	−7	Hoeg et al., 1986
Gemfibrozil	−34	−40	+7	Illingworth et al., 1989
Probucol	−37	−40	−16	Witztum et al., 1989
Neomycin +				
d-Thyroxine	−30	−27	−19	Vogelberg et al., 1982

NR, not reported.

niacin or an HMG CoA reductase inhibitor are the most effective in reducing the LDL cholesterol concentrations. Figure 1 summarizes the ability of selected combinations of lipid-lowering drugs that demonstrated an additive effect on modifying the plasma lipoprotein concentrations. Combinations of bile acid sequestrants with niacin or the HMG CoA reductase inhibitors lovastatin and simvastatin were particularly effective. The LDL cholesterol concentrations were reduced in these studies from 32 to 66% with an average reduction exceeding 50%. In addition, most of these combinations of drugs had at least the theoretic advantage of increasing the HDL cholesterol. The effects on HDL cholesterol concentrations ranged from a –2% to a +33% change with an average increase of nearly +19%. The most striking effects on the plasma lipoprotein concentrations were observed using triple drug therapy (Malloy et al., 1987). In this study of 21 heterozygous familial hypercholesterolemic patients, the combination of colestipol (30 g/day), niacin (mean dose 5.5 g/day), and lovastatin (40 mg/day) significantly reduced the total and LDL cholesterol concentrations by 55% and 61%, respectively. The maximum response in an individual patient was a 79% reduction in the LDL cholesterol concentration. The HDL cholesterol was also significantly affected with an average increase of 32%. Therefore, combination of these lipid-lowering drugs can profoundly modify the plasma lipoprotein profile in even those heterozygous familial hypercholesterolemic patients who have been notoriously resistant to treatment.

III. ADVERSE EFFECTS

As with any medical intervention, the use of hypolipidemic medications can lead to side effects. The most frequently encountered problems are mild, self-limited, and annoying (Table 2). However, as discussed below, serious and potentially life-threatening adverse effects have also been observed (Mullin et al., 1989; Marias and Larson, 1990). In addition, lipid-lowering medications may lead to interference with the efficacy of other medications or even have additive effects on the induction of adverse side effects (Table 3). The difficulties that can arise with the use of hypolipidemic medications not only trouble the patient, but they also reduce the compliance which, in turn, limits the effectiveness in preventing premature cardiovascular disease. Therefore, familiarity with the side effect profile of the individual drugs and means of reducing these symptoms are important in the management of the hypercholesterolemic patient.

The most serious adverse effects have been observed with the use of niacin and lovastatin. Niacin was originally discovered to reduce blood cholesterol

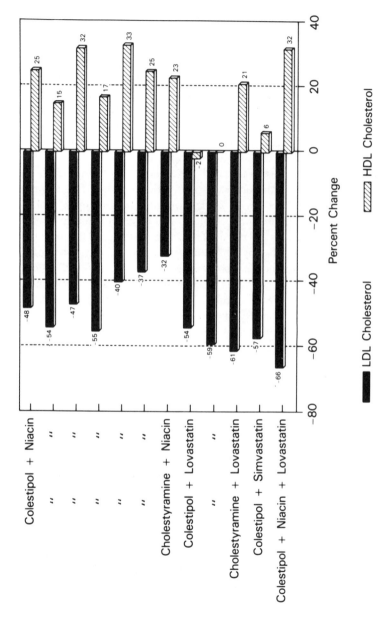

Figure 1 The effects of selected drug combinations on LDL and HDL cholesterol concentrations. The study results shown in this figure represent the percent change in LDL and HDL cholesterol concentrations in clinical trials that demonstrated an additive effect on plasma lipoprotein concentrations.

Table 2 The Hypolipidemic Drugs: Side Effects, Costs, and Contraindications

Drug	Cost/month	Side effects	Contraindications
Niacin 0.5–1.5 g bid plain sustained release	 $ 3.90 4.26	skin flushing · headache · pruritus · hyperglycemia · hyperuricemia · abdominal pain · insomnia	· diabetes · gout · peptic ulcers · asthma · hepatic disease
Colestipol 5–15 g bid packets powder	 36.58 27.38	· constipation	· use of coumarins · fasting hypertri- glyceridemia (>250 mg/dl)
Cholestyramine packets powder bar	 55.91 58.34 64.80	· constipation	· use of coumarins · fasting hypertri- glyceridemia (>250 mg/dl)
Gemfibrozil 300–600 mg bid	 22.28	· abdominal pain · diarrhea · reduced libido · myositis · increased appetite · nausea	· use of coumarins · cholelithiasis · hepatitis
Lovastatin 20–40 mg qd or bid	 46.88	· gastrointestinal upset · hepatitis · myopathy · sleep disturbances	· fertile women open to pregnancy · renal disease · hepatic disease · intestinal disease
Clofibrate 1 g bid	 22.10	· same as gemfibrozil	· same as gemfibrozil
Probucol 0.5 g bid	 43.90	· diarrhea · nausea	· cardiac arrhythmia · prolonged QT interval

The average wholesale price to pharmacists for a 30 supply of a minimum is based upon the 1989 Federal Red Book values. The listed adverse effects are the most common or the most important ones, and the contraindications are relative rather than absolute.

Table 3 Interaction of the Hypolipidemic Drugs with Other Drugs

Hypolipidemic drug	Adverse effect	Second drug
Bile acid sequestrants (colestipol and cholestyramine)	impaired GI absorption	coumarins thiazides digoxin synthroid beta blockers phenobartibal penicillin tetracycline steroids phenylbutazone
Probucol	QT interval prolongation	antiarrhythmic drugs
Lovastatin	myopathy	niacin gemfibrozil cyclosporine erythromycin

concentrations by serendipity (Altschul et al., (1955). Subsequent investigations conducted in the 1950s and early 1960s (Parsons and Flinn, 1957; Parsons, 1961; Christensen et al., 1961) indicated that the doses required to get a lipid-lowering effect were occasionally associated with the development of hepatitis. Hepatoxicity is rare with ingestion of less than 3 grams of niacin given as monotherapy, but it has been observed in patients with preexisting liver disease at doses as low as 1.5 grams of niacin per day (Litin and Anderson, 1989) and has caused fulminant hepatic failure (Clementz and Holmes, 1987; Mullin et al., 1989). One patient taking 6 grams of plain niacin tablets per day ran out of his prescribed medication while on vacation. Shortly after substituting his usual regimen with a sustained release form of the medication, he developed hepatic failure requiring liver transplantation. A recent report also indicates that combination of niacin with gemfibrozil may precipitate hepatitis (Litin and Anderson, 1989). It is not yet clear whether combination drug therapy leads to increased risk of niacin-induced hepatotoxicity, but this possibility should be considered when prescribing combination therapy. Although niacin has been associated with these severe adverse effects, clinically significant hepatotoxicity is rare. Over a 5-year period, none of the 1119 patients that were randomized to receive niacin (average dosage 2.5 g/day) experienced hepatic failure (Coronary Drug Project, 1975). Hyperuricemia with podagra, hyperglycemia, and asymptomatic rises in the serum transaminases were observed more frequently in niacin-treated patients than in the placebo group in this large, prospective, multi-centered clinical trial. However, no life-threatening adverse effects were observed. In fact, the reduced incidence of nonfatal myocardial infarction that was observed in the Coronary Drug Project was followed by a significant 11% reduction in all-cause mortality (Canner et al., 1976). In addition, niacin combined with colestipol has been demonstrated to reduce the extent of angiographically defined coronary atherosclerosis (Blankenhorn et al., 1987). Therefore, niacin can continue to be used as a hypolipidemic medication, but its use should be avoided in patients with underlying liver disease or suspected alcohol abuse. In addition, caution should be used in combining niacin with any other hypolipidemic medications except for the bile acid sequestrants.

Several potential adverse effects have been of concern with the inhibitors of cholesterol biosynthesis. The experience with the development of ichthyosis (Anchor et al., 1961) and cataracts (Laughlin and Carey, 1962) with triparanol (MER-29) in the early 1960s has led to intensive assessments of these as well as other theoretic adverse effects of these compounds (Hoeg and Brewer, 1987; Tobert, 1988a). As monotherapy, few adverse side effects have been observed with these compounds. Less than 2% of patients receiving lovastatin, the first HMG CoA reductase inhibitor that has been widely used, have experienced the most frequent side effects of myopathy and hepatitis. However, it appears that myopathy may be more frequently observed when lovastatin is combined with other prescription medications. Myopathy has been described with the use of lovastatin combined with cyclosporine in transplant recipients (East et al., 1988; Norman et al., 1988; Tobert, 1988b). Cyclosporine itself has been implicated in the development of symptomatic myopathy (Noppen et al., 1987; Fernandez-Sola et al., 1990). Therefore, combination of lovastatin with cyclosporine may enhance a cyclosporine-mediated predispositon towards myopathy. Of more general interest, however, is the possibility that combination of lovastatin with more commonly prescribed medications may also lead to symptomatic myopathy. Patients receiving erythromycin (East et al., 1988; Ayanian et al., 1988; Corpier et al., 1988), niacin (Tobert, 1988; Norman et al., 1988; Reaven and Witztum, 1988), and gemfibrozil (Tobert, 1988; Marias and Larson, 1990) in combination with lovastatin have developed myopathy. In some instances the myopathy developed into frank rhabdomyolysis leading to acute renal failure necessitating transient use of hemodialysis (Marias and Larson, 1990). More than 1 million patients have received prescriptions for lovastatin, and as the clinical experience widens, further rare, but significant, adverse effects may be observed. Physicians suspecting potential drug–drug interactions and hypolipidemic therapy side effects should report them to the manufacturer and to the Food and Drug Administration to permit the documentation necessary to fully interpret the risk-benefit of hypolipidemic therapy in specific clinical contexts.

IV. SELECTING A DRUG COMBINATION

Several factors are involved in prescribing combination therapy to treat hyperlipidemia. Table 4 lists the most clinically relevant questions that should be asked before initiating combination hypolipidemic drug treatment. First, it is critical that the patient be given an adequate trial of dietary and pharmacological treatment with a single agent. Most hypercholesterolemic patients will not require more than one hypolipidemic medication, and a 3–6-month treatment period with diet and drug monotherapy is indicated. The exception to this approach is the patient with familial hypercholesterolemia. These patients generally manifest total and LDL cholesterol concentrations in excess of 300 mg/dl and 225 mg/dl, respectively. An accelerated course of therapy is indicated with these patients since they will almost always require combination of diet with two or more hypolipidemic drugs. Also, it is not mandatory that the maximal dosage of each drug be used before a second medication is added. For instance, a second medication such as a bile acid sequestrant can be added to a 1.5 g/day niacin regimen. This limits the adverse effects of niacin and still permits an additive or synergistic response with a bile acid sequestrant.

If the patient is hypertriglyceridemic, a bile acid sequestrant should not be used as the initial medication since these compounds may exacerbate hypertri-

Table 4 Questions to Ask Before Initiating Combination Drug Therapy for Hypercholesterolemia

---

1. Has there been an adequate diet/monotherapy drug trial? At least two to three lipoprotein determinations at monthly intervals should be obtained prior to initiating combination drug treatment.
2. Does the patient have fasting hypertriglyceridemia? Bile acid sequestrants should not be used as the initial drug in these patients, but it may be used as an additional agent.
3. Are there any contraindications to the use of the hypolipidemic drug combination?
4. Is the patient taking other medications that would interact with the hypolipidemic drugs?
5. Are the direct drug costs as well as the indirect costs (blood work, office visits, ophthalmological testing) an obstacle to treatment?

---

glyceridemia. Niacin or gemfibrozil would be preferable agents in the patient that has both elevated LDL cholesterol and an increased concentration of fasting triglycerides. However, once one of these other drugs has been initiated, addition of a bile acid sequestrant has been shown to improve the lipoprotein concentrations.

Relative contraindications exist for most of the major lipid-lowering medications (Table 2). In addition, there may other potential drug–drug interactions that must be considered if the patient is also taking other prescription drugs (Table 3). Finally, cost may be a consideration of many patients (Table 2). A 30-day supply of the minimal dose of hypolipidemic medications ranges from $3.90 for plain niacin to as much as $64.80 (cost to pharmacist) for the cholestyramine bar form. One possible advantage of combination drug therapy is that lower dosages of the more expensive medications can be used to achieve the goal lipid response.

As outlined in Figure 1, the most effective combination drug therapies all include the use of a bile acid sequestrant. Combinations of either colestipol or cholestyramine with niacin, gemfibrozil, or an HMG CoA reductase inhibitor all significantly reduce the LDL cholesterol concentration. Only colestipol + lovastatin did not significantly increase the HDL cholesterol concentrations. Therefore, one of these combinations would be worthwhile in selected hypercholesterolemic patients. The specific combination in a given patient will need to be individualized based upon concurrent drug use, contraindications, and cost.

V. CONTROVERSIES AND FUTURE DIRECTIONS

Although a great deal of information is rapidly being generated about lipid-lowering drugs used both as monotherapy and in combination, a great deal remains unknown. The vast majority of combination drug studies which have focused upon the treatment of hypercholesterolemia have been conducted in markedly hypercholesterolemic patients. These studies have almost uniformly avoided patients with other metabolic conditions. Studies are currently underway to assess the effects of medications as monotherapy as well as in combination therapy to treat hyperlipidemia in commonly encountered diseases such as diabetes mellitus as well as in patients with compromised renal function. The selection for most studies has also been directed toward patients with an elevated LDL cholesterol concentration. What should be done with the hypertriglyceridemic patient and patients with depressed HDL cholesterol concentrations? The Helsinki Heart Study indicated that the dyslipoprotein-emia reflected by fasting hypertriglyceridemia may also be amenable to pharmacological intervention (Frick et al., 1987). The relative protection from cardiovascular disease endpoints in this trial suggested that pharmacological intervention was possibly mediated by affecting the HDL cholesterol concentrations. These findings suggest that other lipoprotein endpoints may eventually be of clinical utility.

Perhaps constituents within the lipoprotein particles other than the cholesterol and triglyceride moieties will become more clinically useful in making therapeutic decisions. Recently a variety of apolipoproteins and lipoproteins have been observed to correlate with symptomatic cardiovascular disease (Brewer et al., 1989). Apolipoproteins A-I and B (Macjiecko et al., 1983; Brunzell et al., 1984; Miller, 1987; Alaupovic et al., 1988) have been particularly good candidates for therapeutic targets. These apolipoproteins are the principal apolipoproteins on HDL and LDL, respectively. In addition, determination of the concentrations of these apolipoproteins may provide more precise detection for patients at risk for premature cardiovascular disease. Determination of another lipoprotein particle, Lp(a), may also provide clinically relevant cardiovascular disease risk information that may not be reflected in the currently utilized lipid determinations (Kostner et al., 1981; Utermann, 1989). The use of new drugs or combinations of medications to modify the concentrations of these constituents will become active areas of investigation. In addition, it will be necessary to demonstrate the efficacy of modifying these other parameters in the context of the development of cardiovascular disease. Either cardiovascular morbidity-mortality endpoints or at least some surrogate such as coronary arteriographic assessment will be required to translate any changes in biochemical parameters into effects on the progression of atherosclerosis. Therefore, future effort in selecting different patient populations with different lipoprotein-apolipoprotein biochemical profiles may lead to more targeted pharmacological intervention. Strategies which effectively utilize complementary mechanisms of actions that are available with combination drug therapy in these patient populations are underway.

REFERENCES

Alaupovic, P., McConathy, W. J., Fesmire, J., Tavella, U. M., and Bard, J. M. (1988). Profiles of apolipoproteins and apolipoprotein B-containing lipoproteins with ischemic heart disease and coronary atherosclerosis. *Am. Heart J.* **113**:589–597.

Altschul, R., Hoffer, A., and Stephen, J. D. (1955). Influence of nicotinic acid on serum cholesterol in man. *Arch. Biochem.* **54**:558–559.

Anchor, R. W. P., Winkelmann, R. K., and Perry, H. O. (1961). Cutaneous effects from use of triparonol (MER-29): Preliminary data on ichthyosis and loss of hair. *Mayo Clinic Proc.* **36**:217–228.

Angelin, B., Eriksson, and M. Einarsson, K. (1986). Combined treatment with cholestyramine and nicotinic acid in heterozygous familial hypercholesterolemia: Effects on biliary lipid composition. *Eur. J. Clin. Invest.* **16**:391–396.

Ayanian, A. Z., Fuchs, C. S., and Stone, R. M. (1988). Lovastatin and rhabdomyolysis. *Ann. Intern. Med.* **109**:597–598.

Blankenhorn, D. M., Nessim, S. A., Johnson, R. L., Sanmarco, M. E., Azen, S. P., and Cashin-Hemphill, L. (1987). Beneficial effects of combined colestipol-niacin therapy on coronary atherosclerosis and coronary venous bypass grafts. *JAMA* **251**:365–374.

Brewer, H. B., Jr., Gregg, R. E., and Hoeg, J. M. (1989). Apolipoproteins, lipoproteins, and atherosclerosis. In *Heart Disease*. Edited by E. Braunwald. New York, W. B. Saunders Company, pp. 121–136.

Brunzell, J. D., Sniderman, A. D., Albers, J. J., and Kwiterovich, P. O. (1984). Apoproteins B and A-I and coronary artery disease in humans. *Arteriosclerosis* **4**:79–83.

Canner, P. L., Berge, K. G., Wenger, N. K., Stamler, J., Friedman, L., Prineas, R. J., and Friedewald, W. (1976). Fifteen year mortality in Coronary Drug Project patients: Long-term benefit with niacin. *J. Am. Coll. Cardiol.* **8**:1245–1255.

Christensen, N. A., Achor, R. W., Berge, K. G., and Mason, H. L. (1961). Nicotonic acid treatment of hypercholesterolemia, comparison of plain and sustained action preparations, and report of two cases of jaundice. *JAMA* **177**:546–550.

Clementz, G. L., and Holmes, A. W. (1987). Nicotinic acid-induced fulminant hepatic failure. *J. Clin. Gastroenterol.* **9**:582–584.

Coronary Drug Project Research Group. (1975). Clofibrate and niacin in coronary heart disease. *JAMA* **231**:360–381.

Corpier, C. L., Jones, P. H., Suki, W. N., Lederer, E. D., Quinones, M. A., Schmidt, S. W., and Young, J. B. (1988). Rhabdomyolysis and renal injury with lovastatin use. *JAMA* **260**:239–241.

Curtis, L. D., Dickson, A. C., Ling, K. L. E., and Betteridge, J. (1988). Combination treatment with cholestyramine and bezafibrate for heterozygous familial hypercholesterolemia. *BMJ* **297**:173–175.

Das, G. (1986). Colestipol and clofibrate combination therapy for hypercholesterolemia. *Curr. Ther. Res.* **40**:1114–1120.

Dujovne, C. A., Krehbiel, P., Decoursey, S., Jackson, B., Chernoff, S. B., Pitterman, A., and Garty, M. (1984). Probucol with colestipol in the treatment of hypercholesterolemia. *Ann. Intern. Med.* **100**:477–482.

Dujovne, C. A., Krehbiel, P., and Chenoff, S. B. (1986). Controlled studies of the efficacy and safety of combined probucol-colestipol therapy. *Am. J. Cardiol.* **57**:36H–42H.

East, C., Alivizatos, P. A., Grundy, S. M., Jones, P. H., and Farmer, J. A. (1988).

Rhabdomyolysis in patients receiving lovastatin after cardiac transplantation. *N. Engl. J. Med.* **318**:47–48.

Expert Panel. (1988). Report of the National Cholesterol Education Program on detection, evaluation, and treatment of high blood cholesterol in adults. *Arch. Intern. Med.* **148**:36–69.

Fernandez-Sola, J., Campistol, J., Casademont, J., Grau, J. M., and Urbano-Marquez, A. (1990). Reversible cyclosporine myopathy. *Lancet* **i**:362–363.

Frederickson, D. S., Levy, R. I., and Lees, R. S. (1967). Fat transport in lipoproteins: An integrated approach to mechanisms and disorders. *N. Engl. J. Med.* **276**:34–44, 94–103, 148–156, 215–228, 273–281.

Frick, M. H., Elo, O., Haapa, K. A., Heinonen, O. P., Heinsalmi, P., Helo, P., Huttunen, J. K., Kaitaniemi, P., Koskinen, P., Manninen, V., Maenpaa, H., Malkonen, M., Manttari, M., Norola, S., Pasternack, A., Pikkaraienen, J., Romo, M., Sjoblom, T., and Nikkila, E. A. (1987). Helsinki Heart Study. Primary prevention trial with gemfibrozil in middle aged men with dyslipidemia. *N. Engl. Med.* **317**:1237–1245.

Goldstein, J. L., Hazzard, W. R., Schrott, H. G., Bierman, E. L., Motulsky, A. G., Levinski, M. J., and Campbell, E. D. (1973a). Hyperlipidemia in coronary heart disease: I. Lipid levels in 500 survivors of myocardial infarction. *J. Clin. Invest.* **52**:1533–1543.

Goldstein, J. L., Schrott, H. G., Hazzard, W. R., Bierman, E. L., Motulsky, A. G., Campbell, E. D., and Levinski, M. J. (1973b). Hyperlipidemia in coronary heart disease: II. Genetic analysis of lipid levels in 176 families and delineation of a new inherited disorder, combined hyperlipoproteinemia. *J. Clin. Invest.* **52**:1544–1568.

Goldstein, J. L., and Brown, M. S. (1989). Familial hypercholersterolemia. In *The Metabolic Basis of Inherited Disease*. 6th Ed. Edited by C. R. Scriver, A. L. Beaudet, W. S. Sly, and D. Valle; consulting editors, J. B. Stanbury, J. B. Wyngaarden, and D. S. Frederickson. New York, McGraw-Hill Information Services Company, pp. 1215–1250.

Heller, F. R., Desager, J. P., and Hervengt, C. (1981). Plasma lipid concentration and lecithin:cholesterol acyltransferase activity in normolipidemic subjects given fenofibrate and colestipol. *Metabolism* **30**:67–71.

Hoeg, J. M., and Brewer, H. B. Jr. (1987). 3-Hydroxy-3-methylglutaryl-coenzyme A reductase inhibitors in the treatment of hypercholesterolemia. *JAMA* **258**:3532–3536.

Hoeg, J. M., Maher M. M., Bailey K. R., Zech L. A., Gregg R. E., Sprecher D. L., and Brewer, H. B., Jr. (1985). Effects of combination cholestyramine-neomycin treatment on plasma lipoprotein concentrations in type II hyperlipoproteinemia. *Am. J. Cardiol.* **55**:1282–1286.

Hoeg, J. M., Maher, M. B., Bou, E., Zech, L. A., Bailey, K. R., Gregg, R. E., Sprecher, D. L., Susser J. K., Pikus, A. M., and Brewer, H. B., Jr. (1984). Normalization of plasma lipoprotein concentrations in patients with type II hyperlipoproteinemia by combined use of neomycin and niacin. *Circulation* **70**:1004–1011.

Hoeg, J. M., Maher, M. B., Bailey, K. R., and Brewer, H. B. (1986). The effects of mevinolin and neomycin alone and in combination on plasma lipid and lipoprotein concentrations in type II hyperlipoproteinemia. *Atherosclerosis* **60**:2009–2014.

Hunninghake, D. B., Probstfeld, J. L., Crow, L. O., and Isaacson, S. O. (1981a). Effect of colestipol and clofibrate on plasma lipid and lipoproteins in type IIA hyperlipoproteinemia. *Metabolism* **30**:605–609.

Hunninghake, D. B., Bell, C., and Olson, L. (1981a). Effect of colestipol and clofibrate, singly and in combination, on plasma lipid and lipoproteins in type IIB hyperlipoproteinemia. *Metabolism* **30**:610–615.

Illingworth, D. R., Phillipson, B. E., Rapp, J. H., and Connor, W. E. (1981). Colestipol plus nicotinic acid in treatment of heterozygous familial hypercholesterolemia. *Lancet* **1**:296–298.

Illingworth, D. R. (1984). Mevinolin plus colestipol in therapy for severe heterozygous familial hypercholesterolemia. *Ann. Intern. Med.* **101**:598–604.

Illingworth, D. R., and Bacon, S. (1989). Influence of lovastatin plus gemfibrozil on plasma lipids and lipoproteins in patients with heterozygous familial hypercholesterolemia. *Circulation* **79**:590–596.

Kane, J. P., Malloy, M. J., Tun, P., Phillips N. R., Friedman D. D., Williams M. L., Rowe J. S., and Havel, R. J. (1981). Normalization of low density lipoprotein levels in heterozygous familial hypercholesterolemia with a combined drug regimen. *N. Engl. J. Med.* **304**:251–258.

Kostner, G., Avogaro, P., Cazzolato, G., Marth, E., Bittolo-Bon, G., and Quinici, G. B. (1981). Lipoprotein Lp(a) and the risk for myocardial infarction. *Atherosclerosis* **38**:51–61.

Kuo, P. T., Kostis, J. B., Moreya, A. E., and Hayes, J. A. (1981). Familial type II hyperlipoproteinemia with coronary heart disease: Effect of diet-colestipol-nicotinic acid treatment. *Chest* **79**:286–291.

Laughlin, R. C., and Carey, T. F. (1962). Cataracts in patients treated with triparanol. *JAMA* **181**:339–340.

Leren, T. P., Hjermann, I., Berg, K., Leren, P., Foss, O. P., and Viksmoen, L. (1988). Effects of lovastatin alone and in combination with cholestyramine on serum lipids and apolipoproteins in heterozygotes for familial hypercholesterolemia. *Atherosclerosis* **73**:135–141.

Litin, S. C., and Anderson, C. F. (1989). Nicotinic acid-associated myopathy: A report of three cases. *Am. J. Med.* **83**:481–483.

Mabuchi, H., Sakai, T., Sakai, Y., Yoshimura, A., Watanabe, A., Wakasugi, T., Koizumi, J., and Takeda, R. (1983). Reduction of serum cholesterol in heterozygous patients with familial hypercholesterolemia: Additive effects of compactin and cholestyramine. *N. Engl. J. Med.* **308**:609–613.

Macjiecko, J. J., Holmes, D. R., Kottke, B. A., Zinsmeister, A. K., Dinh, D. M., and Mao, S. J. T. (1983). Apolipoprotein A-I as a marker of angiographically assessed coronary artery disease. *N. Engl. J. Med.* **309**:385–389.

Malloy, M. J., Kane, J. P., Kunitake, S. T., and Tun, P. (1987). Complementarity of colestipol, niacin, and lovastatin in treatment of severe familial hypercholesterolemia. *Ann. Intern. Med.* **107**:616–623.

Marias, G. E., and Larson, K. K. (1990). Rhabdomyolysis and acute renal failure induced by combination lovastatin and gemfibrozil therapy. *Ann. Intern. Med.* **112**:228–230.

Miller, N. E. (1987). Association of high-density lipoprotein subclasses and apolipoproteins with ischemic heart disease and coronary atherosclerosis. *Am. Heart J.* **113**:589–597.

Mullin, G. E., Greenson, J. K., and Mitchell, M. C. (1989). Fulminant hepatic failure after ingestion of sustained-release nicotinic acid. *Ann. Intern. Med.* **111**:253–255.

Nessim, S. A., Chin, H. P., Alaupovic, P., and Blankenhorn, H. H. (1983). Combined therapy of niacin, colestipol, and fat-controlled diet in men with coronary bypass. *Arteriosclerosis* **3**:568–573.

Noppen, M., Velkeriers, B., Dierckx, R., Bruyland, M., and Vanhaelst, L. (1987). Cyclosporine and myopathy. *Ann. Intern. Med.* **107**:945–946.

Norman, D. J., Illingworth, D. R., Munson, J., and Hosenpud, J. (1988). Myolysis and acute renal failure in a heart-transplant recipient receiving lovastatin. *N. Engl. J. Med.* **318**:46–48.

Packard, C. J., Stewart, J. M., Morgan, G., Lorimar, A. R., and Shepherd, J. (1980). Combined drug therapy for familial hypercholesterolemia. *Artery* **7**:281–289.

Parsons, W. B., Jr., and Flinn, J. H. (1957). Success of niacin and failure of nicotimamide in reducing plasma cholesterol levels in patients with hypercholesterolemia. *Circulation* **16**:499.

Parsons, W. B., Jr. (1961). Studies of nicotinic acid use in hypercholesterolemia: Changes in hepatic function, carbohydrate intolerance, and uric acid metabolism. *Arch. Intern. Med.* **107**:653–667.

Reaven, P., and Witztum, J. L. (1988). Lovastatin, nicotinic acid, and rhabdomyolysis. *Ann. Intern. Med.* **109**:597–598.

Series, J. J., Caslake, M. J., Kilday, C., Cruickshank, A., Demant, T., Lorimer, A. R., Packard, C. J., and Shepherd, J. (1989). Effects of combined therapy with bezafibrate and cholestyramine on low-density lipoprotein metabolism in type IIa hypercholesterolemia. *Metabolism* **38**:153–158.

Stone, N. J., Levy, R. I., Fredrickson, D. S., and Verter, J. (1974). Coronary artery disease in 116 kindred with familial type II hyperlipoproteinemia. *Circulation* **49**:476–488.

Tobert, J. A. (1988a). Efficacy and long-term adverse effect pattern of lovastatin. *Am. J. Cardiol.* **62**:28J–34J.

Tobert, J. A. (1988b). Rhabdomyolysis in patients receiving lovastatin after cardiac transplantation. *N. Engl. J Med.* **318**:48.

Utermann, G. (1989). The mysteries of lipoprotein (a). *Science* **246**:904–910.

Vogelberg, K. H., Koschinsky, T., Hein, H., and Gries, F. A. (1982). Effect of neomycin sulphate alone and in combination with d-thyroxine on serum lipoprotein in hypercholesterolemic subjects. *Eur. J. Clin. Pharmacol.* **22**:33–38.

Weisweiler, P. (1988). Simvastatin plus low-dose colestipol in the treatment of severe familial hypercholesterolemia. *Curr. Ther. Res.* **44**:802–806.

Weisweiler, P., Merk, W., Jacob, B., and Schwandt, (1986). Fenofibrate and colestipol: Effects on serum and lipoprotein lipids and apolipoproteins in familial hypercholesterolemia. *Eur. J. Clin. Pharmacol.* **30**:191–194.

Weisweiler, P. (1989). Low-dose colestipol plus fenofibrate: Effects on plasma lipoproteins, lecithin:cholesterol acyltransferase, and postheparin lipases in familial hypercholesterolemia. *Metabolism* **38**:271–275.

Witztum, J. L., Simmons, D., Steinberg, D., Beltz, W. F., Weinreb R., Young, S. G., Lester, P., Kelly, N., and Juliano, J. (1989). Intensive combination drug therapy of familial hypercholesterolemia with lovastatin, probucol, and colestipol hydrochloride. *Circulation* **79**:16–28.

11

Dietary Treatment of Hypercholesterolemia

Wahida Karmally and Henry N. Ginsberg

Columbia University College of Physicians and Surgeons
New York, New York

I. INTRODUCTION

The role of diet in the prevention, development, and treatment of atherosclerotic cardiovascular disease cannot be overemphasized (Committee on Diet and Health, 1989). Animal studies relating dietary fat and cholesterol to the development of arterial lesions similar to those found in human atherosclerosis date back nearly a century. Epidemiological observations followed soon after, suggesting that in countries where the native population consumed low fat, low cholesterol diets, the incidence of arteriosclerosis was much reduced. World War II, with its concomitant shortage of meat, eggs, and dairy products in Europe, was associated with reduced rates of death from atherosclerotic cardiovascular disease (Vartiainen and Kanerva, 1947).

The well-designed epidemiological studies of the past 30 years (Stamler et al., 1985; Anderson et al., 1987) clearly implicated both plasma total and LDL cholesterol as risk factors for coronary artery disease and HDL cholesterol as a protective factor against such disease. The relationship between diet and atherosclerosis and the link between dietary fat, particularly saturated fat intake, and plasma lipid levels has been less well accepted. A review of the literature, however, should make it clear that such a relationship does exist. The studies by Keys and his colleagues demonstrating the association of dietary fat and both plasma cholesterol levels and cardiovascular mortality are central to a rationale for dietary therapy of hyperlipidemia (Keys, 1970, 1980). Those studies receive strong support from the Ni-Hon-San Study (Kagan et al., 1981) in which Japanese men in Japan were compared to cohorts that migrated to Hawaii and to San Francisco. As the Japanese men moved east, their intake of fat increased along with the plasma cholesterol levels and their incidence of coronary disease. On the other hand, Irish brothers living in Boston and Ireland who were eating the same amounts of saturated fats had similar rates of coronary heart disease (Kushi et al., 1985).

The relationship between dietary cholesterol intake and either plasma cholesterol levels or coronary heart disease incidence has been even less well accepted. Many diet studies have failed to show a relationship between increased plasma cholesterol concentrations and additions of dietary cholesterol to diets already containing cholesterol. Studies in which dietary cholesterol has been added to cholesterol-free diets have, however, uniformly shown increased plasma cholesterol levels on the latter diets. Both Hegsted et al. (1965) and Keys et al. (1965) demonstrated effects of dietary cholesterol on plasma cholesterol concentrations. In addition, several long-term follow-up studies have demonstrated increased risk for coronary disease related to dietary cholesterol intake (Stamler and Shekelle, 1988).

Tightly controled trials of different diets in the so-called "metabolic ward studies" have also confirmed that diets high in saturated fats and cholesterol increase plasma total and LDL cholesterol levels. These studies have, however, overwhelmed health professionals with data related to the effects of individual classes of fats (saturated, monounsaturated, polyunsaturated) on plasma levels of individual lipoproteins. In many instances, particularly when concomitant changes in LDL and HDL cholesterol have been observed, these studies have left the practitioner and his or her staff with a feeling of uncertainty. For these reasons, we will briefly review this area before beginning our discussion of dietary therapy of hypercholesterolemia.

II. EFFECTS OF SATURATED FATS ON PLASMA LIPIDS

There is a wealth of data indicating that dietary saturated fat intake is associated with increased plasma levels of total and LDL cholesterol (Hegsted et al., 1965; Keys et al. 1965; Committee on Diet and Health, 1989). While there are some studies in animals indicating individual differences in the effects of individual saturated fatty acids on plasma cholesterol concentrations, much less information is available for humans. Studies by Ahrens et al. (1957), Hegsted et al. (1965), Keys et al. (1965), and Bonanome and Grundy (1988) suggest that stearic acid (18:0) may not have any cholesterol-raising effects. Even if this is correct (and confirmation will have to await further, carefully controlled clinical trials), our present sources of stearic acid (meats) are usually high in other saturated fatty acids. Palmitic acid (16:0), myristic acid (14:0), and lauric acid (12:0) are present in differing proportions in meats, dairy products, and tropical oils, and studies testing whether these fatty acids have differential effects on plasma total and LDL cholesterol may be informative to the food designers. At the moment, overall reductions in an individual's intake of foods containing saturated fats seems the prudent course to follow (Committee on Diet and Health, 1989).

III. EFFECTS OF MONOUNSATURATED FATS ON PLASMA LIPIDS

The recent focus on dietary monounsaturated fats derives from the work by both Keys and his colleagues (Keys, 1970, 1980) indicating that some populations in he Mediterranean area consume large quantities of monounsaturates (18:1) and maintain normal plasma cholesterol levels and low cardiovascular risk profiles. Grundy (1986) and Mattson and Grundy (1985) demonstrated that diets in which monounsaturated fats replaced saturated fats reduced plasma total and LDL cholesterol levels. In addition, their results suggested that unlike polyunsaturates, monounsaturates did not reduce HDL cholesterol. These results have been frequently interpreted to mean that adding monounsaturates to a diet would reduce total and LDL cholesterol levels in the blood: the studies only demonstrated that replacing saturated fats with monounsaturated fats might be equal to replacing saturated fats with polyunsaturated fats. Regarding the issue of the effects of different fatty acids on plasma HDL cholesterol levels, several studies have demonstrated no reduction in HDL levels when diets consistent with the AHA Step 1 diet are used (Vessby et al., 1985; Ginsberg et al., 1990). At this time, based on all available data, there is no reason to suggest that hypercholesterolemic patients add monounsaturated fats to their diets in an attempt to reduce their levels of total and LDL cholesterol. On the other hand, the results of the studies noted above do indicate that monounsaturates may be used as a replacement for saturated fats without any adverse effects on plasma lipid concentrations. Of course, the caloric density of any fat is more than twice that of carbohydrate, and individuals who are "counting calories" should attempt to use carbohydrates to replace fats in their diet.

IV. EFFECTS OF POLYUNSATURATED FATS ON PLASMA LIPIDS

Based on the work of Hegsted et al. (1965) and Keys et al. (1965), many physicians and nutritionists in the 1960s and 1970s were advocating that patients actively consume additional quantities of polynsaturated fats to lower their plasma cholesterol levels. Although some work (Mensink and Katan, 1989) suggests that polyunsaturated fats, like monounsaturated fats, are relatively ineffective, by themselves, in lowering cholesterol (as opposed to their use to replace saturated fats), the overall evidence is still in favor of polyunsaturated fats as having an important role in any cholesterol-lowering diet. Of concern, however, are the data indicating that polyunsaturates may, in addition to lowering LDL cholesterol, also reduce HDL cholesterol. Most of the studies suggesting such activity are, however, confounded by either marked concomitant reductions in total and saturated fats or by the use of very large amounts of polyunsaturated fats (Vessby et al., 1985). In fact, when diets consistent with the AHA Step 1 diet are used (Vessby et al. 1985; Ginsberg et al., 1990) or when subjects are followed over longer periods of time (Thueesen et al., 1986; Kromhout et al., 1987), HDL cholesterol levels appear to be unchanged. In addition, it is not at all clear why a reduction in HDL cholesterol induced by a low fat diet should be viewed as detrimental. This view is based on an extrapolation from cross-sectional data, within single populations consuming average (high fat) diets. There are no data addressing the incidence of coronary heart disease in a population where a low fat diet–induced fall in HDL cholesterol has occurred. In contrast, populations (either entire countries or subgroups within a country) who consume low fat diets have low rates of coronary disease (Keys, 1970, 1980). Overall, less emphasis should be placed on diet-induced changes in HDL cholesterol until more long-term data are available. The recommendation that consumption of polyunsaturated fatty acids not exceed 10% of total calories is a very conservative approach derived from a lack of long-term data from populations consuming more than 10% of calories as polyunsaturates.

In summary, the efficacy of diets low in saturated fat and cholesterol in lowering serum cholesterol has been shown extensively in clinical, experimental, and epidemiological research (Committee on Diet and Health, 1989). It is therefore essential that dietary approaches to hyperlipidemia be the cornerstone of any therapeutic program initiated to reduce an individual's plasma lipid levels and, concomitantly, their risk for coronary heart disease.

V. INITIATING DIETARY TREATMENT

The dietary factors that contribute significantly to elevation of plasma cholesterol are:

1. High intake of saturated fatty acids
2. High intake of dietary cholesterol
3. Caloric intake in excess of energy requirements and the concomitant obesity

Lowering intake of saturated fat and cholesterol should clearly be the most important focus of any nutritional treatment for hypercholesterolemia. For most people, dietary changes aimed at lowering saturated fat and cholesterol intake will be the only intervention required to lower serum cholesterol levels and thereby lower risk for coronary artery disease (The Expert Panel, 1988). The degree to which an individual's blood cholesterol level drops after initiation of diet therapy depends on their eating pattern before diet modifications are made and their inherent degree of responsiveness. Individuals exhibit great biological variability (Ginsberg et al., 1981; Katan et al., 1986). Usually patients with high cholesterol levels experience the greatest reduction in total and LDL cholesterol.

We need to establish an eating style which contains 7–10% of the calories as saturated fat, not more than 200–300 mg of cholesterol per day, and sufficient calories to maintain ideal body weight. Although there is no known human requirement for saturated fat or cholesterol after the age of 2 years, an attempt to lower the intake of saturated fat and cholesterol even further may affect food palatability and patient adherence to the new dietary regimen.

A. Current Eating Style in America

Recent food consumption data (Bunch, 1985; Marstan and Raper, 1985; Brown et al., 1985; Slattery and Randall, 1988) indicate that the American people are choosing foods that are fresh, lower in fat, and reduced in sugar. The purchase of whole milk and cream has decreased by almost 25% and the use of butter by over one third. The per capita consumption of eggs has dropped by approximately 15%. The consumption of vegetable fats has increased by almost 75%. While the consumption of fresh and frozen vegetables has increased, red meat continues to be a major protein food in the diet. Meat, together with poultry, contributes one third of the total fat in the diet. Most of the saturated fatty acids come from animal products and from tropical oils used in baked goods. Egg yolks are still a major source of cholesterol, contributing 30% of the cholesterol in the diet. Beef, hot dogs, and cold cuts contribute another third of the cholesterol in the diet, while the rest comes from butter, cheese, ice cream, and whole milk. Although consumption of low fat milk and skim milk is increasing, cream products like half and half, sour cream, and heavy cream have also become popular.

The average intake of saturated fatty acids is 14–16% of total calories. Cholesterol intake in adult men is approximately 450 mg/dl, while women consume 350 mg/day. Although the intake of these nutrients has declined considerably over the past 20 years, it is not yet optimum and contributes to the high levels of plasma cholesterol in the American population. In addition, obesity is prevalent due to increased intake of calories and contributes to the development of coronary heart disease (Kannell et al., 1967).

B. Guidelines for a Cholesterol-Lowering Diet Program

The National Cholesterol Education Program has recommended a two-step approach to lower plasma total cholesterol concentrations by progressively reducing intakes of saturated fatty acids and cholesterol and to promote weight loss in overweight patients by reducing total caloric intake.

The Step 1 diet, which is similar to the guidelines recommended by the American Heart Association, is a population-based approach for lowering blood cholesterol. The recommendations (Table 1) include a total fat intake of less than 30% of total calories; an intake of saturated fat less than 10% of

Table 1 Dietary Therapy of High Blood Cholesterol Levels

	Recommended intake	
Nutrient	Step 1 diet	Step 2 diet
Total fat	Less than 30% of total calories	Less than 30% of total calories
Saturated fatty acids	Less than 10% of total calories	Less than 7% of total calories
Polyunsaturated fatty acids	Up to 10% of total calories	Up to 10% of total calories
Monounsaturated fatty acids	10–15% of total calories	10–15% of total calories
Carbohydrates	50–60% of total calories	50–60% of total calories
Protein	10–20% of total calories	10–20% of total calories
Cholesterol	Less than 300 mg/day	Less than 200 mg/day
Total calories	To achieve and maintain desirable weight	To achieve and maintain desirable weight

calories; an intake of polyunsaturated fat up to 10% of calories; and an intake of the rest of fat calories as monounsaturates. Cholesterol intake should be less than 300 mg/day. Dietary treatment should be aimed to achieve and maintain ideal body weight and healthy eating patterns, with a permanent change in eating behavior.

The Step 1 diet (Table 2) should be followed for a minimum of 3 months to maximize the time for the desired response expected with good adherence. If the response is not achieved, the NCEP recommendation is to progress to the Step 2 diet (Table 1). The Step 1 diet should reduce plasma cholesterol levels about 10% from baseline, depending on previous diet pattern and inherent characteristics of responsiveness. Advancement to the Step 2 diet may achieve a further 5% drop in plasma total cholesterol.

The Step 2 diet is recommended if the response to the Step 1 diet is not optimal. It calls for reducing further the saturated fatty acid intake to less than 7% of calories and cholesterol intake to less than 200 mg/day. Both the Step 1 and Step 2 diets recommend that patients achieve and maintain ideal body weight.

The Step 2 diet may require intensive nutritional counseling in order to lower the saturated fat and cholesterol contents of the diet even further without jeopardizing food palatability and acceptability. The total fat intake, however, can be maintained at 30% of total calories (Table 1). This would allow the individual to use monounsaturated sources of fat (olive and canola oils) as a replacement for the additional removal of saturated fats, thereby providing satiety attributable to the fat content of the meal.

Table 2 The Step 1 Diet

Fish, chicken, turkey, and lean meats (5–6 oz. a day)	
Choose:	Fish, poultry without skin, lean cuts of beef, lamb, pork or veal, shellfish
Decrease:	Fatty cuts of beef, lamb, pork; spare ribs, organ meats, regular cold cuts, sausage, hot dogs, bacon, sardines, roe, caviar
Skim and low fat milk, cheese, yogurt, and dairy substitutes (at least 2 servings a day)	
Choose:	Skim or 1% fat milk (liquid, powdered, evaporated), low fat buttermilk
	Nonfat (0% fat) or low fat yogurt
	Nonfat or low fat cottage cheese (1% fat)
	Low fat cheeses, farmer or pot cheeses (all of these should be labeled no more than 2–3 g of fat per ounce)
	Sherbert, sorbet, skim milk desserts, calorie-reduced Tofutti (without added fat)

(*continued*)

Table 2 (*continued*)

Decrease:	Whole milk (4% fat): regular, evaporated, condensed; cream, half and half, 2% milk, imitation milk products, most nondairy creamers, whipped toppings
	Whole milk yogurt
	Whole milk cottage cheese (4% fat)
	All natural cheeses (e.g., blue, Roquefort, Camembert, cheddar, Swiss), low fat or "light" cream cheese, low fat or "light" sour cream, cream cheeses, sour cream
	Ice cream

Eggs (No more than 3 egg yolks per week)

Choose:	Egg whites (2 whites equal 1 whole egg in recipes), cholesterol-free egg substitutes
Decrease:	Egg yolks, "Caesar" dressing, "lobster sauce," "hollandaise" made with egg yolks

Fruits and vegetables (fruit, 2–4 servings: vegetables, 3–5 servings)

Choose:	Fresh, frozen, canned, or dried fruits and vegetables
Decrease:	Vegetables prepared in butter, cream, or other high fat sauces

Breads and cereals (6–11 servings a day)

Choose:	Homemade baked goods using unsaturated oils sparingly, angel food cake, low fat crackers, low fat cookies
	Pasta, rice, barley, wheat, oats
	Whole-grain breads and cereals (oatmeal, whole wheat, rye, bran, multigrain, etc.)
Decrease:	Commercial baked goods: pies, cakes, doughnuts, croissants, pastries, muffins, biscuits, high fat crackers, high fat cookies
	Egg noodles and grains prepared with butter sauces
	Breads in which eggs are a major ingredient, granolas made with hydrogenated fats, coconut oil, palm oil, or palm kernel oil

Fats and oils (up to 6–8 tsp/day in prepared foods, salad dressings, or as a spread or as seeds and nuts)

Choose:	Baking cocoa
	Unsaturated vegetable oils: corn, olive, rapeseed (canola oil), safflower, sesame, soybean, sunflower, rice bran
	Margarine or shortenings made from one of the unsaturated oils list above, diet margarine
	Mayonnaise, salad dressings made with unsaturated oils listed above, low fat dressings
	Seeds and nuts
Decrease:	Chocolate
	Butter, coconut oil, palm oil, palm kernel oil, lard, bacon fat, cottonseed oil, peanut oil
	Dressings made with sour cream
	Coconut, Brazil, macadamia, cashew nuts

The choices in the eating plans for Step 1 and Step 2 diets would differ in the amounts and selections of food that are major sources of saturated fatty acids and/or cholesterol (meat, poultry, seafood, milk and other dairy foods, fats and oils, and egg yolks).

Patients who need to progress to the Step 2 diet would benefit from intensive counseling by a registered dietitian who has expertise in counseling the patient with cardiovascular disease. Registered dietitians can be identified by calling the local hospital, the affiliate of the American Heart Association, or the American Dietetic Association.

Patients being treated with either the Step 1 or Step 2 diets should have serum cholesterol levels measured after 3–4 weeks, and again after 3 months of treatment. A person who has been successful in reaching desired goals for cholesterol lowering by diet should be followed every 3–4 months thereafter with blood tests and visits with someone trained to assist in diet therapy (for the Step 1 diet) or a registered dietitian (for the Step 2 diet).

C.   Dietary Recommendations

The diet recommended to lower blood cholesterol must:

1.   Be nutritionally balanced, providing the essential nutrients, as per the Recommended Dietary Allowances.
2.   Include a variety of foods, including (a) whole grain products, whole grain breads and cereals containing vitamins, minerals, protein and fiber; (b) fruits and vegetables providing beta carotene, vitamin C, folic acid, soluble and insoluble fiber, and minerals; (c) legumes providing protein, fiber, vitamins, and minerals; (d) poultry without skin, all kinds of fish, lean cuts of meat containing heme iron (a highly biologically available iron source) and nonfat milk and milk products, which are excellent sources of calcium and protein. Nuts which have mainly unsaturated fat may be included in small amounts (because of their caloric content).
3.   Lower the total fat intake to less than 30% of fat calories so that the intake of saturated fat is reduced. The average current intake of total fat is approximately 38% of total caloric intake.
4.   Lower the saturated fatty acids to less than 10% of calories. This would mean that most people on the typical American diet would have to lower their saturated fat intake by one third to meet the requirements of the AHA/NCEP Step 1 eating plan. The rest of the 30% fat allowance may be distributed between polyunsaturated fatty acids and monosaturated fatty acids. The polyunsaturates can be increased to a level of 10% of calories. The current American diet includes approximately 7% of calories as polyunsaturates.

5. Reduce dietary cholesterol. A cholesterol intake of less than 300 mg per
    day is recommended as the initial step (Step 1 NCEP and AHA) in the
    dietary management of high LDL cholesterol levels. Further reductions
    to less than 200 mg per day are required for the Step 2 diet.

D. Nutrient Classes

Saturated Fatty Acids

The foods that contribute to saturated fatty acid intake are (1) red meats such
as beef, veal, lamb, pork, processed meat products, and poultry with skin; (2)
milk and other dairy products; and (3) certain tropical vegetable fats such as
coconut oil, palm kernel oil, and palm oil (Table 3). The saturated fatty acid
content of coconut oil is 87%. Fats that have a high percentage of saturated fat
are solid at room temperature and are used in commercial baking of cakes,
pastries, cereals, and granola. The "nondairy" creamers and dairy substitutes
for whipped cream and sour cream, which may be labeled as containing "no
cholesterol" because they are derived from plants, are usually made with
coconut or palm oil. These vegetable fats are frequently used commercially
because they are inexpensive and resist oxidation (which extends shelf life).

A food labeled as "cholesterol-free" should not be assumed to be acceptable. The label of such foods must be checked for ingredients so that the fat
content and type can be ascertained. The most important message to the
patient is that we need to consider two components in foods, namely fats and
cholesterol. While some foods may not have cholesterol, they may have large
quantities of fat, e.g., vegetable oils, nuts, and seeds. On the other hand, not
all foods that have cholesterol have excessive fat. A food that is considered to
be part of a heart-healthy regimen must be evaluated for its fat content, its
saturated fat content, and its cholesterol content.

Although the different saturated fatty acids, ranging in length from 8 to 18
carbon atoms, do, as a group, raise plasma LDL levels, each acid may vary in
its hypercholesterolemic effect. Keys and co-workers (Keys et al., 1965)
concluded that lauric acids (12:0), myristic acid (14:0), and palmitic acid
(16:0) had almost the same effect on blood cholesterol by raising it by about
2.7 mg/dl for each percent of their calories in the diet. On the other hand,
Hegsted et al., (1965) found that each saturated fatty acid varied in its effect
on blood cholesterol levels, and that stearic acid (18:0) did not influence the
plasma cholesterol level.

Polyunsaturated Fatty Acids

These are divided into two major categories—the omega-6 and omega-3 fatty
acids. The main omega-6 fat is linoleic acid, which is an essential fatty acid
and is present in large amounts in safflower, sunflower, soybean and corn oil

Table 3 Fat and Cholesterol Contents of Selected Foods

Food	Amount	Total fats(g)	SFA(g)	MUFA(g)	PUFA(g)	Choleste-rol(mg)
Corn oil	1 Tbsp	13.6	1.7	3.3	8.0	0
Safflower oil	1 Tbsp	13.6	1.2	1.6	10.1	0
Sunflower oil	1 Tbsp	13.6	1.4	2.7	8.9	0
Olive oil	1 Tbsp	13.5	1.8	9.9	1.1	0
Canola oil	1 Tbsp	13.6	0.9	7.6	4.5	0
Sesame oil	1 Tbsp	13.6	1.9	5.4	5.7	0
Soybean oil	1 Tbsp	13.6	2.0	3.2	7.9	0
Peanut oil	1 Tbsp	13.5	2.3	6.2	4.3	0
Cottonseed oil	1 Tbsp	13.6	3.5	2.4	7.1	0
Rice bran oil	1 Tbsp	13.6	2.7	5.3	4.8	0
Margarine, soft tub	1 Tbsp	14.1	2.1	4.5	4.5	0
Margarine, stick	1 Tbsp	14.1	2.1	5.4	3.3	0
Chicken fat	1 Tbsp	12.8	3.8	5.7	2.7	11
Lard	1 Tbsp	12.8	5.0	5.8	1.4	12
Beef tallow	1 Tbsp	12.8	6.4	5.3	0.5	14
Palm oil	1 Tbsp	13.6	6.7	5.0	1.3	0
Butter	1 Tbsp	11.5	7.1	3.3	0.4	31
Palm kernel oil	1 Tbsp	13.6	11.1	1.5	0.2	0
Coconut oil	1 Tbsp	13.6	11.8	0.8	0.2	0
Almonds	½ oz	7.3	0.7	4.8	1.5	0
Walnuts	½ oz	8.0	0.5	1.8	5.3	0
Peanuts	½ oz	7.0	0.9	3.5	2.2	0
Cashew nuts	½ oz	6.5	1.3	3.9	1.1	0
Macadamia nuts, oil roasted	½ oz	10.9	1.6	8.6	0.2	0
Brazil nuts	½ oz	9.4	2.2	3.2	3.4	0
Sesame seeds	½ oz	16.0	2.3	6.2	7.2	0
Milk, skim	8 oz	0.4	0.3	trace	trace	4
Milk, 1% fat	8 oz	2.6	1.6	0.8	0.1	10
Milk, 2% fat	8 oz	4.7	2.9	0.1	0.2	18
Milk, whole	8 oz	8.9	5.6	2.6	0.3	35
Milk, butter-milk	8 oz	2.2	1.3	0.6	0.1	9
Milk, human	8 oz	10.8	4.9	4.1	1.2	34
Milk, goat	8 oz	10.1	6.5	2.7	0.4	28
Yogurt, plain whole milk	8 oz	7.4	4.8	2.0	0.2	29

(continued)

Table 3 (*continued*)

Food	Amount	Total fats(g)	SFA(g)	MUFA(g)	PUFA(g)	Choleste-rol(mg)
Yogurt, plain low fat	8 oz	3.5	2.3	1.0	0.1	14
Cottage cheese, 1%	4 oz	1.2	0.7	0.3	0.1	5
Mozzarella, part skim	1 oz	4.5	2.9	1.3	0.1	16
Mozzarella, whole	1 oz	6.1	3.7	1.9	0.8	22
Sour cream	1 oz	5.9	3.7	0.8	0.1	12
Feta	1 oz	6.0	4.2	1.3	0.2	25
American pro-cessed	1 oz	8.9	5.6	2.5	0.3	27
Brie	1 oz	7.9	4.9	NA	NA	28
Swiss	1 oz	7.8	5.0	2.1	0.3	26
Parmesan grated	1 oz	8.5	5.4	2.5	0.2	22
Cream cheese	1 oz	9.9	6.2	2.8	0.4	31
Ricotta, whole milk	4 oz	14.7	9.4	4.5	0.5	58
Egg, large	1	5.6	1.7	2.3	0.7	210
Beef (round)	3-½ oz[a]	8.0	2.9	3.1	0.3	82
Lamb (leg)	3-½ oz[a]	8.2	3.0	3.4	0.5	89
Pork (fresh)	3-½ oz[a]	10.5	3.6	4.8	1.3	92
Veal (lean)	3-½ oz[a]	6.6	1.8	2.4	0.6	128
Beef liver	3-½ oz[a]	4.9	1.9	0.7	1.0	389
Turkey (light without skin)	3-½ oz[a]	3.2	1.0	0.6	0.1	69
Turkey (dark without skin)	3-½ oz[a]	7.2	2.4	1.6	2.1	85
Chicken (light without skin)	3-½ oz[a]	4.1	1.1	1.2	0.8	75
Chicken (dark without skin)	3-½ oz[a]	7.1	2.1	3.0	2.0	117
Duck (flesh only)	3-½ oz[a]	11.2	4.2	3.1	1.2	89
Haddock	3-½ oz[a]	0.9	0.2	0.2	0.2	74
Cod	3-½ oz[a]	0.9	0.2	0.1	0.2	55
Snapper	3-½ oz[a]	1.7	0.4	0.3	0.6	47
Tuna, bluefin	3-½ oz[a]	6.3	1.6	2.1	1.8	49
Salmon, coho	3-½ oz[a]	7.4	1.2	2.1	2.2	87

(*continued*)

Table 3 (*continued*)

Food	Amount	Total fats(g)	SFA(g)	MUFA(g)	PUFA(g)	Choleste-rol(mg)
Lobster, northern	3-½ oz[a]	0.6	0.1	0.1	0.1	72
Crab, blue	3-½ oz[a]	1.8	0.2	0.2	0.6	100
Shrimp, mixed species	3-½ oz[a]	1.1	0.3	0.2	0.4	195
Clam, mixed species	3-½ oz[a]	2.0	0.2	0.2	0.5	67
Tuna, white	3-½ oz[a]	2.2	0.6	0.6	0.1	42

[a]Cooked.
Source: Composition of Food Agriculture Handbooks 8–1,3,4,5,10,13,15, U.S. Department of Agriculture.

(Table 3). The oils in most cold water fish are major sources of omega-3 fatty acids: eicosapentaenoic acid (EPA) and docosahexaenoic acid (DHA). These fatty acids are effective in lowering triglyceride levels when fed in large amounts. They have not been shown to be helpful in lowering LDL cholesterol levels. Fish oil capsules marketed by different companies usually contain one third of their fat content as omega-3 fatty acid and are not recommended for the treatment of hypercholesterolemia. However, both high fat fish such as salmon, mackerel, and bluefish that are rich in omega-3 fatty acids and low fat fish like sole, flounder, cod, and halibut should be included in the diet plan because they are good sources of protein and can be useful substitutes for meat and cheese, which are high in saturated fatty acids.

Monounsaturated Fatty Acids

These are mainly present as oleic acid in olive oil and canola oil (low erucic acid rapeseed oil). Monounsaturated fats should make up 10–15% of calories. The current American diet supplies as much oleic acid as is recommended, but the oleic acid is usually derived from animal fats, which are also high in saturates. When the intake of animal fat is decreased, vegetable oils and nuts can be included in the meal plan to increase the monounsaturated fat intake.

Dietary Cholesterol

Cholesterol from food sources is supplied only by animal foods (Table 3). The organ meats (brain, liver, kidney, sweetbreads) are very rich sources of cholesterol. Animal meat (both muscle and fat) contains cholesterol. There is no significant difference in the cholesterol content of beef, lamb, pork, chicken, or turkey. Fish (except some shellfish such as shrimp) are lower in cholesterol than meat or poultry.

Reduction in the consumption of egg yolks, organ meats, dairy foods, and meats will lower intake of cholesterol. Humans appear to respond to the cholesterol in the diet with a modest and variable response indicating that they are less sensitive to cholesterol in the diet (Keys, 1984). It has been suggested that an increase of cholesterol of 100 mg per 1000 calories could raise the blood cholesterol level between 5 and 10 mg/dl.

Although blood cholesterol had fractions of very low density, low density, and high density lipoprotein cholesterol, dietary cholesterol is not comprised of these fractions. Dietary cholesterol and cholesterol synthesized in the body are mixed together in the liver and are apportioned into the lipoprotein fractions both in the liver and in the blood.

Protein

The intake of protein that is recommended is about 15% of total caloric intake. This level of intake still meets the RDA (recommended dietary allowance) for a female consuming 1200 kcal/day. The sources of protein should be from a variety of low fat animal foods (Table 4) and plant foods such as legumes and grains. The amount of lean animal foods recommended could be a maximum of 5–6 oz. per day. High protein foods are usually associated with high fat content. The exceptions are egg whites and isolated soy protein and casein supplements. High protein diets used in weight-reducing fad diet programs can have significant adverse effects on serum cholesterol levels because of the simultaneous increase in saturated fat and cholesterol intake.

Carbohydrates

The carbohydrate content of the therapuetic diet will be approximately 55% of the total calories. Dietary carbohydrates include simple sugars (the monosaccharides and mainly the disaccharide sucrose used in the preparation of food)

Table 4 Low Fat Cuts of Red Meat

Beef	Veal	Pork	Lamb
Round	All fat trimmed	Tenderloin leg	Leg
Sirloin	cuts except com-	(fresh)	Arm
Chuck	mercially ground	Shoulder (arm or	Loin
Loin	and breast of veal	picnic)	

and the complex carbohydrates (both digestible starch and the indigestible fibers). The recommendation is to eat more of the complex carbohydrates which are nutrient-rich and less of the simple carbohydrates which are devoid of other nutrients and provide only "empty" calories.

The indigestible carbohydrates are also known as dietary fiber. There are two different kinds of fiber in foods; one is "insoluble" in the gastrointestinal track. This type of fiber provides bulk and aids in the movement of food and water through the intestine. It is found in food sources such as whole wheat, whole grain cereals (*caution:* granolas made with animal fats and/or vegetable shortenings are high in saturated fatty acids), corn, and vegetables. Insoluble fiber may protect and help in the treatment of diseases of the intestinal tract, i.e., constipation, diverticulosis, hemorrhoids, and cancer of the colon and rectum.

The other type of fiber is souble in the intestinal tract. Rich sources of soluble fiber are oatmeal, oat bran, legumes containing gums like β-glucan (dried peas and beans), psyllium seeds, and some fruits, like grapefruit and apple, that contain pectin. Soluble fiber has been shown to lower LDL cholesterol, control diabetes by slowing absorption of glucose, and aid in appetite control by creating satiety. Some studies have suggested that large amounts of oat bran (providing 15–25 g of soluble fiber) eaten daily can lower plasma cholesterol by 3–15%. Saturated fat intake was reduced concomitantly in the studies showing the larger effects on plasma cholesterol concentrations. Adding soluble fiber containing foods to the diet could be a valuable adjunct to a low saturated fat, low cholesterol diet. Since eating large quantities of fiber can cause gastrointestinal side effects, it is important to add fiber-rich foods slowly to the diet to help the body adjust and improve tolerance. It is also important to optimize the fluid intake when high fiber diets are consumed.

Alcohol

Although there are epidemiological data suggesting that modest alcohol consumption is associated with higher levels of blood HDL cholesterol and reduced rates of cardiovascular disease, alcohol is not recommended in the prevention or treatment of coronary heart disease. Even moderate consumption can have an effect on increasing blood pressure, triglyceride levels, weight gain, and heart enlargement.

Coffee

Recent research data from several countries has associated excessive coffee (both regular and decaffeinated) drinking with increased LDL cholesterol levels. However, the risk for coronary artery disease remains to be established for the level and type of coffee consumption in the United States. Here moderation is the key word, with the added caution that only nonfat or 1% fat milk be used with it. Tea drinking appears to have no correlation with serum cholesterol levels and coronary artery disease (Tuomilehto et al., 1987).

Supplements

Products like fish oil capsules and soy lecithin which are promoted as cholesterol-lowering agents by health food stores have been found to have no therapeutic value in the treatment of high total and LDL cholesterol levels.

Lecithin is a phospholipid that is an important component of cell membranes and the outer surface of lipoproteins in the plasma. Lecithin supplement is isolated from soybeans which contain mono and polyunsaturated fatty acids. It can, therefore, have a cholesterol-lowering effect if it is substituted (in large quantities) for saturated fat in the diet. However, this would be an expensive way of including unsaturated fatty acids in the diet. Small amounts of lecithin, taken as a supplement, have no effect on plasma lipid and lipoprotein levels.

Fish oils containing omega-3 fatty acids have been shown to lower triglycerides in the blood, possibly by suppressing VLDL production in the liver. Several studies, however, have not demonstrated a significant effect of fish oil supplements in lowering LDL cholesterol levels. It is important to remember that commercial fish body oil preparations have calories, like any other fat, and usually have cholesterol. Fish liver oils not only increase the fat and cholesterol content of the diet but also have large amounts of vitamins A and D. If consumed over long periods of time, toxic symptoms with damage to the liver may occur.

E. Special Considerations

Hypertriglyceridemic Individuals

Patients with hypertriglyceridemia could be benefited by various strategies: weight reduction, exercise, abstaining from alcohol, and lowering of total and saturated fat intake (Step 1 Diet). For borderline to moderately severe hypertriglyceridemia (250–750 mg/dl), the main approaches should be the Step 1 diet, weight reduction, increases in physical activity, and treatment of the underlying problem which may be alcoholism, diabetes mellitus, hypothyroidism, chronic renal disease, and liver disease.

Severe hypertriglyceridemia and chylomicronemia (plasma levels of triglyceride > 1000 mg/dl) should be treated with a very low fat diet (10–20% of total calorie intake as fat) to prevent the patient from getting pancreatitis. These patients should also be told that if they are very sensitive to fatty foods, one meal comprising of prime ribs, baked potato topped with sour cream, and cheesecake can precipitate an attack of pancreatitis. Fish oils as a supplement to a low fat diet may help further reduce serum triglyceride levels in some patients (Karmally et al., 1989).

Elderly

Evidence from more recent long-term follow-up of the Framingham study support the view that reduction of high blood cholesterol levels in the elderly will prevent coronary heart disease (Kannell and Gordon, 1978). The NCEP guidelines recommend that clinical judgment be used in dealing with individual patients, particularly the elderly. The Step 1 guidelines, which emphasize a less aggressive approach to diet treatment, is appropriate in elderly patients. For patients who have lactose intolerance, "lactaid" or "lactrase" treated low fat dairy foods should be recommended to optimize calcium intake.

Children

Blood cholesterol levels become a serious concern in children if there is a strong family history of coronary heart disease. The AHA states that it is safe to implement the Step 1 diet guidelines for children over the age of 2 years. It is important to ensure that the child receives sufficient calories for normal growth and development. Total calories and protein intake should not be compromised when the goal is to lower saturated fat and cholesterol intake. The child's diet should be altered very slowly in order to obtain maximum compliance and to initiate lifelong changes in habits.

Pregnant Women

The rise in serum cholesterol and triglycerides during pregnancy are not generally of clinical importance. However, women who have hyperlipidemia prior to pregnancy should continue with a cholesterol-lowering diet regimen that provides a well-balanced diet with adequate nutrition, as per needs of pregnancy (Committee on Diet and Health, 1989).

F.   Initiating the Diet Treatment Program

The physician needs to set the stage for dietary treatment because the success of diet therapy greatly depends on the physician's attitude and motivating skills. The physician's positive attitude toward nutrition intervention can influence the patient's attitude toward making dietary changes. Referring the patient to a registered dietition would be the preferred route to facilitate diet modification and nutritional counseling necessary to help patients make permanent changes in his or her eating style. However, instruction of the patient in the Step 1 diet can be accomplished with the leadership of the physician and his or her staff of registered nurses, physicians' assistants, or other office personnel who have been trained to do nutritional assessments and dietary counseling. Assessment of patient compliance is essential to determine if the diet changes are optimum to maximize their effects of LDL cholesterol. Besides self-reporting, collateral reports provided by family members or friends who attend the counseling sessions and objective measurements of serum cholesterol and body weight are recommended.

Nutritional counseling is initiated after a complete assessment of the patient's social and personal factors. A questionnaire that provides information on the patient's usual eating patterns (food preparation techniques, mealtime practices, restaurant eating), previous experiences with dietary change, and social support should be completed by the patient prior to the counseling session. This information will help to identify the areas that need modification and provide positive feedback when the eating style conforms to the diet therapy goals.

Individual dietary assessment of free-living outpatients can be done by having the patient keep records of everything ingested on 4 consecutive days (2 weekdays and 2 weekend days). A 7-consecutive-day food record and a food-frequency questionnaire are alternative approaches to ascertaining dietary intake. Recalls of food eaten in the previous 24 hours may not give the true picture of the diet because of individual variability in recall accuracy. Although food frequency methods have been established to be reliable and valid, the ever-increasing complexity of the available food supply will lead to long tedious lists of foods for the patient to check. Four-consecutive-day food records are acceptable for estimating intake of calories, cholesterol, fat, and saturated fat (Jackson et al., 1986). Patients are instructed to write down the time food is ingested and the type and the amount eaten (in household measures). The food intake records may be assessed qualitatively to understand the patient's eating style and to monitor dietary compliance. Quantitative analysis can be done using databases with more than 1000 foods available for use with microcomputers.

When diet-related behaviors have to be modified, psychosocial, cultural, and situational factors are involved. More than just eating behaviors may be involved (Danish et al., 1986). For example, making a switch to margarine made with unsaturated oils instead of butter, which is preferred by other household members, may include:

1. Understanding food labels to make the right choice.
2. Changes in routine shopping habits, which may include butter and frozen convenience foods containing butter and other saturated fats.

3. Time needed for shopping and cooking. The patient may depend on a family member to do food shopping and cooking.
4. Dealing with family members who use butter in food preparation
5. Experimenting with different unsaturated oils and/or margarine to find a suitable replacement for butter.

Nutritional counseling is described as a two-part process (Danish, 1975). First of all, it is important to develop rapport, empathy, and a trusting relationship before implementation of strategies leading to behavioral change. In order to establish the relationship as a "helper," it is necessary to know the patient's interest, understanding of nutrition, approach to making food choices in relation to high blood cholesterol, and concerns about making choices.

The next process would be goal setting. This strategy is a useful aid to realistic dietary and behavioral changes, and should be directed at the patient's health problem. Many patients can state general concepts that they have heard from the media or from a health care provider, but they may not understand the application of these concepts to making healthy food choices.

G. Guidelines for Nutritional Counseling

1. The setting for effective counseling in a medical treatment area is attractive, comfortable, and conducive to confidentiality.
2. Good communication leads to a harmonious and understanding relationship. The patient needs to understand the purpose of the counseling and the approaches to making permanent dietary changes. These will include: (a) understanding patient's current eating style and the behavior associated with eating and (b) making dietary changes aimed at lowering blood cholesterol in a step-by-step manner.
3. The counselor should help the patient identify goals through the following steps: (a) understanding that the blood cholesterol is elevated, probably because the current eating style is high in saturated fat, cholesterol, and/or calories; (b) identifying behaviors such as shopping for groceries, cooking methods, eating habits that lead to an increased consumption of fat and cholesterol; and (c) helping the patient choose one behavior that would be easiest to change. The patient may find it just as easy to walk to work along a street where there is a coffee shop that sells fresh plain raisin bagels instead of the usual shop to get a buttered corn muffin. If the patient is successful in making this change and enjoys it, the change could become a permanent feature of the patient's eating style.

The behavior chosen for change should be realistic, specific, and flexible. Goals that are absolute may make the patient feel that he/she is a total failure if there is just one lapse in behavior. For example, if the patient sets a goal that a daily chocolate snack will be eliminated from the diet, it may be difficult to achieve the goal. It would be more realistic if the initial goal is to substitute fruit for two of the chocolate snacks during the week.

The patient should be made to realize that there will be problems along with successes. Problems should be discussed at the counseling sessions in order to learn how to approach them. At times, patients will cancel their appointments if they are made to feel that they are unable to reach a certain goal; for them this would be a sign of failure.

4. Education is an important component of counseling. The patient has to have knowledge about the composition of foods, heart-healthy food preparation methods, and behavioral approaches to making dietary changes. It is important to teach only what is necessary for that particular individual, using a few guidelines for each session. Since people learn in different ways, written materials and simple visual aids may help significantly in the teaching process.

Another technique that can be utilized is role playing to help the patient deal with social situations that are causing difficulties (Raab and Tillotson, 1983). The patient may have difficulty getting unsaturated oil for salad in a restaurant or the patient may be unable to communicate with a spouse who believes it is wholesome to cook with butter. This spouse could also be invited to a food demonstration which focuses on recipe modification to make the meal lower in saturated fat and cholesterol.

Encouraging the patient to have family and friends involved in healthy eating could remove some of the roadblocks to adherence. People generally consider eating a social event. The patient should be encouraged to bring the spouse or any significant person—a friend or a relative—who can provide the support while the behavioral changes are being made.

Most people can adapt better when introduced to a progressive change in eating style. Permanent change is much more likely if alterations in well-established eating styles are made gradually and comfortably. The patient may be more able to accept selecting leaner cuts and smaller portions of meat than trying to make to changes in all food groups at the same time. Furthermore, giving information on fat and cholesterol content of foods can facilitate making healthy choices.

Establishing continuity by phone, mail, or visits is important for successful counseling. At follow-up sessions with the patient, the progress towards meeting goals should be addressed in a positive way, concentrating initially on the successful changes and the techniques used to make these changes. It is also important to discuss the difficulties, if any, the patient has encountered in making choices. Adherence can be estimated by measuring blood cholesterol levels at 4–6 weeks and again at 3 months. It is important to remember that biological variability, as well as external factors such as seasonal change, can affect blood cholesterol levels. Hence, there may be a delay between a dietary change and a biological change. Food intake may be assessed qualitatively to see if the patient has been successful in selecting low fat choices. Food intake may also be assessed quantitatively using a nutrition software program. If the goal is to lose weight, the patient can be weighed at each visit, or the patient can be asked to self-monitor weight and report it by telephone or mail.

H. Cooking Tips and Recipe Modification

Methods that require little or no fat are preferred. Foods could be prepared in an interesting manner with the right combination of herbs and spices even if they are steamed, broiled, baked, grilled, microwaved with no fat, or sautéed with very little unsaturated fat.

Serve smaller portions of meat (3 ounces per person) or meatless or "low meat" dishes. Part of the meat in mixed dishes could be replaced by mushrooms, eggplant, or legumes. Instead of meat, such as hot dogs or hamburgers, fresh tuna or salmon or vegetable kabobs could be grilled at a barbecue. Also, meat could be browned in a skillet and fat drained before making a pasta sauce.

Low fat (1% fat) or nonfat dairy products could be used in place of heavy cream in cooking or at the table. Nonfat dairy desserts and water ices could be served with fresh fruit. Nonfat yogurt could be used in recipes that call for sour cream. Two egg whites could be substituted for one whole egg, and one cup of butter or shortening could be replaced by 3/4 cup unsaturated oil in baking. The American Heart Association's cookbooks have a variety of interesting recipes that could help lower saturated fat and cholesterol intake.

I. Guidelines for Eating Out

Dining out can be a pleasure if you plan ahead. Menu descriptions that have lots of saturated fat and cholesterol may be described as buttered, butter sauce, buttery, sautéed, fried, crispy, creamed, cream sauce, in its own gravy, hollandaise, lobster sauce, au gratin, parmesan, cheese sauce, escalloped, basted, hash, prime, or a casserole (see AHA Dining Out Guide).

Most restaurants will feature items on the menu suitable for the diet regimen. The waiter or waitress will usually be helpful in describing how the dishes are prepared. In difficult situations, the patients could tell the restaurant management they are allergic to animal fats (butter, cream) and that their menu choice should be prepared with an unsaturated oil (olive, canola, corn, etc.)

The following tips will help lower fat and cholesterol intake:

1. Choose from a variety of vegetables, fruits, and salads so long as they are not marinated in oils or served with cream or butter sauce.
2. Request that dressings be served separately so that small amounts can be used on the salad.
3. Select more fish and other seafood and poultry without skin in place of red meats such as beef, veal, lamb, and pork.
4. An appetizer serving of meat may be an interesting accompaniment to a pasta with marinara sauce or a rice vegetable dish.
5. Try eating fresh bread without butter.
6. Choose more fresh fruits, angel food cake, sorbets, and fewer high fat desserts.

VI. SUMMARY

The practical approach to dietary treatment is to apply heart-healthy recommendations to individual food patterns of patients. This means translating the nutritional principles described above into food choices relevant to the individual, so that drastic changes do not have to be made in order to follow a heart-healthy eating plan. Several minor changes in the right direction can have a significant cumulative effect on the attainment of the goals of treatment. Helping people make healthy food choices without a series of "don'ts," but rather with positive messages such as "choose more of" or "try for a change" or "experiment with," will be more effective. The diet that is described as percentages of energy derived from fat, carbohydrate, and protein to maintain the concept of balance is meaningless to an individual who buys food and not nutrients in a supermarket. Moreover, the concept of a balance of nutrients may not be achieved in restaurants, where meals may have a higher fat content than foods prepared at home. Here, again, the individual should be taught to monitor his daily fat and cholesterol intake so that the higher fat meals can be balanced with meals that are lower in fat, particularly saturated fat and cholesterol.

The physician plays an important role either as a primary counselor or as a supporter of the patient's efforts to make changes in his or her eating styles. If the physician emphasizes the importance of the low saturated fat, low cholesterol diet as the primary strategy in treating hypercholesterolemia, the patient will believe that diet modification is an essential and necessary therapeutic measure. The majority of individuals would much rather modify their diet than take medications. It is the role of the physician and his or her staff, and the registered dietitian, to assist the patient in reaching that goal.

REFERENCES

Ahrens, E. H., Jr., Hirsch, J., Insull, W., Jr., Tsaltas, T. T., Blomstrand, R., and Peterson, M. L. (1957). The influence of dietary fats on serum-lipid levels in man. *Lancet* **1**:943–953.

Anderson, K. M., Castelli, W. P., and Levy, D. (1987). Cholesterol and mortality. 30 years of follow-up from the Framingham Study. *JAMA* **257**:2176–2180.

Bonanome, A., and Grundy, S. M. (1988). Effect of dietary stearic acid on plasma cholesterol and lipoprotein levels. *N. Engl. J. Med.* **318**:1244–1248.

Brown, W. V., Ginsberg, H., and Karmally, W. (1985). Diet and the decrease of coronary heart disease. *Am. J. Cardiol.* **54**:27C–29C.

Bunch, K. L. (1985). Consumption trends favor fresh, low fat and sweet. *National Food Review,* USDA, Unit **2**:1–5.

Committee on Diet and Health, Food Nutrition Board, Commission on Life and Sciences, National Research Council. (1989). Report of Diet and Health. Implications for reducing chronic disease risk. Washington, DC, National Academy Press.

Danish, S. J., Lang, D., et al. (1986). Nutrition counseling skills: Continuing education for the dietician. *Topics in Clinical Nutrition* **1**:25–32.

Danish, S. J. (1975). Developing helping relationships in dietetic counseling. *J. Am. Diet. Assoc.* **67**:107–110.

The Expert Panel. (1988). Report of the National Cholesterol Education Program Expert Panel on detection, evaluation and treatment of high blood cholesterol in adults. *Arch. Intern. Med.* **148**:36–69.

Ginsberg, H. N., Barr, S. L., Gilbert, A., Karmally, W., Deckelbaum, R., Kaplan, K., Ramakrishnan, R., Holleran, S., and Dell, R. B. (1990). Reduction of plasma cholesterol levels in normal men on an American Heart Association Step-One diet or a Step 1 diet with added monounsaturated fat. *N. Engl. J. Med.* **322**:574–579.

Ginsberg, H., Le, NA, Mays, C., et al. (1981). Lipoprotein metabolism in nonresponders to increased dietary cholesterol. *Arteriosclerosis* **1**:463–470.

Grundy, S. M. (1986). Comparison of monounsaturated fatty acids and carbohydrates for lowering plasma cholesterol. *N. Engl. J. Med.* **314**:745–748.

Hegsted, D. M., McGandy, R. B., Myers, M. L., and Stare, F. J. (1965). Quantitative effects of dietary fat on serum cholesterol in man. *Am. J. Clin. Nutr.* **17**:281–295.

Jackson, B., Dujovne, C. A., et al. (1986). Methods to assess relative reliability of diet records: Minimum records for monitoring lipid and caloric intake. *J. Am. Diet Ass.* **86:**1531–1535.

Kagan, A., McGee, D. L., Yano, K., Rhoads, G. G., and Nomura, A. (1981). Serum cholesterol and mortality in a Japanese-American population: The Honolulu Heart Program. *Am. J. Epidemiol.* **114:**11–20.

Kannell, W. B., LeBauer, E. J., et al. (1967). Relation of body weight to development of coronary heart disease. The Framingham Study. *Circulation* **25:**734–744.

Kannell, W. B., and Gordon, T. (1978). Evaluation of cardidovascular risk in the elderly. The Framingham Study. *Bull, NY Acad. Med.* **54:**573–591.

Karmally, W., Goldberg, I., and Ginsberg, H. N. (1989). Normalization of plasma triglycerides and high density lipoprotein cholesterol by omega-3-fatty acid supplementation of a low fat diet in a patient with lipoprotein lipase deficiency. *Arteriosclerosis* **9:**709A.

Katan, M. B., Beynen, A. C., DeVries, J. H. M., and Nobels, A. (1986). Existence of consistent hypo- and hyperresponders to dietary cholesterol in man. *Am. J. Epidemiol.* **123:**221–234.

Keys, A. (1970). Coronary heart disease in seven countries. *Circulation Suppl.* **41:**I 1–1211.

Keys, A. (1980). *Seven Countries: A Multivariate Analysis of Death and Coronary Heart Disease.* Cambridge, MA, Harvard University Press.

Keys, A. (1984). Serum cholesterol response to dietary cholesterol. *Am. J. Clin. Nutr.* **40:**351–359.

Keys, A., Anderson, J. T., and Grande, F. (1965). Serum cholesterol response to changes in the diet. IV. Particular saturated fatty acids in the diet. *Metabolism* **14:**776–787.

Kushi, L. H., Lew, R. A., Stare, F. J., Ellison, C. R., el Lozy, M., Bourke, G., Daly, L., Graham, I., Hickey, N., Mulcahy, R., and Kevaney, J. (1985). Diet and 20-year mortality from coronary heart disease. The Ireland-Boston Diet-Heart Study. *N. Engl. J. Med.* **312:**811–818.

Kromhout, D., Arntzenius, A. C., Kempen-Voogd, N., Kempen, H. J., Barth, J. D. van der Voort, H. A., and van der Velde, E. A. (1987). Long-term effects of linoleic acid-enriched diet, changes in body weight and alcohol consumption on serum total and HDL-cholesterol. *Atherosclerosis* **66:**99–105.

Marstan, R., and Raper, N. (1985). Nutrient content of the food supply. *National Food Review,* USDA, Unit **2:**6–12.

Mattson, F. H., and Grundy, S. M. (1985). Comparison of effects of dietary saturated, monunsaturated, and polyunsaturated fatty acids on plasma lipids and lipoproteins in man. *J. Lipid Res.* **26:**194–202.

Mensink,R.P., and Katan, M. B. (1989). Effect of a diet enriched with monounsaturated or polyunsaturated fatty acids on levels of low-density and high-density lipoprotein cholesterol in healthy women and men. *N. Engl. J. Med.* **321:**436–441.

Raab, C., and Tillotson,J.L.(eds.)(1983).Heart to Heart. A Manual on Nutrition Counseling for the Reduction of Cardiovascular Disease Risk Factors. U.S. Department of Health and Human Services. Dallas, TX, American Heart Association, NIH Publication No. 83–1528.

Slattery, M. L., and Randall, D. E. (1988). Trends in coronary heart disease mortality and food consumption in the United States between 1909 and 1980. *Am. J. Clin. Nutr.* **47:**1060–1067.

Stamler, J., Wentworth, D., and Neaton, J. D. (1985). Is the relationship between serum cholesterol and risk of permature death from coronary heart disease continuous and graded? Findings in 356,222 primary screenees of the Multiple Risk Factor Intervention Trial (MRFIT). *JAMA* **256:**2823–2828.

Stamler, J., and Shekelle, R. (1988). Dietary cholesterol and human coronary heart disease. The epidemiologic evidence. *Arch. Pathol. Lab. Med.* **112:**1032–1040.

Thueesen, L., Henriksen, L. B., and Engby, B. (1986). One-year experience with a low-fat, low-cholesterol diet in patients with coronary heart disease. *Am. J. Clin. Nutr.* **44:**212–219.

Tuomilehto, J., Tanskanen, A., Pietinen, P., Aro, A., Salonen, J. T., Happonen, P., Nissinen, A., and Puska, P. (1987). Coffee consumption is correlated with serum cholesterol in middle-age Finnish men and women. *J. Epid. Comm. Health* **41:**237–242.

Vartiainen, I., and Kanerva, K. (1947). Arteriosclerosis and war-time. *Ann. Med. Int. Fenn.* **36:**748–758.

Vessby, B., Lithell, H., Boberg, J. (1985). Reduction of low density and high density lipoprotein cholesterol by fat-modified diets. *Hum. Nutr. Clin. Nutr.* **36C:**203–211.

Index

About the Editor

BASIL M. RIFKIND is Deputy Associate Director of Hypertension, Arteriosclerosis, and Lipid Metabolism Program, Division of Heart and Vascular Diseases of the National Heart, Lung, and Blood Institute (NHLBI), National Institutes of Health (NIH), Bethesda, Maryland; Chief, Lipid Metabolism—Atherogenesis Branch, Division of Heart and Vascular Diseases, NHLBI, NIH; and Project Officer, Lipid Research Clinics Program, Division of Heart and Vascular Diseases, NHLBI, NIH. A Fellow of the Royal College of Physicians and Surgeons and a member of the Royal College of Physicians, Dr. Rifkind received the M.D. degree (1972) from the University of Glasgow, Glasgow, Scotland.